Jorge Martinez, M.D.
Radiology

VIRTUAL COLONOSCOPY

VIRTUAL COLONOSCOPY

Judy Yee, MD
PROFESSOR AND VICE CHAIR
DEPARTMENT OF RADIOLOGY
UNIVERSITY OF CALIFORNIA, SAN FRANCISCO
CHIEF OF RADIOLOGY
SAN FRANCISCO VA MEDICAL CENTER
SAN FRANCISCO, CALIFORNIA

With contributions by

Gregory M. Galdino, MD
BOARD CERTIFIED RADIOLOGIST, PRIVATE PRACTICE
JACKSON RADIOLOGY ASSOCIATES
JACKSON, TENNESSEE

Wolters Kluwer Health | Lippincott Williams & Wilkins
Philadelphia • Baltimore • New York • London
Buenos Aires • Hong Kong • Sydney • Tokyo

Acquisitions Editor: Lisa McAllister
Managing Editor: Kerry Barrett
Project Manager: Rosanne Hallowell
Manufacturing Manager: Kathleen Brown
Marketing Manager: Angela Panetta
Creative Director: Doug Smock
Cover Designer: Andrew Gatto
Production Services: Laserwords Private Limited, Chennai, India

530 Walnut Street
Philadelphia, PA 19106 USA
LWW.com

Printed in the United States

Library of Congress Cataloging-in-Publication Data

Yee, Judy.
Virtual colonoscopy / Judy Yee, with contributions by Gregory M. Galdino.
p. ; cm.
Includes bibliographical references and index.
ISBN-13: 978-0-7817-5770-6
1. Colon (Anatomy)–Tomography. I. Galdino, Gregory M. II. Title.
[DNLM: 1. Colonography, Computed Tomographic–methods. 2. Colonic Neoplasms–radiography. 3. Colonoscopy–methods. WI 520 Y42v 2008]
RC804.T65Y44 2008
616.3′407545–dc22

2007022717

---

10 9 8 7 6 5 4 3 2 1

This book is dedicated to my husband David
and to my daughter Taylor
who have provided me with untiring support,
encouragement,
and laughter along the way.

CONTENTS

FOREWORD

Virtual colonoscopy is coming of age. It is accepted by almost everyone—patients, physicians, and some third-party payers—as an elegant, noninvasive, highly accurate diagnostic approach for the detection of colonic polyps and cancer. With the new multirow detector computed tomography (CT) scanners, the procedure is much easier on patients, and can be performed within one breath-hold and without anesthesia. The various software programs provide much-improved, simultaneous, correlated viewing of prone, supine, 2D, and fly-through images. With CAD (computer-aided detection) programs and fecal tagging becoming available in the near future (eliminating the need for vigorous colonic cleansing), virtual colonoscopy will undoubtedly become the universally accepted, generally reimbursed screening method that will greatly reduce the mortality from colorectal cancer. Optical, conventional colonoscopy will still remain the approach for the removal of polyps, biopsy, and introduction of stents.

Virtual Colonoscopy is a very much needed contribution to educating radiologists and other physicians about this procedure. Dr. Yee is a pioneer and one of the few most experienced radiologists of virtual colonoscopy who has personally significantly advanced the field. Dr. Yee has succeeded in putting all her vast expertise into this opus, making *Virtual Colonoscopy* the most complete and up-to-date book on the subject. It provides the epidemiological background of colorectal cancer with a review of current screening approaches, offering a guide through patient preparation, CT technique, interpretation methods, various pitfalls, colonic and extracolonic findings that need reporting, as well as expected future developments. This permits the reader to become versed in all aspects of virtual CT colonoscopy.

The provision of multiple electronic data sets (available on-line at http://www.yeevirtualcolonoscopy.com) adds to the book's value by taking advantage of modern technological interactive instruction; hands-on practicing on the computer is worth a thousand learned paragraphs.

It is indeed a pleasure and honor to be invited to write the Foreword for this book, undoubtedly a classic in the making.

ALEXANDER MARGULIS, MD
Clinical Professor of Radiology
Weill Medical College
Cornell University
New York, New York

PREFACE

Virtual colonoscopy (also known as computed tomography colonography [CTC]) was first introduced in 1994, and since then has undergone remarkable evolution into a technique that is poised to change the way we screen for colorectal cancer. It has already been integrated into daily use at sites throughout the United States and internationally as a less invasive diagnostic tool for evaluation of the colon. Key developments of CTC over the last decade include the use of multidetector CT scanners allowing thinner and faster slice acquisition, improved and easier-to-use two- and three-dimensional displays with higher resolution, the use of electronic carbon dioxide insufflation for more reliable distention of the colon, and the introduction of computer-aided detection. Minimal and noncathartic tagging protocols are being developed for use with electronic subtraction to help eliminate one of the major barriers to widespread colon cancer screening. Practice guidelines for the performance of CTC in adults have been issued by the American College of Radiology with specific metrics and accreditation requirements to follow.

This well-illustrated book is comprehensive yet practical, and provides both an overview of colorectal cancer screening as well as a thorough description of all facets of CTC. There are more than 700 illustrations included. The first chapter reviews staging, pathophysiology, and risk factors for development and possible strategies for prevention of colorectal cancer. The advantages and disadvantages of the fecal occult blood test, fecal immunochemical test, flexible sigmoidoscopy, double contrast barium enema, and colonoscopy are presented. The remaining chapters are devoted to CTC. Important practical tips are provided on how to effectively cleanse and distend the colon in order to obtain optimum CTC images. Instructions are provided on how to perform time-efficient and accurate interpretations. Normal colorectal anatomy and both the common and uncommon appearances of polyps and cancer on two- and three-dimensional images are reviewed with multiple examples shown. The wide range of pitfalls that are encountered on CTC are presented, along with teaching points as to how to avoid them. The results of published validation trials and the incidence and impact of extracolonic findings are presented. The essential elements of a CTC report and how to effectively communicate the results of CTC are reviewed with sample reports provided. Various strategies that have been developed for tagging and the current status of computer-aided detection (CAD) as well as future challenges are reviewed.

Interactive training is such an important part of developing the skills required for interpreting CTC. To this end we are including access to CTC teaching cases that you can download from the Internet and then install at your own site using various software platforms. This will enable you to start to learn the critical interactive computer workstation skills needed to detect lesions on CTC. A detailed answer key is included and may be used to check your personal results after you have reviewed the cases.

The diagnosis and management of colorectal cancer requires a multidisciplinary approach; this book is intended for radiologists, gastroenterologists, colorectal surgeons, and general practitioners as well as fellows, residents, medical students, and researchers in these specialties. This book is the culmination of many years of experience in collaborating with my outstanding radiology and nonradiology colleagues who have all worked so hard to make an impact by trying to prevent this largely preventable malignancy.

I would like to thank all the trainees and faculty at the University of California, San Francisco, and the San Francisco VA Medical Center who have worked with me on CTC. You have inspired me to keep forging ahead in this field and to try to make a difference. I thank the staff at Wolters Kluwer/Lippincott Williams & Wilkins, especially Kerry Barrett and Lisa McAllister, for their patience and help. Finally but most importantly, this book would not have been possible without the support and understanding of my husband David and my daughter Taylor.

VIRTUAL COLONOSCOPY

CHAPTER 1 COLORECTAL CANCER SCREENING

Judy Yee

Cancer of the colorectum is the third most common cancer in men and women in the United States. Colorectal cancer is the second leading cause of cancer-related deaths in this country. The estimated number of new cases and deaths due to colorectal cancer in 2007 are 153,790 and 52,180 respectively.[1] Colorectal cancer represents approximately 11% of new cancer cases and approximately 10% of all deaths due to cancer.[1] There is an overall lifetime risk of 6% for the development of colorectal cancer with a lifetime risk of 2.5% for dying from this malignancy.[2]

The incidence of colorectal cancer increases with increasing age. Overall, this malignancy affects men and women equally.[3] It is particularly important to remember that most cases of colorectal carcinoma (approximately 75%) occur sporadically in average-risk patients who have no known risk factors.[3]

There have been favorable trends noted with a general decrease in both colorectal cancer incidence and mortality rates since the 1970s. Colorectal cancer incidence rates have been found to stabilize since the mid 1990s.[1] Five-year survival rates have increased by approximately 12% over the last 20 years.[1,4] Improved survival rates are at least in part related to increased screening for polyps, with their subsequent removal preventing progression to malignancy. Colorectal cancers are also diagnosed at an earlier stage when they are more likely curable and treatments have also improved. Although these trends are encouraging, the total impact of earlier diagnosis and treatment on this disease has been limited. Currently, only approximately 39% of cases of colorectal carcinoma are diagnosed when the disease is localized within the bowel wall.[1] Approximately 20% of patients will already have distant metastases from colorectal carcinoma at the time of the initial diagnosis of the disease.[1,4]

Colorectal cancer is predominantly a preventable disease if precursor adenomatous polyps are identified and then removed. However, current screening rates in the United States remain low. In one study, only 17% of individuals aged 50 or older had undergone fecal occult blood testing (FOBT) in the previous year and only 9% had undergone sigmoidoscopy in the previous 3 years.[5] National Health Interview Surveys found that the use of FOBT increased from 18% for men and 21% for women in 1987 to 29% for men and 26% for women in 1998.[6]

This chapter discusses the epidemiology, staging, and pathophysiology of colorectal cancer as well as risk factors for development. The advantages and disadvantages of the currently recommended available screening tests for colorectal carcinoma are described. Knowledge of the characteristics of this malignancy as well as the current tools used to detect it are necessary for understanding the role of virtual colonoscopy (computed tomographic colonography) in screening for colorectal cancer.

STAGING

Staging of colorectal cancer is related to the extent of tumor through the layers of the colon wall, extension outside the colon locally, and the degree of metastases to lymph nodes and other organs. Survival rates correlate directly with the stage of the disease. There are several systems used for staging colorectal cancer including the Dukes', Astler-Coller, and TNM/American Joint Committee on Cancer (AJCC) systems. The Dukes and the Astler-Coller systems stage colorectal carcinoma using A through C, with the Astler-Coller system being more complex with an additional stage D and the use of subdivisions. The TNM/AJCC system is the most detailed staging system and delineates the extent of the primary tumor (T), the involvement of lymph nodes (N), and whether distant metastasis is present or not (M). The T categories of colorectal carcinoma detail the extent of spread of tumor through the layers of the bowel wall starting with the innermost layer to the outermost layer in the following order: mucosa, submucosa, muscularis propria, subserosa, and serosa. The N categories describe the spread of tumor to lymph nodes and if present, the number of involved lymph nodes. The M categories tell whether there is spread of malignancy to distant sites such as the liver, lungs, or nonregional lymph nodes (see Tables 1.1 and 1.2).[7]

TABLE 1.1 TNM Classification of Colorectal Carcinoma

Primary Tumor (T)

Tx: Primary tumor cannot be assessed because of incomplete information
T0: No evidence of primary tumor
Tis: Carcinoma *in situ* or intramucosal carcinoma
T1: Tumor invades submucosa
T2: Tumor invades muscularis propria
T3: Tumor invades the subserosa but not into neighboring organs or tissues
T4: Tumor directly invades other organs or nearby tissues

Regional Lymph Nodes (N)

Nx: Regional lymph nodes cannot be assessed because of incomplete information
N0: No regional lymph node involvement
N1: Tumor in 1 to 3 regional lymph nodes
N2: Tumor in 4 or more regional lymph nodes

Distant Metastasis (M)

Mx: Distant metastasis cannot be assessed because of incomplete information
M0: No distant metastasis
M1: Distant metastasis present

PATHOPHYSIOLOGY

Most colorectal malignancies are adenocarcinomas and arise from precursor tubular adenomatous polyps.[8] Histologically polyps with a villous component have an even higher chance of transforming into a malignancy. It can take a relatively long time of up to 10 years for an adenomatous polyp, particularly those smaller than 10 mm in diameter, to transition into an invasive malignancy.[2] Therefore, colorectal cancer is a malignancy that is ideally suited for screening with the intent to prevent its occurrence by removing the precursor lesion. The prevalence of adenomatous polyps increases with increasing age. At age 50, approximately 25% of individuals will have an adenomatous polyp of any size. By age 80, approximately 50% to 60% of individuals will harbor an adenomatous polyp.[2] Overall, only 3% to 5% of individuals with adenomatous polyps will develop malignancy.[9] Although it is difficult to know exactly which adenomas will undergo malignant transformation, it has been found that the risk of malignancy is related to polyp size. Only approximately 1% of adenomas smaller than 10 mm are found to contain malignancy.[10] However, adenomatous polyps between 10 and 15 mm in size have an up to 15% chance of transforming into a malignancy within 10 years[11] (see Table 1.3).

RISK FACTORS

There are known risk factors for the development of colorectal carcinoma. A large majority of cases of colorectal carcinoma occur in individuals aged 50 and older. Therefore, screening for colorectal cancer in asymptomatic individuals with no known risks for colorectal carcinoma is recommended starting at age 50.

Familial factors associated with an increased risk for the development of colorectal carcinoma include familial adenomatous polyposis (FAP) and Gardner syndrome. Hereditary nonpolyposis colorectal carcinoma (HNPCC) is another familial risk factor.[12] Increased risk for developing colorectal carcinoma has also been found in the Ashkenazi Jewish population.

A personal or close family history of adenomatous polyps or colorectal carcinoma will increase an individual's risk for subsequent development of this malignancy. First-degree relatives of patients with colonic adenomas have been found to carry a 1.3- to 1.6-fold increased risk for the development of colorectal carcinoma.[13] Studies have also found that the risk of colorectal cancer in

TABLE 1.2 Stage Grouping of Colorectal Carcinoma

Stage	Tumor (T)	Node (N)	Metastasis (M)	Dukes[a]	MAC[b]
0	Tis	N0	M0	—	—
I	T1	N0	M0	A	A
	T2	N0	M0	A	B1
IIA	T3	N0	M0	B	B2
IIB	T4	N0	M0	B	B3
IIIA	T1–T2	N1	M0	C	C1
IIIB	T3–T4	N1	M0	C	C2/C3
IIIC	Any T	N2	M0	C	C1/C2/C3
IV	Any T	Any N	M1	—	D

[a]Dukes B is a composite of better (T3 N0 M0) and worse (T4 N0 M0) prognostic groups, as is Dukes C (any T N1 M0 and any T N2 M0).
[b]MAC is the modified Astler-Coller classification.
Used with the permission of the American Joint Committee on Cancer (AJCC). *The original source for this material is the AJCC cancer staging manual*, 6th ed. Chicago: Springer-Verlag New York; www.springer-ny.com, 2002.

TABLE 1.3 Evolution of Colonic Polyps

Polyp Size	Chance of Being an Adenoma (%)	Chance of Being Malignant Now (%)	If Adenoma, Chance of Being Malignant in 10 Years (%)	Overall Chance of Being Malignant in 10 Years (%)
<5 mm	30	<0.01	<5	1
5–9 mm	50	<1	5–10	2–5
10–15 mm	80	1–5	10–15	5–10

(Adapted from Ferrucci JT. Colon cancer screening with virtual colonoscopy: Promise, polyps, politics. *AJR Am J Roentgenol.* 2001;177(5):975–988.)

family members is increased even further when patients are diagnosed before the age of 60.[14,15] Individuals with a first-degree relative with colorectal cancer have a twofold to fourfold increased risk for the development of colorectal carcinoma.[16] In women, a personal history of ovarian, endometrial, or breast carcinoma is associated with an increased incidence of colorectal carcinoma. Chronic inflammatory bowel disease of long duration, typically over 10 years, is related to an increased risk for colorectal cancer development.

Various environmental factors have also been linked with the development of colorectal carcinoma including a diet high in fats or red meat and low in fiber. Inactivity and being significantly overweight have been linked to increased risk for development of colon cancer.[17] Smoking and moderate-to-heavy alcohol use have also been found to enhance the risk for developing colorectal cancer.[13]

In women, multiple studies have found a decreased risk for developing colorectal cancer with the use of hormone replacement therapy. A meta-analysis of epidemiologic studies of colorectal cancer found a 20% reduction in the development of colorectal cancer in postmenopausal women who had used hormone replacement therapy.[27] In a randomized controlled trial evaluating healthy postmenopausal women, colorectal cancer rates were reduced by 37% in those who received hormone replacement therapy.[28] However, the National Polyp Prevention Trial found no significant decrease in colorectal cancer recurrence in women with known colorectal adenomas taking hormone replacement therapy, although there was a significant risk reduction for recurrence of distal adenomas in users.[29] Routine use of hormone replacement therapy in women is not recommended because of an associated increased risk of breast cancer, stroke, and pulmonary embolism.

PREVENTION

Approximately 90% of all cases of colorectal cancer are preventable.[1] To decrease the likelihood of developing colorectal carcinoma, the American Cancer Society recommends the consumption of healthy foods, particularly vegetables and fruits, maintaining a physically active lifestyle, and a healthy weight, as well as limiting alcohol intake.[1] There have been multiple published studies evaluating the effect of different vitamins and medications in helping to prevent the development of colorectal carcinoma. Folic acid[18,19] and calcium supplements[20,21] have been found in some studies to reduce the occurrence of colorectal cancer. Although the exact mechanism is unclear, calcium is thought to bind to bile acids within the bowel lumen and thereby inhibit the carcinogenic effects of the bile acids.[21] Aspirin and nonsteroidal anti-inflammatory drugs (NSAIDs) have also been found to decrease the likelihood of developing colorectal adenomas and carcinoma.[22–26] They inhibit both cyclooxygenase-1 (COX-1) and cyclooxygenase-2 (COX-2) which are enzymes involved in the synthesis of prostaglandin. COX-2 has been found to be elevated in up to 90% of sporadic colon carcinomas and 40% of colonic adenomas.[25] A large randomized trial found that a low dose of 81 mg of aspirin daily had a moderate preventive effect on colonic adenomas after a few years of usage.[22]

CURRENT GUIDELINES

The best strategy for prevention of colorectal cancer is early screening. Screening allows the detection and removal of premalignant adenomatous polyps, thereby preventing progression of the adenoma–carcinoma sequence. It also allows for earlier diagnosis of colorectal cancer at a stage when the tumor is most curable. Screening leads to decreased morbidity and mortality from colorectal cancer.[30] Current guidelines from the United States Preventive Services Task Force and the American Cancer Society recommend that screening for average-risk patients should begin at age 50.[31,32]

Colorectal cancer screening may be performed using several existing algorithms (see Table 1.4). The American Cancer Society recommends screening of average-risk adults aged 50 and older with one of the following options: (a) annual FOBT or fecal immunochemical testing (FIT), (b) flexible sigmoidoscopy every 5 years, (c) annual FOBT or FIT plus flexible sigmoidoscopy every 5 years (this combination is preferred over either test alone), (d) double-contrast barium enema (DCBE) every 5 years, or (e) conventional colonoscopy every 10 years.[33] The digital rectal examination is not recommended as a screening tool for colorectal cancer, since <10% of cancers may be detected using this test.[1,31] All of the currently suggested colorectal cancer screening tools offer specific benefits and limitations.

TABLE 1.4 American Cancer Society Recommendations for Colorectal Cancer Screening in Average-Risk Adults Beginning at Age 50

Test	Frequency
1. Fecal occult blood test (FOBT), or fecal immunochemical test (FIT)	Annual
2. Flexible sigmoidoscopy	Every 5 years
3. FOBT or FIT and flexible sigmoidoscopy	Annual FOBT or FIT and flexible sigmoidoscopy every 5 years
(Of the above options, the combination of FOBT or FIT annually plus flexible sigmoidoscopy every 5 years is preferable.)	
4. Double-contrast barium enema	Every 5 years
5. Colonoscopy	Every 10 years

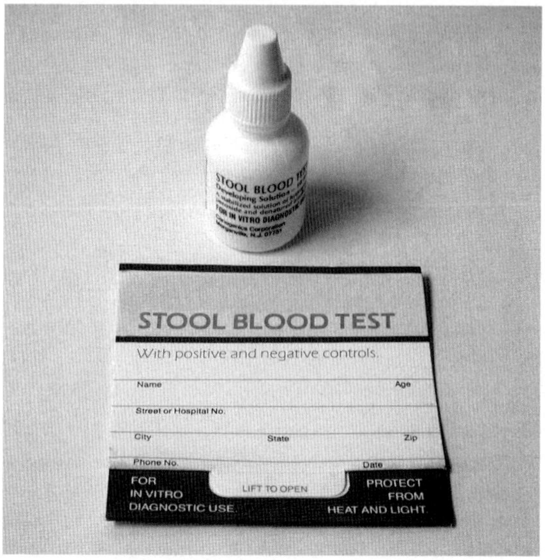

FIGURE 1.1 Fecal occult blood test is performed using this guaiac-impregnated card that turns blue in the presence of hemoglobin when a drop of hydrogen peroxide developer is added.

FECAL OCCULT BLOOD TEST AND FECAL IMMUNOCHEMICAL TEST

FOBT has been in use for more than three decades and is the least expensive of all the currently recommended screening tests for colorectal cancer (see Fig. 1.1). FOBT was first introduced as a colon cancer screening tool in 1967 by Greegor.[34] FOBT is a noninvasive screening tool that does not require the patient to first undergo bowel cleansing. Stool samples are tested for blood leaked by cancers or polyps. Blood is detected when heme oxidizes a colorless substance (α-guaiaconic acid) into a blue color (guaiacum blue) on a test card. The recommended approach to screening involves testing three stool specimens on consecutive days (yields up to 89%–100% sensitivity with final card, specificity decreases from 97% to 94% from first to final card).[35,36] This is preferred rather than a single in-office FOBT that yields a 25% to 40% sensitivity and 96% specificity.[37] Rehydration of the sample during processing increases sensitivity to 60% but lowers specificity to 90%.[38,39]

More recently, in a large study of 2,885 asymptomatic patients who underwent FOBT followed by endoscopy, the sensitivity of a single rehydrated guaiac test for detecting advanced neoplasia was only 24% with a specificity of 94%.[40] FOBT has also been shown to have very low positive predictive values (2.2%–11%)[37] and to result in a large number of false positives, which may lead to unnecessary invasive procedures for additional patient evaluation.

In spite of its questionable performance, FOBT is the best-studied colorectal cancer screening option regarding its impact on mortality. Randomized controlled trials have found an overall 15% to 33% reduction in mortality due to colorectal cancer with annual or biennial FOBT.[41–46]

Dietary restriction for a period of at least 72 hours is required before performing the guaiac-based FOBT. False-positive test results may occur following the ingestion of particular foods containing peroxidase (red meat, turnips, horseradish, broccoli, cabbage) or with particular medications that can cause gastrointestinal blood loss (aspirin and NSAIDs). Other causes of gastrointestinal bleeding (hemorrhoids, diverticulosis, peptic ulcer disease) and rehydration of the stool specimen during the processing may also increase the number of false-positive results. False-negative results occur in individuals who ingest vitamin C and antioxidants. Patients who excrete only small amounts (<20 mL/day) of blood from cancers and polyps may also have a false-negative FOBT.[47,48]

In April 2002, the American Cancer Society's Colorectal Cancer Advisory Group found evidence that the FIT provided advantages over FOBT and hence it should be included in their guideline of recommendations for colorectal cancer screening.[49] The FIT directly detects human hemoglobin in the stool using antihemoglobin antibodies. Monoclonal or polyclonal antibodies are used to detect the intact globin protein of hemoglobin. Labeled antibody attaches to the globin antigen and gives a positive test result. A positive FIT is specific for lower gastrointestinal tract bleeding since the globin protein does not remain intact when it passes through the upper gastrointestinal tract. Similar to FOBT, stool samples are collected at home and no bowel cleansing is needed. Patient compliance may be improved because patients do not need to undergo dietary restrictions before the test. Additionally, only one or two stool samples are required as compared with three for FOBT. However, the benefits of this new test must be considered along with a relatively higher cost. The Medicare payment for FOBT is \$4.50, whereas the cost of the FIT is approximately \$30.

Some studies have also found that immunochemical tests are more sensitive and specific than guaiac-based FOBT.[41,50,51] Allison et al. evaluated 8,104 patients and compared two types of guaiac FOBT with the FIT and found that FIT had a 69% sensitivity for colorectal carcinoma detection as compared with only 37% sensitivity for the most widely used type of FOBT.[41] Morikawa et al. studied 21,805 asymptomatic patients with the FIT and colonoscopy and found that FIT was positive in 1,231 cases (5.6%).[51] The sensitivity of FIT for detecting invasive carcinoma was 66% and for detecting advanced neoplasia was 27%. FIT was also found to detect advanced neoplasia better in the distal colon. Other studies have not identified a clear improvement in detection rates. Ko et al. compared FOBT and FIT in a Veterans Affairs clinic.[52] The positivity rate was 9% for both the FOBT group (122/1396) and for the FIT group (128/1410). Seventeen percent (12/69) of patients with a positive FIT had an adenoma >1 cm or a colorectal carcinoma as compared with 30% (19/64) of patients for FOBT. It was concluded that overall FIT and FOBT had comparable performance.

FLEXIBLE SIGMOIDOSCOPY

Flexible sigmoidoscopy was first introduced in 1976.[3] A flexible sigmoidoscope allows direct visualization of the distal 60 cm of the colorectum (see Fig. 1.2). The flexible sigmoidoscope allows a more complete evaluation of the distal colon than the rigid sigmoidoscope with less patient discomfort. Patients are required to undergo a bowel-cleansing enema before sigmoidoscopy. On the morning of the procedure one or two saline enemas are administered. Typically the procedure takes approximately 10 to 20 minutes and no sedation is administered. Various health care providers routinely perform flexible sigmoidoscopy including gastroenterologists, surgeons and other physicians, nurses, and physician assistants.

There are four case–control studies that have found that sigmoidoscopy with polypectomy reduces colorectal cancer mortality by 60% to 70% when considering the distal colon and by 30% when considering the entire colon.[53–56] The sensitivity of flexible sigmoidoscopy for detecting polyps in the distal colon ranges between 68% and 78%[57,58] with a specificity of up to 99%.[59] Lesions in the proximal or right colon, which are increasing in prevalence,[57,60–64] are missed entirely by the sigmoidoscope. In fact, 46% to 52% of asymptomatic subjects with advanced proximal neoplasms were found to have no distal polyps, which would have yielded a negative sigmoidoscopy.[64] An association of older age and female gender with suboptimal reach of the flexible sigmoidoscope has also been found.[65] Walter et al. found that in men, inadequate sigmoidoscopy occurred in 10% in those aged between 50 and 59 and increased progressively to 22% in those aged 80 or older. In women, inadequate examinations occurred in 19% of those aged between 50 and 59 and increased to 32% in those aged 80 and older.[65]

Sigmoidoscopy is associated with a small risk of perforation (1 to 2 per 10,000 examinations) with slightly higher perforation rates if biopsy or polypectomy is performed.[66] Rarely significant postpolypectomy hemorrhage, and even death, can result from sigmoidoscopy.[58] Poor compliance has been encountered with flexible sigmoidoscopy and because no sedation is typically administered patients undergoing flexible sigmoidoscopy will experience some pain. Initial results from the Prostate, Lung, Colorectal, and Ovarian (PLCO) Cancer Screening Trial found gender differences for follow-up testing, with women being more likely to refuse repeat sigmoidoscopy at a 3-year follow-up than men.[67]

The combination of FOBT with sigmoidoscopy has been found to increase the detection of colorectal cancer by a factor of 3 to 4.[68,69] However, a significant percentage of neoplasia is missed. In a large prospective study of 2,885 patients by Lieberman et al., the combination of one-time screening using FOBT with sigmoidoscopy detected only 75.8% of patients with advanced neoplasia.[40] *Advanced neoplasia* was defined as a large adenoma measuring 10 mm or larger, a villous adenoma, an adenoma with high-grade dysplasia, or an invasive carcinoma. Although no randomized trials have documented the impact of combined FOBT and sigmoidoscopy on colorectal cancer mortality, nonrandomized studies suggest a 43% reduction in mortality rate.[70] The results of the PLCO study, which is a randomized controlled trial evaluating the effectiveness of sigmoidoscopy every 5 years in patients receiving FOBT, are pending with results on mortality expected in 2008.[71,72]

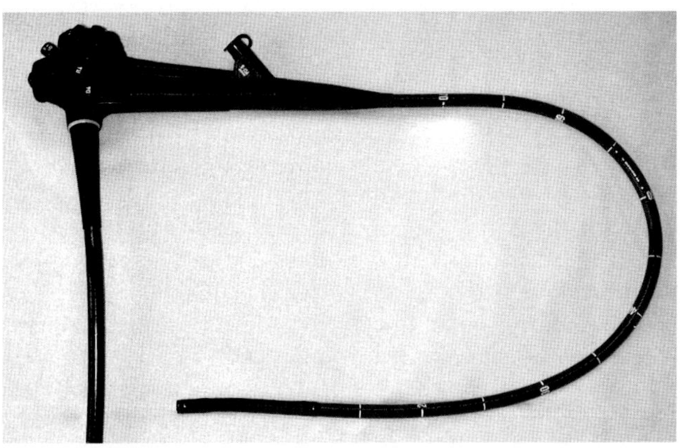

FIGURE 1.2 Flexible sigmoidoscopy is performed using a flexible 60-cm endoscope.

DOUBLE-CONTRAST BARIUM ENEMA

The double-contrast barium enema (DCBE) is endorsed by the American Cancer Society and other organizations as a valid option for colorectal cancer screening. Currently, Medicare reimburses for the DCBE used for colorectal cancer screening in both average-risk and high-risk patients. DCBE allows complete radiologic examination of the colon. Following the retrograde administration of

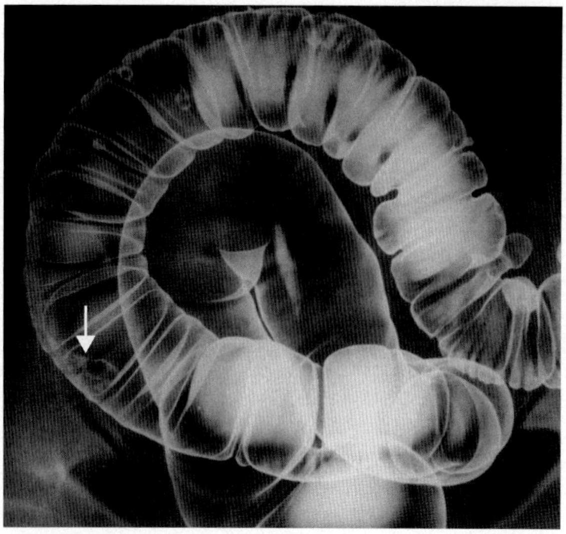

FIGURE 1.3 Double-contrast barium enema shows a large polyp located in the sigmoid that is coated by barium. Several small diverticula are also present scattered throughout the sigmoid.

barium into the colon, the barium is drained and air is instilled to distend the colon, allowing visualization of the mucosa and potential lesions which are outlined by a barium coating (see Fig. 1.3). Patients are required to undergo a low-fiber or liquid diet starting 24 hours before the test. During the afternoon or evening before the barium enema, patients ingest a laxative, typically a saline cathartic such as sodium phosphate or magnesium citrate. Bisacodyl tablets and suppository are included as part of the cleansing regimen and commercially prepackaged bowel-cleansing kits containing these components are available. The procedure takes approximately 20% to 30 minutes in total and typically <5 minutes of fluoroscopy time.[73] No sedation is administered and some patients may experience pain or embarrassment.[74] An antispasmodic agent such as glucagon may be given intravenously.

A drawback to the DCBE is that although it is considered a total colon examination, it may not image the entire colon in approximately 5% to 10% of cases and another examination such as colonoscopy or virtual colonoscopy may be needed. Ionizing radiation is required for imaging and the radiation dose that patients are exposed to during the DCBE is approximately 300 to 500 mrem. However, there is no direct evidence that radiation exposures in this dosage range significantly increase the risk of cancer. An uncommon complication of DCBE is colonic perforation. In a survey of 759 radiologists who performed a total of 738,216 barium enemas, the perforation rate was found to be low at only 1 in 25,000 and the mortality rate was even lower at 1 in 56,786.[75]

The performance of the DCBE has been found to be variable. The sensitivity of DCBE has been found to range between 70% and 90% for large polyps measuring >1 cm. Less optimal performance had been found with sensitivities between 50% and 80% for polyps measuring <1 cm and 55% to 85% for Dukes' stage A and B cancers.[76–78] Other studies have found colorectal cancer miss rates of approximately 18% for the DCBE.[79–81] More recently, in the United States National Polyp Study, patients who had undergone previous colonoscopy and polypectomy were studied by DCBE and colonoscopy. DCBE was found to have low sensitivity for detecting polyps when compared with colonoscopy. For adenomas larger than 10 mm, the sensitivity was only 48%. For adenomas <5 mm and between 6 and 10 mm, the sensitivity was 32% and 53%, respectively. Overall specificity was found to be 82% to 88%.[82] However, decreased sensitivity for the smaller adenomas may not be clinically important. In a national survey of radiologists and primary care physicians regarding colorectal cancer screening with the DCBE, 75% of radiologists said that the DCBE is a "very effective" colorectal cancer screening procedure as compared with 33% of primary care physicians. Fifteen percent of radiologists reported an increase in the volume of DCBEs performed over the last 3 years.[83] Although there are no controlled studies demonstrating the effectiveness of DCBE for decreasing colorectal cancer mortality, it remains a recommended screening option since indirect evidence shows a benefit from detection of similar polyps and early cancers by other screening tests.

COLONOSCOPY

Colonoscopy was first introduced in the early 1970s and is often considered to be the gold standard for colon evaluation (see Fig. 1.4). The colonoscope allows direct visualization of the mucosal surface and permits biopsy and removal of suspicious lesions. Dietary restriction is required starting 24 hours before the procedure and patients are instructed to remain on a clear liquid diet. Colonic cleansing is achieved by ingestion of either a large volume of polyethylene glycol lavage solution or a saline cathartic during the early evening of the day before the test. Patients usually receive multidrug intravenous sedation for colonoscopy and must be accompanied by another person on the day of the procedure since they cannot drive a vehicle after the procedure and must be escorted home. Colonoscopy takes approximately 20 to 30 minutes, but can take much longer for trainees. The reported rate of failed or incomplete colonoscopy is variable, ranging between 2% to 25%, and depends on operator experience and adequacy of bowel cleansing.[3,84–86] Following the actual procedure, recovery time for the patient is approximately 2 to 3 hours.

The effectiveness of colonoscopy as a screening tool is derived from indirect evidence such as from studies that have shown that polyp detection and removal decreases the incidence of colorectal cancer, that identifying early-stage cancers reduces mortality, and that colonoscopy is able to detect most of these lesions.[30,87] An observational study by Winawer et al. was performed evaluating 1,418 patients who underwent colonoscopy during which one or more colorectal adenomas were removed.[30] Periodic colonoscopy was performed during an average

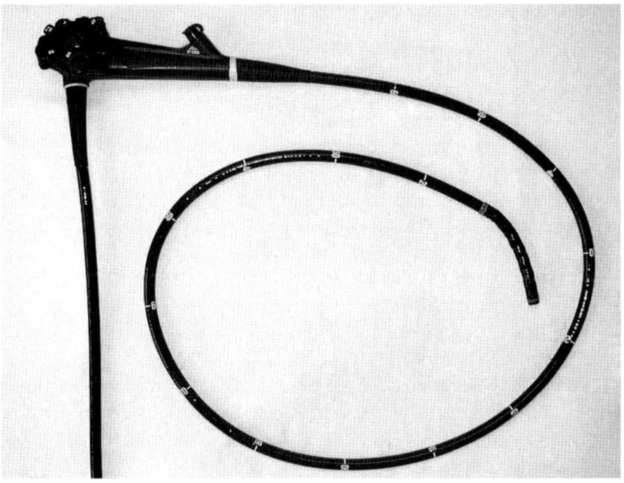

FIGURE 1.4 Colonoscopy is performed using a flexible 160-cm endoscope.

follow-up period of 5.9 years and the incidence of colorectal cancer was determined. Only five asymptomatic early-stage colon cancers were identified upon follow-up of the patient cohort. It was concluded that polypectomy resulted in a lower incidence of colorectal carcinoma. There are no randomized controlled trials demonstrating that colonoscopy reduces the incidence of colorectal cancer. Results from a case-controlled study suggest that colonoscopy reduces the risk of mortality from colorectal cancer (odds ratio = 0.41) and the risk for developing colorectal cancer by 50%.[88] Lieberman et al. evaluated the role of colonoscopy for colon cancer screening in 3,121 asymptomatic Veteran Affairs patients.[57] Advanced disease was found in 10.5% of them. Patients with distal colonic adenomas were found to be more likely to have advanced proximal neoplasia. Fifty-two percent of 128 patients with advanced proximal neoplasia did not have distal adenomas. It was concluded that colonoscopic screening can detect advanced colonic neoplasms in asymptomatic patients and that many of these neoplasms would not be detected using sigmoidoscopy. Imperiale et al. studied 1,994 adults who underwent colonoscopic screening and identified advanced neoplasms in 5.6% of them.[64] Of those patients with advanced proximal neoplasms, 46% did not have a distal polyp. If colonoscopy had been performed only in patients with distal polyps that would have been identified by sigmoidoscopy, approximately half of the cases of advanced proximal neoplasia would not be detected.

Although colonoscopy is used as the reference standard for other colon screening tools, it has also been found to miss lesions.[79,89,90] Rex et al. performed a study using back-to-back colonoscopy and determined the sensitivity of colonoscopy to be 94% for adenomas that are 10 mm or larger, 87% for 6 to 9 mm adenomas, and 73% for adenomas <5 mm.[90] The specificity of colonoscopy is reported to be as high as 99%.[59] The sensitivity of colonoscopy for the detection of large adenomas was found to be lower in a recent study where virtual colonoscopy and colonoscopy performance were compared using a segmental unblinding methodology. In fact, virtual colonoscopy outperformed colonoscopy where the per-polyp sensitivity for the detection of large polyps was found to be 92.2% for virtual colonoscopy and 88.2% for optical colonoscopy.[91]

Widespread use of colonoscopic screening has been limited by cost and low compliance. Poor patient tolerance of the bowel-cleansing regimen required before colonoscopy has been a significant barrier as well as the perception of colonoscopy as an invasive procedure. In fact, when physicians, nurses, and their spouses were invited for free screening colonoscopy, less than 15% accepted.[92] In a study of 1,136 gastroenterologists, 68% felt that the recommendations for colorectal cancer screening by the American Cancer Society were adequate. However, only 38% strictly followed the recommendations, 39% partially, and 23% did not follow them at all.[93] Approximately 25% of patients who underwent colonoscopy found it to be distressing and uncomfortable in a study by Durdey et al.[94]

Colonoscopy also carries the risk of perforation (1 per 1,000 for diagnostic colonoscopy, 1 per 500 for therapeutic colonoscopy), postpolypectomy hemorrhage (3/1,000 have major bleeding), infection, and arrhythmias.[3] There is a very small risk of death from the procedure of 1 to 3 per 10,000. Respiratory depression may occur secondary to the sedation. Although colonoscopy is the most accurate screening examination available, doubts have been raised as to whether the potential benefits may not justify the additional risks to patients.[31]

FECAL DNA TESTING

Assays of DNA markers in stool represent a potential noninvasive alternative method to screen for colorectal cancer. Specific DNA mutations or modifications in cells exfoliated from colorectal cancers and adenomatous polyps may be used as screening markers. Guaiac FOBT and IFT have limitations because early-stage colorectal cancers and adenomatous polyps typically do not bleed frequently, whereas DNA is shed continuously into the lumen. Amplification tests such as polymerase chain reaction are then employed so that even trace amounts of DNA may be detected.

Single-marker assays are unlikely to have clinical relevance because most colorectal cancers are not associated with one molecular mutation. Ahlquist et al. evaluated a multitarget assay panel that targeted point mutations at 15 mutational sites on *K-ras, APC*, and *p53* genes, all of which are implicated in colorectal cancer oncogenesis. BAT-26 deletion, a microsatellite instability marker commonly found in proximal tumors, and highly amplifiable DNA were also included in the assay panel. A blinded study was performed in 22 patients with colorectal carcinoma, 11 patients with large adenomas and 28 patients with endoscopically normal colons. Sensitivity was 91% for cancers and 82% for large adenomas with a specificity of 93%.[95]

Subsequent studies evaluating multitarget assays have had less optimal results with a range of sensitivity for detection of colorectal cancer between 26% and

71% although with high specificity ranging between 93% and 100%. Dong et al. evaluated 51 patients with colorectal cancer using an assay targeting alterations in K-ras, p53 and BAT-26 deletion and found a sensitivity of 71%.[96] Rengucci et al. analyzed samples from 46 patients with colorectal cancer targeting K-ras, p53, and microsatellite instabilities. Results were poor and showed an overall sensitivity for fecal DNA markers of 26%.[97] Another study of 52 patients by Tagore et al. evaluated alterations in K-ras, APC, p53, BAT-26 deletion and long DNA demonstrated a sensitivity of 63% for colorectal carcinoma and 57% for adenomas with high-grade dysplasia.[98]

Multitarget panel assays must undergo additional investigation in large asymptomatic screening patient cohorts before any recommendations may be made. Advantages of fecal DNA marker testing include its noninvasiveness, the lack of a need for dietary restriction or bowel cleansing, and the need for only one stool sample. Disadvantages include the need for an entire bowel movement to be sent for testing, current suboptimal performance results and high cost. Currently, fecal DNA assays are relatively expensive and cost between $500 and $800 per test.[99]

REFERENCES

1. Jemal A, Siegel R, Ward E, et al. Cancer statistics, 2007. *CA Cancer J Clin*. 2007;57:43–66.
2. American Cancer Society. *Cancer Facts and Figures 2004*. Atlanta, GA: American Cancer Society; 2004.
3. Winawer SJ, Fletcher RH, Miller L, et al. Colorectal cancer screening: clinical guidelines and rationale. *Gastroenterology*. 1997;112:594–642.
4. Winawer SJ, Fletcher RH, Rex D, et al. Colorectal cancer screening and surveillance: clinical guidelines and rationale-update based on new evidence. *Gastroenterology*. 2003;124:544–560.
5. Anderson LM, May DS. Has the use of cervical, breast and colorectal cancers screening increased in the Unites States? *Am J Public Health*. 1995;85:840–842.
6. Breen N, Wagener DK, Brown ML, et al. Progress in cancer screening over a decade: results of cancer screening from the 1987, 1992, and 1998 National Health Interview Surveys. *J Natl Cancer Inst*. 2001;93:1704–1713.
7. Greene FL, Page DL, Fleming ID, et al., *AJCC Cancer Staging Manual*, 6th edition. New York: Springer-Verlag; 2002:113–119.
8. Bond JH. Clinical evidence for the adenoma-carcinoma sequence, and the management of patients with colorectal adenomas. *Semin Gastrointest Dis*. 2000;11:176–184.
9. Eide TJ. Natural history of adenomas. *World J Surg*. 1991;15:3–6.
10. Muto T, Bussey HJR, Morson BC. The evolution of cancer of the colon and rectum. *Cancer*. 1975;36:2251–2270.
11. Ferrucci JT. Colon cancer screening with virtual colonoscopy: promise, polyps, politics. *Am J Roentgenol*. 2001;177(5):975–988.
12. Johns Le, Houlston RS. A systematic review and meta-analysis of familial colorectal cancer. *Am J Gastroenterol*. 2001;96:2992–3003.
13. Lynch KL, Ahnen DJ, Byers T, et al. First-degree relatives of patients with advanced colorectal adenomas have an increased prevalence of colorectal cancer. *Clin Gastroenterol Hepatol*. 2003;1:69–70.
14. Winawer SJ, Zauber AG, Gerdes H, et al. Risk of colorectal cancer in the families of patients with adenomatous polyps. *N Engl J Med*. 1996;334:82–87.
15. Ahsan H, Neugut AI, Garbowski GC, et al. Family history of colorectal adenomatous polyps and increased risk for colorectal cancer. *Ann Intern Med*. 1998;128:900–905.
16. Lieberman DA, Prindiville S, Weiss DG, et al. VA Cooperative Study Group 380. Risk factors for advanced colonic neoplasia and hyperplastic polyps in asymptomatic individuals. *JAMA*. 2003;29:2959–2967.
17. Sandler RS. Epidemiology and risk factors for colorectal cancer. *Gastroenterol Clin North Am*. 1996;25:717–735.
18. Choi SW, Mason JB. Folate and carcinogenesis: an integrated scheme. *J Nutr*. 2000;130:129–132.
19. Ulvik A, Evensen ET, Lien EA, et al. Smoking, folate and methylenetetrahydrofolate reductase status as interactive determinants of adenomatous and hyperplastic polyps of colorectum. *Am J Med Genet*. 2001;101:246–254.
20. Wu K, Willett WC, Fuchs CS, et al. Calcium intake and risk of colon cancer in women and men. *J Natl Cancer Inst*. 2002;94:437–446.
21. Baron JA, Beach M, Mandel JS, et al. Calcium Polyp Prevention Study Group. Calcium supplements for the prevention of colorectal adenomas. *N Engl J Med*. 1999;340:101–107.
22. Baron JA, Cole BF, Sandler RS, et al. A randomized trial of aspirin to prevent colorectal adenomas. *N Engl J Med*. 2003;348:891–899.
23. Sandler RS, Halbi S, Baron JA, et al. A randomized trial of aspirin to prevent colorectal adenomas in patients with previous colorectal cancer. *N Engl J Med*. 2003;348:883–890.
24. Coogan PF, Rosenberg L, Louik C, et al. NSAIDS and risk of colorectal cancer according to presence or absence of family history of the disease. *Cancer Causes Control*. 2000;11:249–255.
25. Janne PA, Mayer RJ. Chemoprevention of colorectal cancer. *N Engl J Med*. 2000;342:1960–1968.
26. Gupta RA, Dubois RN. Colorectal cancer prevention an d treatment by inhibition of cyclooxygenase-2. *Nat Rev Cancer*. 2001;1:11–21.
27. Grodstein F, Newcomb PA, Stampfer MJ. Postmenopausal hormone therapy and the risk of colorectal cancer: a review and meta-analysis. *Am J Med*. 1999;106:574–582.
28. Writing Group for the Women's Health Initiative Investigators. Risks and benefits of estrogen plus progestin in healthy postmenopausal women: principal results from the women's health initiative randomized controlled trial. *JAMA*. 2002;288:321–333
29. Woodson K, Lanza E, Tangrea JA, et al. Hormone replacement therapy and colorectal adenoma recurrence among women in the Polyp Prevention Trial. *J Natl Cancer Inst*. 2001;93:1799–1805.
30. Winawer SJ, Zauber AG, Ho MN, et al. The National Polyp Study Workgroup. Prevention of colorectal cancer by colonoscopic polypectomy. *N Engl J Med*. 1993;329:1977–1981.
31. United States Preventative Services Task Force. Screening for colorectal cancer: recommendation and rationale. *Ann Intern Med*. 2002;137:129–131.
32. Centers for Disease Control and Prevention (CDCP). *Behavioral risk factor surveillance system survey data*. Atlanta, GA: U.S. Department of Health and Human Services, Centers for Disease Control and Prevention; 1999.
33. www.cancer.org/docroot/CRI/content/CRI_2_4_3X_Can_colon_and_rectum_cancer_be_found_early.asp?rnav=cri, accessed May 25, 2007.
34. Greegor DH. Diagnosis of large-bowel cancer in the asymptomatic patient. *JAMA*. 1967;201:943–945.

35. Nakama H, Yamamoto M, Kamijo N, et al. Colonoscopic evaluation of immunochemical fecal occult blood test for detection of colorectal neoplasia. *Hepatogastroenterology*. 1999;46:228–231.
36. Yamamoto M, Nakama H. Cost-effectiveness analysis of immunochemical occult blood screening for colorectal cancer among three fecal sampling methods. *Hepatogastroenterology*. 2000;47:396–399.
37. Bini EJ, Rajapaksa RC, Weinshel EH. The findings and impact of nonrehydrated guaiac examination of the rectum (FINGER) study: a comparison of 2 methods of screening for colorectal cancer in asymptomatic average-risk patients. *Arch Intern Med*. 1999;159:2022–2026.
38. Ransohoff DF, Lang CA. American College of Physicians. Screening for colorectal cancer with the fecal occult blood test: a background paper. *Ann Intern Med*. 1997;126:811–822.
39. Wagner J, Tunis S, Brown M. Cost-effectiveness of colorectal cancer screening in average-risk adults. In: Young G, Rozen P, Levin B, et al. eds. *Prevention and Early Detection of Colorectal Cancer*. London: WB Saunders; 1996:321–356.
40. Lieberman DA, Weiss DG. One-time screening for colorectal cancer with combined fecal occult-blood testing and examination of the distal colon. *N Engl J Med*. 2001;345:555–560.
41. Allison JE, Tekawa IS, Ransom LJ, et al. A comparison of fecal occult-blood tests for colorectal-cancer screening. *N Engl J Med*. 1996;334:155–159.
42. Ahlquist DA, Wieand HS, Moertel CG, et al. Accuracy of fecal occult blood screening for colorectal neoplasia. A prospective study using Hemoccult and HemoQuant tests. *JAMA*. 1993;269:1262–1267.
43. Levin B, Hess K, Johnson C. Screening for colorectal cancer. A comparison of 3 fecal occult blood tests. *Arch Intern Med*. 1997;157:970–976.
44. Hardcastle JD, Chamberlain JO, Robinson MH, et al. Randomised controlled trial of faecal-occult-blood screening for colorectal cancer. *Lancet*. 1996;348:1472–1477.
45. Kronborg O, Fenger C, Olsen J, et al. Randomised study of screening for colorectal cancer with faecal-occult-blood test. *Lancet*. 1996;348:1467–1471.
46. Mandel JS, Bond JH, Church TR, et al. Reducing mortality from colorectal cancer by screening for fecal occult blood. Minnesota Colon Cancer Control Study. *N Engl J Med*. 1993;328:1365–1371.
47. Doran J, Hardcastle JD. Bleeding patterns in colorectal cancer: the effect of aspirin and the implications for faecal occult blood testing. *Br J Surg*. 1982;69:711–713.
48. Greegor DH. Detection of silent colon cancer in routine examination. *CA Cancer J Clin*. 1969;19:330–337.
49. Smith RA, Cokkinides V, Eyre HJ. American Cancer Society guidelines for the early detection of cancer, 2003. *CA Cancer J Clin*. 2003;53:27–43.
50. Young GP, St John JB, Winawer SJ, et al. Choice of fecal occult blood tests for colorectal cancer screening: recommendations based on performance characteristics in population studies. *Am J Gastroenterol*. 2002;97:2499–2507.
51. Morikawa T, Kato J, Yamaji Y, et al. A comparison of the immunochemical fecal occult blood test and total colonoscopy in the asymptomatic population. *Gastroenterology*. 2005;129:422–428.
52. Ko CW, Dominitz JA, Nguyen TD. Fecal occult blood testing in a general medical clinic: comparison between guaiac-based and immunochemical-based tests. *Am J Med*. 2003;115:111–114.
53. Selby JV, Friedman GD, Quesenberry CP Jr, et al. A case-control study of screening sigmoidoscopy and mortality from colorectal cancer. *N Engl J Med*. 1992;326:653–657.
54. Newcomb PA, Norfleet RG, Storer BE, et al. Screening sigmoidoscopy and colorectal cancer mortality. *J Natl Cancer Inst*. 1992;84:1572–1575.
55. Muller AD, Sonnenberg A. Protection by endoscopy against death from colorectal cancer. A case-control study among veterans. *Arch Intern Med*. 1995;155:1741–1748.
56. Kavanagh AM, Giovannucci EL, Fuchs CS, et al. Screening endoscopy and risk of colorectal cancer in United States men. *Cancer Causes Control*. 1998;9:455–462.
57. Lieberman DA, Weiss DG, Bond JH, et al. Veterans Affairs Cooperative Study Group 380. Use of colonoscopy to screen asymptomatic adults for colorectal cancer. *N Engl J Med*. 2000;343:162–168.
58. Atkin WS, Hart A, Edwards R, et al. Uptake, yield of neoplasia, and adverse effects of flexible sigmoidoscopy screening. *Gut*. 1998;42:560–565.
59. Ransohoff DF, Sandler RS. Clinical practice. Screening for colorectal cancer. *N Engl J Med*. 2002;346:40–44.
60. Nelson RL, Persky V, Turyk M. Time trends in distal colorectal cancer subsite location related to age and how it affects choice of screening modality. *J Surg Oncol*. 1998;69:235–238.
61. Kee F, Wilson RH, Gilliland R, et al. Changing site distribution of colorectal cancer. *Br Med J*. 1992;305:158.
62. Mamazza J, Gordon PH. The changing distribution of large intestinal cancer. *Dis Colon Rectum*. 1982;25:558–562.
63. Rex DK, Johnson DA, Lieberman DA, et al. American College of Gastroenterology. Colorectal cancer prevention 2000: screening recommendations of the American College of Gastroenterology. *Am J Gastroenterol*. 2000;95:868–877.
64. Imperiale TF, Wagner DR, Lin CY, et al. Risk of advanced proximal neoplasms in asymptomatic adults according to the distal colorectal findings. *N Engl J Med*. 2000;343:169–174.
65. Walter LC, deGarmo P, Covinsky KE. Association of older age and female sex with inadequate reach of screening flexible sigmoidoscopy. *Am J Med*. 2004;116:174–178.
66. Nelson RL, Abcarian H, Prasad ML. Iatrogenic perforation of the colon and rectum. *Dis Colon Rectum*. 1982;25:305–308.
67. Weissfeld JL, Ling BS, Schoen RE, et al. Adherence to repeat screening flexible sigmoidoscopy in the prostate, lung, colorectal, and ovarian (PLCO) cancer screening trial. *Cancer*. 2002;94:2569–2576.
68. Berry DP, Clarke P, Hardcastle JD, et al. Randomized trial of the addition of flexible sigmoidoscopy to faecal occult blood testing for colorectal neoplasia population screening. *Br J Surg*. 1997;84:1274–1276.
69. Rasmussen M, Kronborg O, Fenger C, et al. Possible advantages and drawbacks of adding flexible sigmoidoscopy to hemoccult-II in screening for colorectal cancer. A randomized study. *Scand J Gastroenterol*. 1999;34:73–78.
70. Winawer SJ, Flehinger BJ, Schottenfeld D, et al. Screening for colorectal cancer with fecal occult blood testing and sigmoidoscopy. *J Natl Cancer Inst*. 1993;85:1311–1318.
71. Kramer BS, Gohagan J, Prorok PC, et al. A National Cancer Institute sponsored screening trial for prostatic, lung, colorectal, and ovarian cancers. *Cancer*. 1993;71:589–593.
72. Prorok PC, Andriole GL, Bresalier RS, et al. Design of the prostate, lung, colorectal and ovarian (PLCO) cancer screening trial. *Control Clin Trials*. 2000;21:273S–309S.
73. Levine MS, Glick SN, Rubesin SE, et al. Double-contrast barium enema examination and colorectal cancer: a plea for radiologic screening. *Radiology*. 2002;222:313–315.

74. Kim LS, Koch J, Yee J, et al. Comparison of patients' experience during imaging tests of the colon. *Gastrointest Endosc*. 2001;54:67–74.
75. Blakeborough A, Sheridan MB, Chapman AH. Complications of barium enema examinations: a survey of UK Consultant Radiologists 1992 to 1994. *Clin Radiol*. 1997;52:142–148.
76. Hixson LJ, Fennerty MB, Sampliner RE, et al. Prospective study of the frequency and size distribution of polyps missed on colonoscopy. *J Natl Cancer Inst*. 1990;82:1769–1772.
77. Fork FT. Double contrast enema and colonoscopy in polyp detection. *Gut*. 1981;22:971–977.
78. Steine S, Stordahl A, Lunde OC, et al. Double-contrast barium enema versus colonoscopy in the diagnosis of neoplastic disorders: aspects of decision-making in general practice. *Fam Pract*. 1993;10:288–291.
79. Hixson LJ, Fennerty MB, Sampliner RE, et al. Prospective blinded trial of the colonoscopic miss rate of large colorectal polyps. *Gastrointest Endosc*. 1991;37:125–127.
80. Brady AP, Stevenson GW, Stevenson I. Colorectal cancer overlooked at barium enema examination and colonoscopy: a continuing perceptual problem. *Radiology*. 1994;192:373–378.
81. Rex DK, Rahmani EY, Haseman JH, et al. Relative sensitivity of colonoscopy and barium enema for detection of colorectal cancer in clinical practice. *Gastroenterology*. 1997;112:17–23.
82. Winawer SJ, Stewart ET, Zauber AG, et al. National Polyp Study Work Group. A comparison of colonoscopy and double-contrast barium enema for surveillance after polypectomy. *N Engl J Med*. 2000;342:1766–1772.
83. Klabunde CN, Jones E, Brown ML, et al. Colorectal cancer screening with double-contrast barium enema: a national survey of diagnostic radiologists. *Am J Roentgenol*. 2002;179:1419–1427.
84. Anderson ML, Heigh RI, McCoy GA, et al. Accuracy of assessment of the extent of examination by experienced colonoscopists. *Gastrointest Endosc*. 1992;38:560–563.
85. Marshall JB, Barthel JS. The frequency of total colonoscopy and terminal ileal intubation in the 1990's. *Gastrointest Endosc*. 1993;39:518–520.
86. Nelson DB, McQuaid KR, Bond JH, et al. Procedural success and complications of large-scale screening colonoscopy. *Gastrointest Endosc*. 2002;55:307–314.
87. Citarda F, Tomaselli G, Capocaccia R, et al. Efficacy in standard clinical practice of colonoscopic polypectomy in reducing colorectal cancer incidence. *Gut*. 2001;48:812–815.
88. Muller AD, Sonnenberg A. Prevention of colorectal cancer by flexible endoscopy and polypectomy. A case-control study of 32,702 veterans. *Ann Intern Med*. 1995;123:904–910.
89. Bensen S, Mott LA, Dain B, et al. Polyp Prevention Study Group. The colonoscopic miss rate and true one-year recurrence of colorectal neoplastic polyps: Polyp Prevention Study Group. *Am J Gastroenterol*. 1999;94:194–199.
90. Rex DK, Cutler CS, Lemmel GT, et al. Colonoscopic miss rates of adenomas determined by back-to-back colonoscopies. *Gastroenterology*. 1997;112(1):24–28.
91. Pickhardt PJ, Choi JR, Hwang I, et al. Computed tomographic virtual colonoscopy to screen for colorectal neoplasia in asymptomatic adults. *N Engl J Med*. 2003;349:2191–2200.
92. Rex DK, Lehman GA, Ulbright TM, et al. Colonic neoplasia in asymptomatic persons with negative fecal occult blood tests: influence of age, gender, and family history. *Am J Gastroenterol*. 1993;88:825–831.
93. Afridi J, Jafri SF, Marshall JB. Do gastroenterologists themselves follow the American Cancer Society recommendations for colorectal cancer screening? *Am J Gastroenterol*. 1994;89:2184–2187.
94. Durdey P, Weston PMT, Williams NS. Colonoscopy or barium enema as initial investigation of colonic disease. *Lancet*. 1987;2:549–551.
95. Ahlquist DA, Skoletsky JE, Boynton KA, et al. Colorectal cancer screening by detection of altered human DNA in stool: feasibility of a multitarget assay panel. *Gastroenterology*. 2000;119:1219–1227.
96. Dong SM, Traverso G, Johnson C, et al. Detecting colorectal cancer in stool with the use of multiple genetic targets. *J Natl Cancer Inst*. 2001;93:858–865.
97. Rengucci C, Maiolo P, Saragoni L, et al. Multiple detection of genetic alterations in tumors and stool. *Clin Cancer Res*. 2001;7:590–593.
98. Tagore KS, Lawson MJ, Yucaitis JA, et al. Sensitivity and specificity of a stool DNA multitarget assay panel for the detection of advanced colorectal neoplasia. *Clin Colorectal Cancer*. 2003;3:47–53.
99. Agrawal J, Syngal S. Colon cancer screening strategies. *Curr Opin Gastroenterol*. 2004;21:59–63.

CHAPTER 2 EXAMINATION PREREQUISITES

Judy Yee

Computed tomographic (CT) scanners, computer workstations, and graphic software for computed tomographic colonography (CTC) have undergone significant technologic advances over the last 10 years. However, the diagnostic ability of this test still relies on two key examination prerequisites. The colon must be well cleansed and well distended in order to obtain images that are optimally diagnostic. The presence of fluid or solid stool in the colon can compromise the accuracy of CTC and result in both missed lesions and false positives. Suboptimal distension or collapse of the colon can also cause lesions to be overlooked and may also simulate the stenosis of an annular carcinoma. Dual position (supine and prone) scanning is performed so that regions of the colon that have retained material or poor distension on one view may show improved cleansing or distension in the opposing position.

COLONIC CLEANSING

Cleansing of the colon is currently still necessary for CTC. Poor cleansing has been shown to decrease the sensitivity of CTC for the detection of polyps of all sizes.[1] Polyps and cancers may be hidden in residual fluid pools or obscured by large amounts of retained solid material (see Figs. 2.1–2.4). Solid stool may also be mistaken for a sessile polyp, particularly if it is homogeneous in appearance on the two-dimensional CT images and adherent to the colon wall (see Fig. 2.5).

The protocol used for colonic preparation for CTC consists of two parts. The first part requires that the patient undergo dietary limitation and maintain a clear liquid diet starting 24 hours before the CT scan. The second part requires that the patient ingest a laxative that stimulates evacuation of colonic contents. The agents used for bowel cleansing for CTC are similar to those employed for other colon tests such as barium enema and standard colonoscopy. Saline cathartics such as sodium phosphate and magnesium citrate are highly osmotic agents that contain inorganic ions that cause shifting of fluid into the bowel lumen to stimulate peristalsis and emptying of the colon. Polyethylene glycol is an electrolyte lavage solution that is ingested in large volumes causing evacuation of the colon.

Sodium Phosphate

Sodium phosphate (also called phosphosoda) is often employed as a cathartic agent before barium enemas and colonoscopy. It is also one of the laxatives used for bowel cleansing before CTC. The osmotic effects of sodium phosphate cause large outflow from the colon. Sodium phosphate is available in a 45-mL (1.5 oz) bottle either alone or in a kit also containing four (5 mg) bisacodyl tablets and one (10 mg) bisacodyl suppository. Bisacodyl acts as a contact laxative and stimulates parasympathetic reflexes to increase bowel peristalsis.[2]

On the day preceding the CTC, patients are instructed to mix 45 mL (1.5 oz) of sodium phosphate with 120 mL (4 oz) of cool water, which is ingested with an additional 240 mL (8 oz) of water at approximately 5 P.M. It takes approximately 1 hour for the laxative effect to occur and patients are requested to stay near a rest room. Approximately 3 hours later at 8 P.M. the patient ingests the four bisacodyl tablets that take effect after approximately 6 to 12 hours. The bisacodyl suppository is placed in the rectum on the morning of the CT procedure and takes approximately 15 minutes for onset of effect. Patients should be instructed to keep the bisacodyl suppository in a cool environment until ready for use since it may easily melt if kept in a pocket for transporting to the imaging site for patient use.

Sodium phosphate is referred to as a *dry preparation* agent because it leaves little residual fluid in the colon. This can occasionally cause solid material to adhere to the bowel wall in the environment of a dry colon that may simulate a polyp on CTC. Many studies have been performed comparing the efficacy of sodium phosphate versus polyethylene glycol for colonic cleansing before colonoscopy. Some of the published trials have found both purgatives to result in similar bowel cleansing.[3–5] However, other studies have found sodium phosphate to cleanse the colon more effectively than polyethylene glycol.[6–8] In a meta-analysis that included

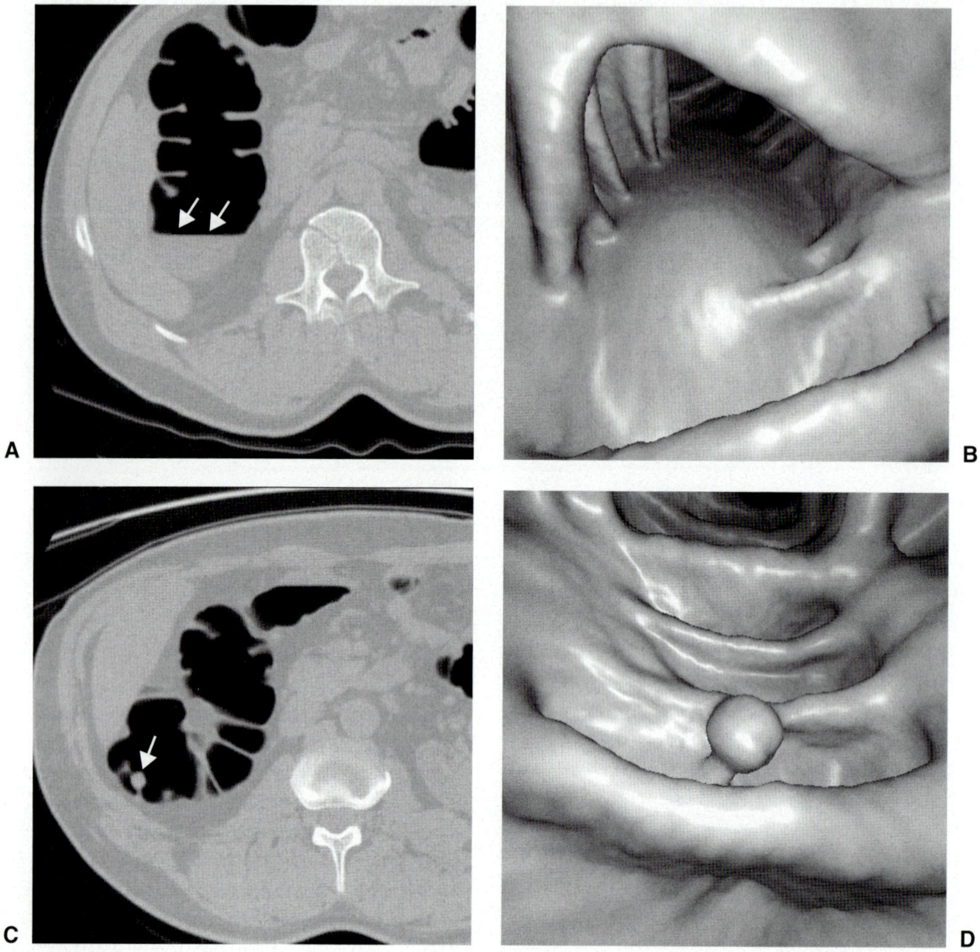

FIGURE 2.1 Layering fluid along the posterior wall of the hepatic flexure on this supine axial view **(A)** and on the three-dimensional endoluminal image **(B)**. The fluid has shifted to reveal a pedunculated polyp on the prone axial view **(C)** and on the corresponding 3D view **(D)**.

eight studies evaluating the effectiveness of sodium phosphate versus polyethylene glycol for cleansing the colon for colonoscopy in a total of 1,286 patients, it was found that there was no statistically significant difference in the quality of bowel cleansing between the two laxatives. However, sodium phosphate was better tolerated by patients and less costly, at a saving of approximately $40 per colonoscopy procedure.[9] In a prospective, blinded randomized trial comparing oral sodium phosphate and polyethylene glycol solutions for bowel preparation before barium enema, no difference was identified in the amount of residual fluid and adequacy of colonic wall coating.[10]

Complications due to the administration of sodium phosphate are uncommon. However, patients may become hypovolemic, and occasionally severe electrolyte abnormalities may occur including hypernatremia, hyperphosphatemia, hypocalcemia, and hypokalemia.[11,12] The administration of sodium phosphate is contraindicated in patients with renal failure, history of electrolyte disturbances, congestive heart failure, ascites, ileus, and bowel obstruction.[13] Patients on diuretic medications should also not receive sodium phosphate. Two doses of sodium phosphate have been prescribed by some physicians and called a *double dose*, consisting of a total volume of 90 mL (3 oz) for bowel cleansing before CTC. One dose is given the evening before the procedure and the second dose is given the morning of the procedure with each dose separated by 10 to 12 hours.[14] Particular caution must be exercised with the use of double dose phosphosoda, given the potential for serious electrolyte abnormalities particularly in the elderly. A warning has been issued by the U.S. Food and Drug Administration (FDA) regarding the potential toxicity of taking sodium phosphate as a bowel cleansing agent before colonoscopy.[15] Recently, the packaging of over-the-counter sodium phosphate was modified in the United States so that a single volume bottle of 90 mL (3 oz) is no longer available. Patients with significant comorbid clinical conditions are advised to avoid the use of sodium phosphate.[16]

Magnesium Citrate

Magnesium citrate is also classified as a saline laxative. It may be employed for bowel cleansing for CTC.

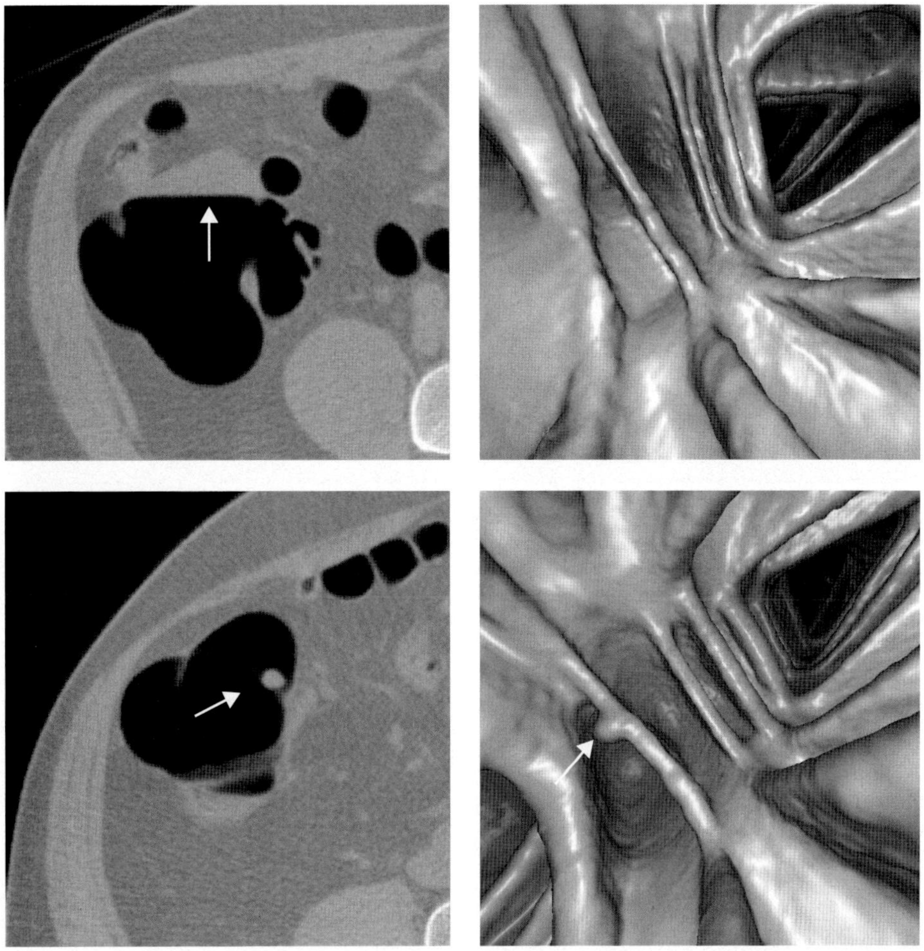

FIGURE 2.2 Prone axial image **(A)** and endoluminal view **(B)** shows residual fluid along the dependent wall. In the supine position, a sessile polyp is apparent on the axial image **(C)** and endoluminal image **(D)** in the same area that was obscured by fluid in the prone position.

Magnesium citrate acts by both preventing resorption of fluid and by stimulating cholecystokinin, which in turn causes small bowel fluid secretion, increased peristalsis and emptying.[17] Magnesium citrate comes packaged in a powder form that the patient reconstitutes with 240 mL (8 oz) of water or as a 300-mL (10-oz) bottle containing a premixed solution ready for ingestion. A typical bowel-cleansing protocol consists of ingestion of magnesium citrate in the late afternoon of the day before the CT at approximately 5 P.M. It is then followed by ingestion of an additional 240 mL (8 oz) of water and the patient is instructed to maintain hydration during the evacuation process. Four bisacodyl tablets and a suppository are administered in addition to the magnesium citrate preparation as described in the preceding text for the sodium phosphate preparation protocol.

Magnesium citrate may be preferred over sodium phosphate in patients who are at risk for electrolyte disturbances. Magnesium citrate is a saline cathartic, but contains much less sodium than sodium phosphate. In its mixed form, magnesium citrate has 12 mg of sodium whereas sodium phosphate contains 5,004 mg of sodium. Magnesium citrate has not been found to cause the same severe electrolyte abnormalities that have been found associated with sodium phosphate. In a study comparing patients who received either magnesium citrate or sodium phosphate, all patients receiving the sodium phosphate preparation were found to have hyperphosphatemia followed by hypocalcemia.[18] A combination of magnesium citrate with a smaller volume of polyethylene glycol has been used successfully as a cleansing regimen for colonoscopy. This was found to improve cleansing and to shorten preparation times.[19]

COLONIC DISTENSION

The colon must be adequately distended in order to allow for the detection of the lesion and to minimize the potential for false-positive lesions (see Figs. 2.6–2.8). Poor distension of a segment of colon may have an appearance similar to an annular carcinoma causing luminal narrowing, particularly on the three-dimensional

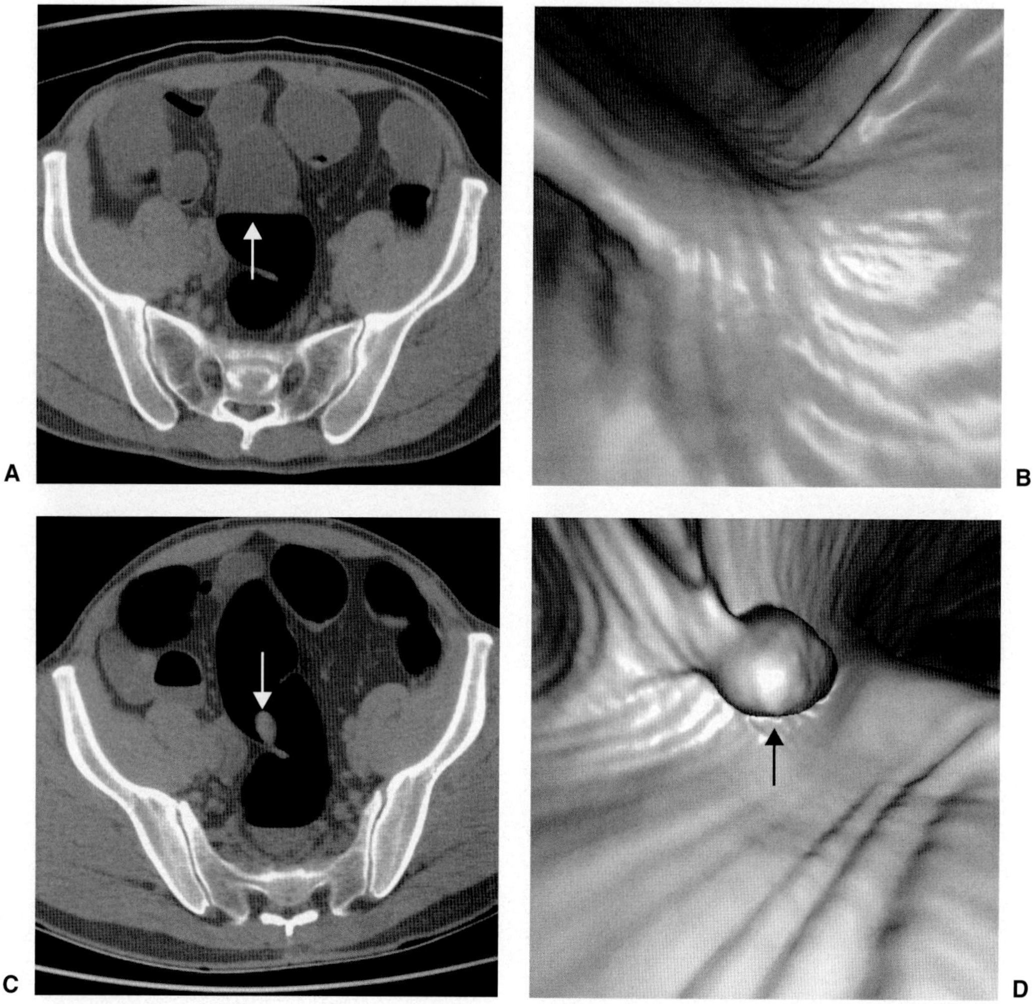

FIGURE 2.3 Large amount of residual fluid is present in the sigmoid colon on the prone axial **(A)** and 3D images **(B)**. A large pedunculated polyp is detected in the supine view on axial **(C)** and 3D views **(D)** after the large fluid pool has moved away. This patient received polyethylene glycol for bowel preparation.

view (see Fig. 2.9). Focal thickening of folds in an area of suboptimal distension may appear polypoid, particularly on two-dimensional images.

HOW TO INSUFFLATE THE COLON

After the patient is placed on the CT table, a rectal tube is inserted for the administration of either room air or carbon dioxide to distend the colon. Placement of the rectal tube may be performed by a trained physician, technologist, or nurse, based on local guidelines. The tip is easily inserted into the rectal vault with the patient in a right side–down decubitus position. Rectal tip placement is facilitated by use of a small amount of lubricant gel. The holes of the rectal tip may become obstructed if too much gel is applied. Lidocaine gel may be used if the patient has anorectal pain or if there is evidence of external hemorrhoids. There are a variety of administration sets that may be used for manual insufflation of gas for CTC. A simple soft rectal tip attached to tubing with an insufflation bulb at the end is adequate and inexpensive. A Foley catheter may also be used, attached to an insufflation bulb.

The colon is insufflated with the patient initially in the right side–down decubitus position, which allows filling of the descending colon and the rectosigmoid. The patient is then rotated into the supine position and additional gas is administered to completely fill the transverse colon and then the right colon. Typically at least 3 L of gas is needed to obtain sufficient colonic distension, and additional gas is required if the patient has difficulty with gaseous retention. Some radiologists will inflate the rectal balloon in order to aid in gaseous and tube retention. However, caution is advised to clear the rectal vault of any lesion first, by performing a rectal examination to help avoid the possibility of causing perforation or significant

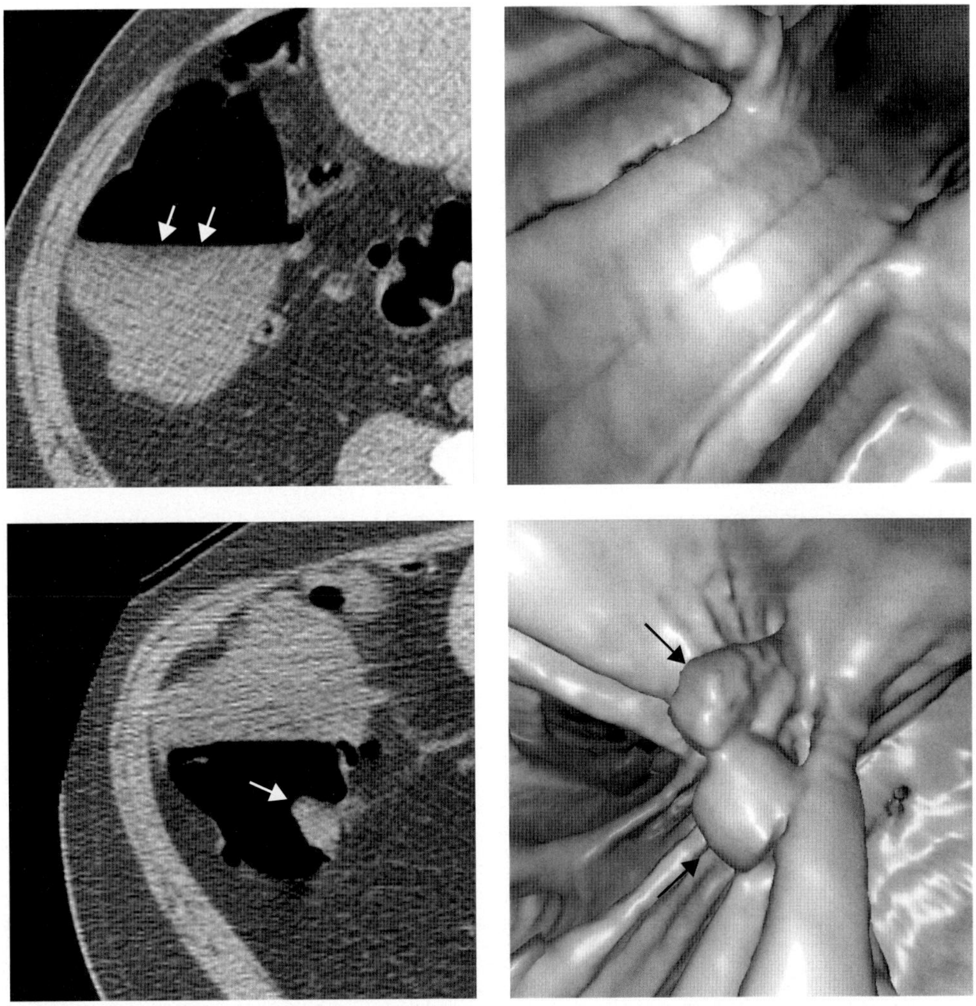

A B C D

FIGURE 2.4 A patient who received polyethylene glycol bowel-cleansing regimen demonstrates a large amount of retained fluid seen in the ascending colon on the supine axial **(A)** and 3D views **(B)**. A polypoid mass that was found to be malignant is revealed on the supine axial **(C)** and 3D views **(D)** when the fluid falls along the dependent wall.

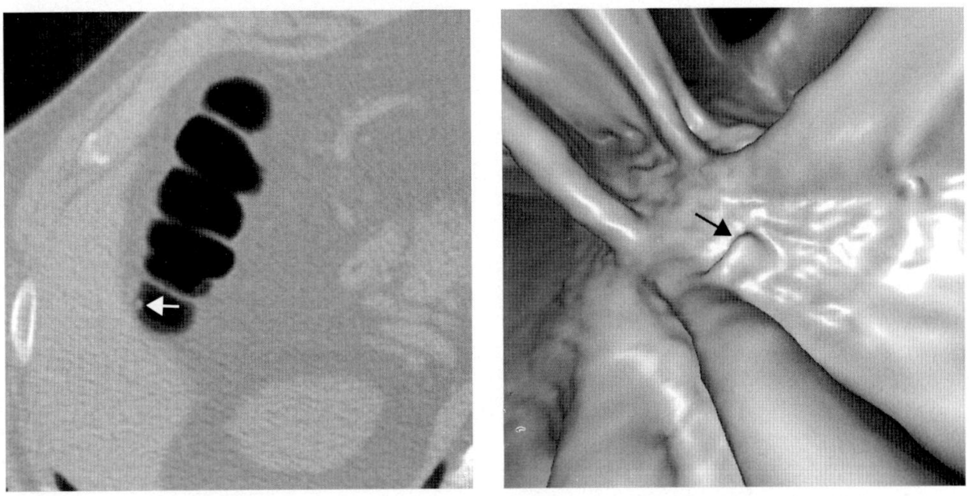

A B

FIGURE 2.5 Supine axial image shows a small polypoid lesion **(A)**. The endoluminal image demonstrates the linear, angular appearance of this lesion that is characteristic of stool **(B)**.

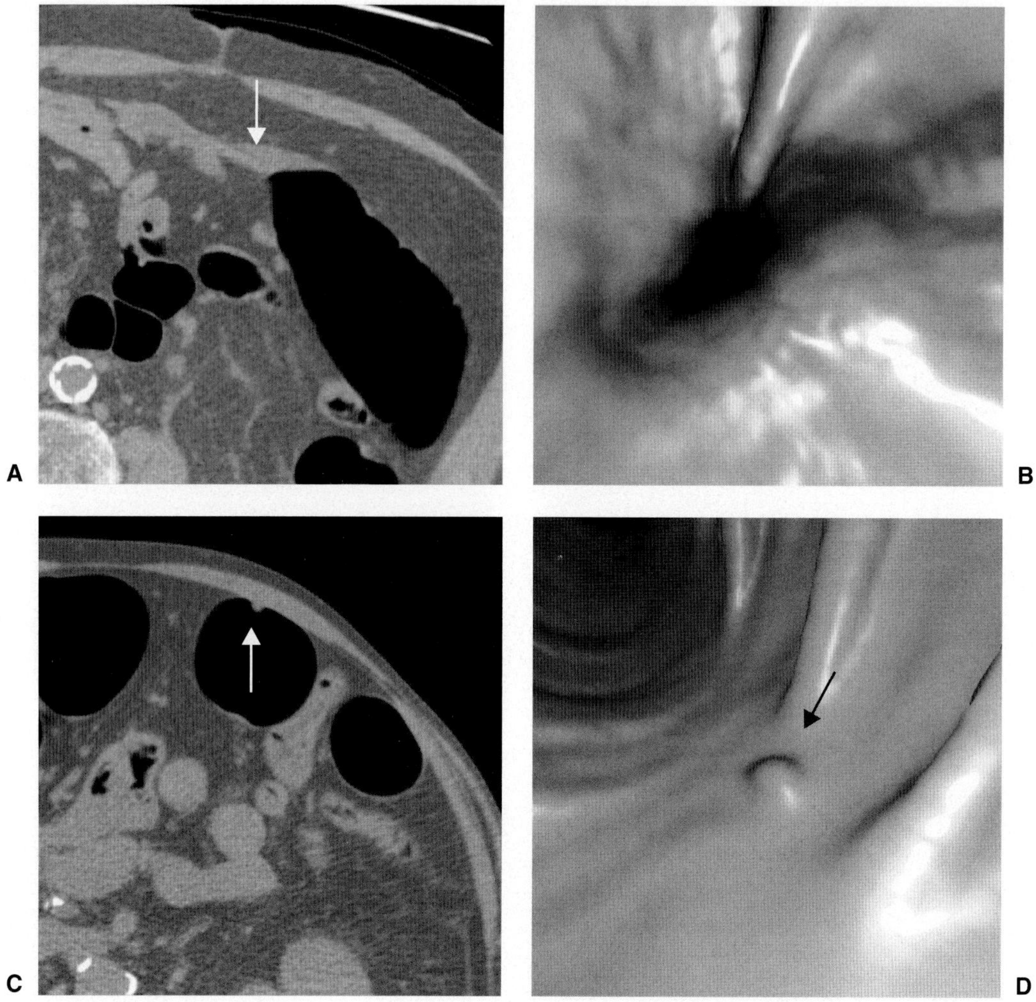

FIGURE 2.6 Collapse of the distal transverse colon is present on the prone axial **(A)** and 3D endoluminal images **(B)**. In the supine position, the transverse colon is optimally distended to show a small polyp along the anterior wall which is well seen on the axial **(C)** and endoluminal views **(D)**.

bleeding. Adequate distension may be obtained in most patients without the use of an inflated rectal balloon.

Insufflation of gas is performed up to maximum patient tolerance or until the patient feels a sense of fullness or mild discomfort in the right abdomen. This will help assure that gas has advanced retrograde to the right colon. When this occurs it is time to obtain a CT scout view of the abdomen and pelvis. If the entire colon is well distended, then the first scan series may be performed. It is important to assure optimum distension of the sigmoid colon since this is the segment that is most likely to have suboptimal distension. Diverticulosis and muscular hypertrophy commonly involve the sigmoid and may contribute to poor distension. However, the sigmoid is also where most colonic polyps and cancers occur. If there is inadequate distension of any colonic segment, then additional gas is administered up to maximum patient tolerance. After the supine scan, the patient is rotated into the prone position and a repeat scout image is obtained. Additional gas insufflation is performed if poorly distended colonic segments are identified. It is helpful to try to lift the abdomen slightly off the CT table when the patient is in the prone position so as to facilitate optimal distension of the transverse colon.[1] This may be achieved by placing a wedge, pillows, or towels underneath the lower chest and pelvic areas and adjusting to the specific patient's body habitus and comfort.

Atmospheric Air

Atmospheric air has been traditionally used for distension of the colon for CTC. Radiologists are familiar with administering room air per rectum through a tube for the air-contrast barium enema examination. Other advantages of employing room air include its easy availability and the absence of additional cost. Atmospheric air is predominantly composed of nitrogen, which is an inert gas so that there is no active diffusion across the colon wall. When the colon is distended with room air, it will remain filled until peristalsis moves the air antegrade and it

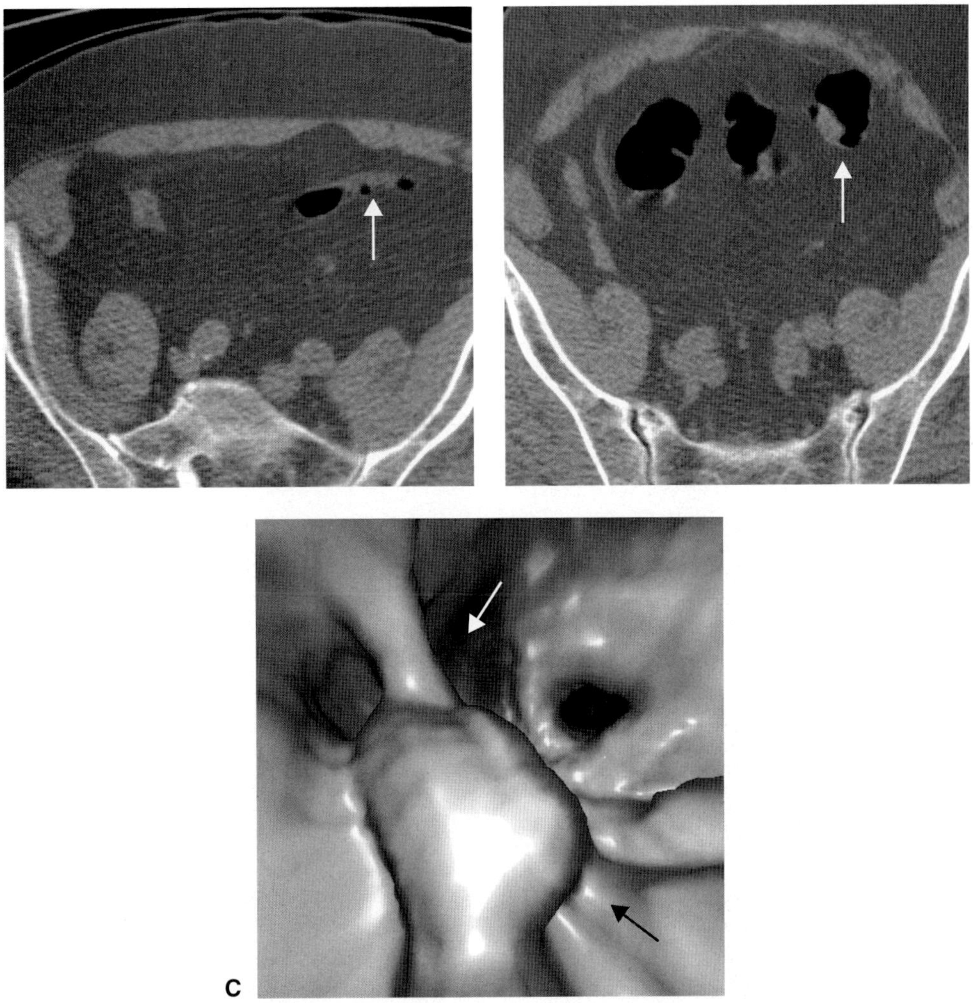

A B C

FIGURE 2.7 Poor distension of the sigmoid is present in the prone position as seen on the axial image **(A)**. When the patient is turned in the supine position a large polyp is identified on the axial image **(B)**, which is seen to be pedunculated on the endoluminal view **(C)**.

is passed distally. Uncommonly, patients may experience severe abdominal pain and may feel bloated for several hours after the CTC examination because of the retention of a large amount of air in the colon. In a study of patient symptoms following air distension of the colon for the barium enema examination, it was found that 7% of patients had severe pain and 13% of patients experienced marked distension.[20]

Carbon Dioxide

Carbon dioxide (CO_2) is an alternative gas used for insufflation of the colon for procedures such as colonoscopy and barium enema. Studies have found that there is decreased patient discomfort with the use of CO_2 for colonic distension. This is thought to be related to the high lipid solubility of CO_2 and its high partial pressure gradient across the wall of the colon so that CO_2 is much more rapidly resorbed than room air. CO_2 is then exhaled through the respiratory system. In a study comparing patient tolerance of CO_2 versus room air in 100 patients undergoing colonoscopy, results showed that there was a statistically significant larger percentage of patients reporting postprocedural pain following room air insufflation. Pain was reported at 1 hour and 6 hours following colonoscopy by 7% and 9% of subjects, respectively insufflated with CO_2 as compared with 45% and 31%, respectively of patients who received air.[21]

Similar results have been obtained in studies evaluating the use of CO_2 as the colonic distending agent for barium enema. In a study of 142 patients undergoing barium enema, approximately half received CO_2 insufflation per rectum and the remaining half received air insufflation. There was a lower incidence of both immediate and delayed pain in patients who received CO_2 insufflation as compared with room air of 12.5% versus 31% and 4.2% versus 12.9% respectively.[22] In another study of patients undergoing barium enema, 86 received room air and 65 received CO_2 for colonic insufflation. Approximately one third of patients who received room

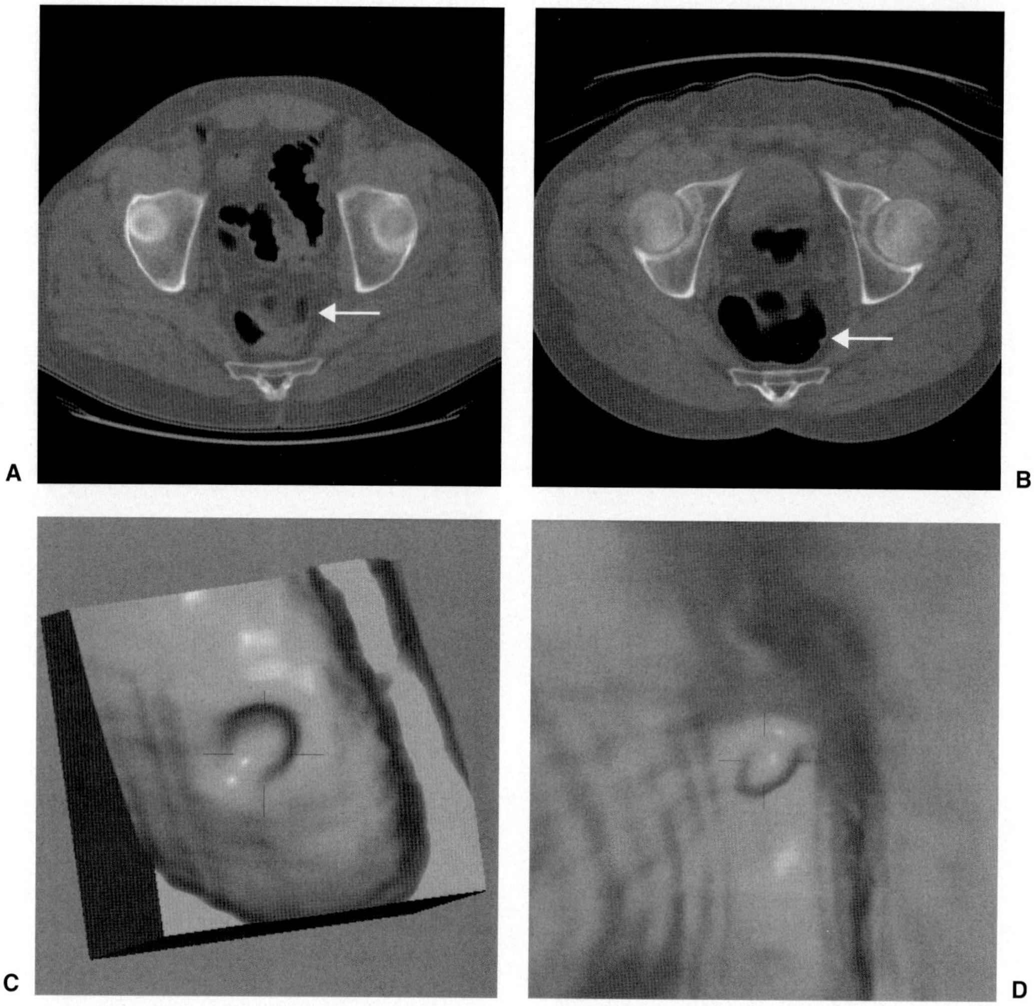

FIGURE 2.8 Collapse of the rectosigmoid junction on the supine axial view **(A)**. Improved distension in this area in the prone position allows diagnosis of a small polyp along the left lateral wall seen on the axial image **(B)**. The small polyp is also well demonstrated on the 3D cube view **(C)** and the endoluminal fly-through image **(D)**.

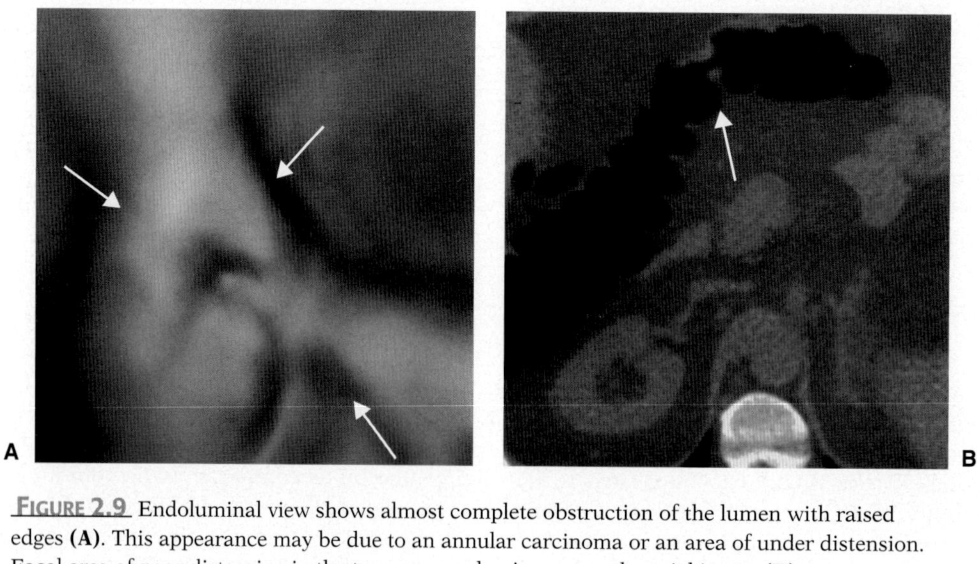

FIGURE 2.9 Endoluminal view shows almost complete obstruction of the lumen with raised edges **(A)**. This appearance may be due to an annular carcinoma or an area of under distension. Focal area of poor distension in the transverse colon is seen on the axial image **(B)**.

air experienced pain, and only 11% of patients with the abdomen were distended with CO_2 complained of pain. Additionally, five patients who received room air reported severe pain but no patients receiving CO_2 complained of severe pain.[23] Three different patient groups undergoing barium enema were evaluated in a study comparing colonic insufflation using air, CO_2, and a 50/50 mixture of the two gases. Colonic mucosal coating with barium was found to be similar in all three groups. Patients who received CO_2 had significantly less immediate and delayed pain as compared to those who had air and less delayed pain as compared to those who had the 50/50 mixture. There was a trend indicating that air alone provided better distension than the other two groups.[24] Manual administration of CO_2 was found to provide suboptimal colonic distension when compared with manual air insufflation in a study of 100 patients undergoing barium enema.[25]

There is increasing experience with the use of CO_2 for colonic distension for CTC. CO_2 may be administered per rectum either manually or using a specific commercially available mechanical device. Our experience has been more consistently reliable optimal colonic distension may be achieved with the mechanical infusion of CO_2 whereas manual administration of CO_2 may lead to less optimal colonic distension. A study by Burling et al. evaluated 47 patients who received automated CO_2 insufflation and 94 patients who received manual CO_2 insufflation for CTC.[26] Results showed that automated CO_2 insufflation significantly improved colonic distension as compared with manual insufflation. The largest benefit was in the sigmoid and descending colons when the patient was supine. Patient acceptance between the two patient groups was similar.

Electronic administration of CO_2 used for colonoscopy has been shown to be safe using a pressure maintained at 35 mm Hg with a CO_2 flow rate of 1 L per minute.[27] The mechanical device for CTC allows instillation of CO_2 at a fixed flow rate of 3 L per minute and up to a maximum pressure of 25 mm Hg. It has been found that starting with a preset pressure of 15 mm Hg and slowly increasing to 25 mm Hg according to patient tolerance allows for excellent optimal colonic distension and excellent patient comfort. Electronic instillation of CO_2 is maintained according to a preset pressure during the acquisition of supine and prone images. A total of approximately 4 L of CO_2 is typically infused for a CTC examination. This is significantly less than the amount of CO_2 insufflated into the peritoneal cavity during a laparoscopic procedure lasting approximately 2 hours, with typical flow rates of 5 to 15 L per minute for a total volume of approximately 40 L of CO_2.[28]

Upon completion of the CT scan, a brief review of supine and prone data sets is recommended to assure adequate diagnostic quality of the images. If there is an area of the colon that is not of diagnostic quality because of poor distension and/or cleansing on both supine and prone images, a limited rescan of the particular segment may be obtained with the patient in a decubitus position. Suboptimal distension is most frequently encountered in the sigmoid colon, especially in older patients who have sigmoid muscular hypertrophy and/or diverticulosis. However, most colorectal polyps and carcinomas are located in the sigmoid and the diagnostic quality of this segment is particularly important.

COLONIC PERFORATION

Perforation of the colon during CTC is very uncommon. To date there are four published case reports documenting colonic perforation following CTC. Three of the patients had an abnormal colon with inflammatory and/or obstructive lesions (ulcerative colitis, Crohn's disease, obstructive carcinoma).[29–31] One patient did not have any known colonic disease, received intravenous antibiotic treatment for the colonic perforation, and did not require surgery.[32]

Colonic perforation is a known risk of conventional colonoscopy and has been reported at an approximate rate of 0.06% to 0.19% of cases.[33–35] Mechanical trauma due to the colonoscope is thought to be the primary cause of perforation. The risk of perforation increases following polypectomy or biopsy. The double-contrast barium enema has been reported to have a risk of perforation ranging between 0.02% and 0.2%.[33] To decrease the likelihood of perforation during barium enema, it is recommended to wait for 7 days following biopsy.[36]

A survey was conducted in 16 medical centers from 5 countries (Working Group on Virtual Colonoscopy) to evaluate the symptomatic perforation rate and the overall significant complication rate of CTC.[37] The group had performed a total of 21,923 CTC studies dating back to 1997. Approximately half the number of the studies were performed for screening and the remaining were diagnostic examinations. Two perforations were identified and both were in patients undergoing diagnostic CTC. Manual room air insufflation was employed in the two patients. One patient was asymptomatic and did not require treatment. The second patient was symptomatic and required treatment. Therefore, the symptomatic perforation rate was determined to be 0.0046% (1/21,923) and the overall perforation rate was 0.0091%. Two other patients developed renal failure related to the bowel preparation and one patient had chest pain. This resulted in a significant complication rate of 0.018% (4/21,923). It was concluded that the safety profile for CTC is very favorable, particularly for asymptomatic screening and distension with automated CO_2.

ANTISPASMODIC AGENTS

A bowel relaxant may be administered before CTC in order to decrease spasm, minimize peristalsis, and increase patient comfort. Glucagon hydrochloride was administered routinely in earlier studies of CTC performed although its effectiveness has not been proved. Hyoscine butylbromide (Buscopan) is used in Europe for both CT and magnetic resonance colonography and has been found in some studies to be more effective than glucagon as a spasmolytic agent and at a cost savings.

Glucagon

Glucagon is a single-chain polypeptide hormone that is normally produced by the pancreatic islet cells of Langherhans. The injectable form is identical to the human form. Its two main actions are elevation of blood glucose level and relaxation of the smooth muscle of the gastrointestinal tract. Glucagon is administered as a hypotonic agent for the stomach, small bowel, and colon for fluoroscopic studies. The effectiveness of glucagon varies according to location and has the maximum effect on the duodenum, followed by the jejunum, and then the stomach. The colon is the least sensitive to glucagon.[38] Patients may uncommonly experience adverse reactions to glucagon such as nausea, vomiting, and headache. Nausea was reported in 4% of patients who received intravenous glucagon before CTC.[39] The use of glucagon is contraindicated in patients with insulinoma, pheochromocytoma, poorly controlled diabetes, and known glucagon hypersensitivity.

Glucagon may also be administered before CTC with the goal of increasing colonic distension and improving patient comfort. Patients included in many of the earlier studies evaluating CTC routinely received 1 mg of glucagon intravenously immediately before the CT scan. This practice was extrapolated from the administration of glucagon before the barium enema examination. Studies have found that glucagon reduces patient discomfort both during and after barium enema.[40,41] Glucagon has also been found to improve the quality of barium enema examinations by improving colonic relaxation and ease of filling.[42] Although glucagon is generally believed to decrease patient discomfort during the barium enema examination, it is still unclear as to whether there is any improvement in bowel distension and polyp detection. In a study of 175 patients undergoing barium enema, approximately half the number of patients received glucagon and the remaining patients did not. Results showed no statistically significant difference when quantifying colonic distension.[41] Another study found that glucagon did not improve the sensitivity or specificity for polyp detection on barium enema.[43] There are significant differences between the barium enema examination and CTC when considering the effectiveness of glucagon. Instillation of liquid barium may cause colonic spasm during the barium enema although this does not occur during CTC. A gas-filled colon is required for a much shorter period of time for CTC due to the very rapid scan time of CTC as compared with the relatively longer procedural time required for barium enema.

Several studies have been published evaluating the effectiveness of glucagon for CTC. Yee et al. performed a study evaluating 60 patients undergoing CTC who received manual air insufflation of the colon.[44] Patients were divided into glucagon and nonglucagon groups. One mg of glucagon was administered intravenously to the 33 patients in the glucagon group. There were no statistically significant differences between the glucagon and nonglucagon groups for segmental as well as overall colonic distension scores in the supine, prone, and combined supine and prone positions. In patients receiving glucagon, 222 segments (84.1%) were considered to be adequately distended. In patients not receiving glucagon, 187 segments (86.6%) were adequately distended. It was also found that the most common segmental locations with inadequate distension were the sigmoid and descending colons. In a study by Morrin et al. 74 patients received intravenous glucagon before CTC and 22 patients did not.[39] Results showed no significant difference in the degree of colonic distension between patients who received glucagon and those who did not (mean distension score = 3.6 vs. 3.9). It was concluded that colonic distension at CTC is improved by dual positioning but not by the administration of intravenous glucagon. The use of glucagon has not been found to improve polyp detection on CTC in an initial study.[45]

Glucagon is not administered routinely for CTC at our institution based on the results of the preceding studies. However, glucagon is given in specific situations where the patient exhibits significant abdominal discomfort or if there is evidence of spasm or poor distension that is not resolved by dual positioning as observed on the scout CT images.

Hyoscine Butylbromide

Hyoscine butylbromide (Buscopan) is an anticholinergic drug that is used in Europe and Asia to induce bowel relaxation. It is clinically used for treatment of irritable bowel syndrome. Buscopan is less costly than glucagon, but it is not licensed for use in the United States. Its mechanism of action is blocking the postganglionic parasympathetic receptors in smooth muscle to induce bowel hypotonia. Buscopan is an anticholinergic agent and is contraindicated in patients with glaucoma, severe prostatic hyperplasia, unstable heart disease, bowel obstruction or ileus, and myasthenia gravis. The administration of anticholinergic agents may cause side effects such as tachycardia, blurry vision, dry mouth, acute urinary retention, and acute dilatation of the stomach.

Conflicting results regarding the effectiveness of Buscopan for colonic distension have been reported in the literature for patients undergoing barium enema. Buscopan was found to be more effective than glucagon for colonic distension in a study evaluating patients who received antispasmodic agents before undergoing double-contrast barium enema.[46] Approximately 5% of patients who received Buscopan complained of blurry vision as a side effect in this study. In another study patients received either intravenous glucagons or oral Buscopan before undergoing barium enema.[41] Results showed no significant difference in colonic distension or abdominal discomfort between the two patient groups.

There have also been controversial results from studies evaluating the utility of Buscopan for CTC. Bruzzi et al. evaluated the efficacy of intravenous Buscopan as a muscle relaxant in CTC.[47] Seventy-three patients were randomized to receive 20 mg Buscopan intravenously ($n = 36$) or no agent ($n = 37$) before CTC. No significant difference was identified between the two groups when evaluating the number of optimally or adequately distended colonic segments. Polyp detection rates were similar between the two groups. In patients with diverticulosis, Buscopan did not have any effect on segments with diverticula, but was associated with improved distension of more proximal segments. The routine administration of Buscopan for CTC was not recommended. In contrast, other studies have documented improved colonic distension following the administration of Buscopan for CTC. Taylor et al. performed a study on 136 patients who were randomized to receive either 20 mg or 40 mg of Buscopan or no spasmolytic before CTC.[48] Results showed that Buscopan improved colonic distension and routine administration was recommended. Improved distension was identified in the cecum, ascending and transverse colons in the supine position, and in the prone ascending and descending colons. The use of a double dose of Buscopan (40 mg) did not have any advantage. In evaluating two types of rectal catheters, this study also found that use of a thin rectal tube is adequate for insufflation of the colon as compared with a balloon catheter. Rogalla et al. showed that there was no significant difference in colon segmental volume and radial distensibility when comparing 80 patients who received intravenous glucagon and 80 patients who received no spasmolytic agent before CTC.[49] However, segmental volume and radial distensibility were significantly larger in the 80 patients who received 20 mg Buscopan intravenously as compared to the patients who did not receive a spasmolytic agent.

REFERENCES

1. Yee J, Kumar NN, Hung RK, et al. Comparison of supine, prone and both supine and prone scans in CT colonography. *Radiology*. 2003;226:653–661.
2. Gelfand DW, Chen MYM, Ott DJ. Preparing the colon for the barium enema examination. *Radiology*. 1991;178:609–613.
3. Golub RW, Kerner BA, Wise WE, et al. Colonoscopic bowel preparations which one? A blinded, prospective, randomized trial. *Dis Colon Rectum*. 1995;38:594–599.
4. Afridi SA, Barthel JS, King PD, et al. Prospective, randomized trial comparing a new sodium phosophate-bisacodyl regimen with conventional PEG-ES lavage for outpatient colonoscopy preparation. *Gastrointest Endosc*. 1995;41:485–489.
5. Marshall JB, Pineda JJ, Barthel JS, et al. Prospective, randomized trail comparing sodium phosphate solution with polyethylene glycol-electrolyte lavage for colonoscopy preparation. *Gastrointest Endosc*. 1993;39:631–634.
6. Cohen SM, Wexner SD, Binderow SR, et al. Prospective, randomized, endoscopic-blinded trial comparing precolonoscopy bowel cleansing methods. *Dis Colon Rectum*. 1994;37:689–696.
7. Kolts BE, Lyles WE, Achem SR, et al. A comparison of the effectiveness and patient tolerance of oral sodium phosphate, castor oil, and standard electrolyte lavage for colonoscopy or sigmoidoscoopy preparation. *Am J Gastroenterol*. 1993;88:1218–1223.
8. Vanner SJ, MacDonald PH, Paterson WG, et al. A randomized prospective trial comparing oral sodium phosphate with standard polyethylene glycol-based lavage solution (Golytely) in the preparation of patients for colonoscopy. *Am J Gastroenterol*. 1990;4:422–427.
9. Hsu CW, Imperiale TF. Meta-analysis and cost comparison of polyethylene glycol lavage versus sodium phosphate for colonoscopy preparation. *Gastrointest Endosc*. 1998;48:276–282.
10. O'Donovan AN, Somers S, Farrow R, et al. A prospective blinded randomized trial comparing oral sodium phosphate and polyethylene glycol solutions for bowel preparation prior to barium enema. *Clin Radiol*. 1997;52:791–793.
11. Ehrenpreis ED, Nogueras JJ, Botoman VA, et al. Serum electrolyte abnormalities secondary to Fleet's phospho-soda colonscopy prep. *Surg Endosc*. 1996;10:1022–1024.
12. Vukasin P, Weston LA, Beart RW. Oral Fleet phospho-soda laxative-induced hyperphosphatemia and hypocalcemic tetany in an adult. *Dis Colon Rectum*. 1997;40:497–499.
13. Fass R, Do S, Hixson LJ. Fatal hyperphosphatemia following Fleet phospho-soda in a patient with colonic ileus. *Am J Gastroenterol*. 1993;88:929–932.
14. Pickhardt P, Choi JR, Hwang I, et al. Computed tomographic virtual colonoscopy to screen for colorectal neoplasia in asymptomatic adults. *Radiology*. 2003;349:2191–2200.
15. Food and Drug Administration. *Science Background: Safety of Sodium Phosphates Oral Solution. Center for Drug Evaluation and Research*. Washington, DC: Food and Drug Administration; 2002.
16. Hookey LC, Depew WT, Vanner S. The safety profile of oral sodium phosphate for colonic cleansing before colonoscopy in adults. *Gastrointest Endosc*. 2002;56:895–902.
17. Bartram CI. Bowel preparation principles and practice. *Clin Radiol*. 1994;49:365–367.
18. Oliviera L, Wexner SD, Daniel N, et al. Mechanical bowel preparation for elective colorectal surgery a prospective, randomized, surgeon-blinded trail comparing sodium phosphate and polyethylene glycol-based oral lavage solutions. *Dis Colon Rectum*. 1997;40:585–591.
19. Sharma VK, Chockalingham SK, Ugheoke EA, et al. Prospective, randomized, controlled comparison of the use of polyethylene glycol electrolyte lavage solution in four-liter versus two-liter volumes and pretreatment with either magnesium citrate or bisacodyl for colonoscopy preparation. *Gastrointest Endosc*. 1998;47:167–171.
20. Skovgaard N, Sloth C, Von Benzon E, et al. The role of carbon dioxide and atmospheric air in double-contrast barium enema. *Abdom Imaging*. 1995;20:436–439.
21. Sumanac K, Zealley I, Fox BM, et al. Minimizing post-colonoscopy abdominal pain by using CO2 insufflation: a prospective, randomized, double-blind, controlled trial evaluating a new commercially available CO2 delivery system. *Gastrointest Endosc*. 2002;56:190–194.
22. Robson NK, Lloyd M, Regan F. The use of carbon dioxide as an insufflation agent in barium enema does it have a role? *Br J Radiol*. 1993;66:197–198.
23. Coblentz CL, Frost RA, Molinaro V, et al. Pain after barium enema: effect of CO2 and air on double-contrast study. *Radiology*. 1985;157:35–36.
24. Holemans JA, Matson MB, Hughes JA, et al. A comparison of air, CO2 and air/CO2 mixture as insufflation agents for double contrast brium enema. *Eur Radiolol*. 1998;8:274–276.
25. Scullion DA, Wetton CWN, Davies C, et al. The use of air or CO2 as insufflation agents for double contrast barium enema: is there a qualitative difference? *Clin Radiol*. 1995;50:558–561.
26. Burling D, Taylor SA, Halligan S, et al. Automated insufflation of carbon dioxide for MDCT colonography: distention and patient experience compared with manual insufflation. *AJR Am J Roentgenol*. 2006;186:96–103.
27. Phaosawasdi K, Cooley W, Wheeler J, et al. Carbon dioxide-insufflated colonoscopy: an ignored superior technique. *Gastrointest Endosc*. 1986;32:330–333.
28. Taskin O, Buhur A, Birincioglu M, et al. The effects of duration of CO2 insufflation and irrigation on peritoneal microcirculation assessed by free radical scavengers and

total glutathione levels during operative laparoscopy. *J Am Assoc Gynecol Laparosc*. 1998;5:129–133.
29. Kamar M, Portnoy O, Bar-Dayan A, et al. Actual colonic perforation in virtual colonoscopy: report of a case. *Dis Colon Rectum*. 2004;47:1242–1246.
30. Coady-Fariborzian L, Angel LP, Procaccino JA. Perforated colon secondary to virtual colonoscopy: report of a case. *Dis Colon Rectum*. 2004;47:1247–1249.
31. Triester SL, Hara AK, Young-Fadok TM, et al. Colonic perforation after computed tomographic colonography in a patient with fibrostenosing Crohn's disease. *Am J Gastroenterol*. 2006;101:189–192.
32. Young BM, Fletcher JG, Earnest F, et al. Colonic perforation at CT colonography in a patient without known colonic disease. *AJR Am J Roentgenol*. 2006;186:119–121.
33. Tran DQ, Rosen L, Kim R, et al. Actual colonoscopy: what are the risks of perforation? *Am J Surg*. 2001;67:845–847.
34. Korman LY, Overholt BF, Box T, et al. Perforation during colonscopy in endoscopic ambulatory surgical centers. *Gastrointest Endosc*. 2003;58:554–557.
35. Anderson ML, Pasha TM, Leighton JA. Endoscopic perforation of the colon: lessons from a 10-year study. *Am J Gastroenterol*. 2000;95:3418–3422.
36. Stevenson G. Normal anatomy and techniques of examination of the colon: barium, CT and MRI. In: Freeny PC, Stevenson GW, eds. *Margulis and Burhenne's Alimentary Tract Radiology*. St. Louis: Mosby; 1994:692–724.
37. Pickhardt PJ. Incidence of colonic perforation at CT colonography: review of existing data and implications for screening of asymptomatic adults. *Radiology*. 2006;239:313–316.
38. Chernish SM, Maglinte DDT. Glucagon: common untoward reactions-review and recommendations. *Radiology*. 1990;177:145–146.
39. Morrin MM, Farrell RJ, Keogan MT, et al. CT colonography: colonic distention improved by dual positioning but not intravenous glucagon. *Eur Radiol*. 2002;12:525–530.
40. Meeroff JC, Jorgens J, Isenberg JI. The effect of glucagon on barium enema examinations. *Radiology*. 1975;115:5–7.
41. Bova JG, Jurdi RA, Bennett WF. Antispasmodic drugs to reduce discomfort and colonic spasm during barium enemas: comparison of oral hyoscyamine, iv glucagon, and no drug. *AJR Am J Roentgenol*. 1993;161:965–968.
42. Harned RK, Stelling CB, Williams S, et al. Glucagon and barium enema examinations: a controlled clinical trial. *AJR Am J Roentgenol*. 1974;126:981–984.
43. Thoeni RF, Vandeman F, Wall SD. Effect of glucagon on the diagnostic accuracy of double-contrast barium enema examinations. *AJR Am J Roentgenol*. 1984;142:111–114.
44. Yee J, Hung RK, Akerkar GA, et al. The usefulness of glucagon hydrochloride for colonic distention in CT colonography. *AJR Am J Roentgenol*. 1999;173:1–4.
45. Yee J, Hung RK, Steinauer-Gebauer AM, et al. Colonic distention and prospective evaluation of colorectal polyp detection with and without glucagon during CT colonography [abstract]. *Radiology*. 1999;213(Suppl):256.
46. Goei R, Nix M, Kessels AH, et al. Use of antispasmodic drugs in double contrast barium enema examination: glucagon or buscopan? *Clin Radiol*. 1995;50:553–557.
47. Bruzzi JF, Moss AC, Brennan DD, et al. Efficacy of IV buscopan as a muscle relaxant in CT colonography. *Eur Radiol*. 2003;13:2264–2270.
48. Taylor SA, Halligan S, Goh V, et al. Optimizing colonic distention for multi-detector row CT colonography: effect of hyoscine butylbromide and rectal balloon catheter. *Radiology*. 2003;229:99–108.
49. Rogalla P, Lembcke A, Ruckert JC, et al. Spasmolysis at CT colonography: butyl scopolamine versus glucagon. *Radiology*. 2005;236:184–188.

CHAPTER 3 OPTIMIZING COMPUTED TOMOGRAPHY TECHNIQUE

Judy Yee

The computed tomography (CT) parameters specifically used to examine the colon for CT colonography (CTC) has evolved with the advancement of CT technology. Helical CT allows volumetric data acquisition and is a requirement for CTC. Helical scanning is based on slip-ring CT technology, which couples continuous motion of the gantry with synchronous table feed.

Single-detector CT enables the performance of CTC. However, multidetector computed tomography (MDCT) is preferred for optimizing the acquisition of data and improving the performance of CTC. Each detector acts as a single unit in single-detector CT and section thickness is determined by the collimation of the x-ray beam. MDCT segments the detectors in the z-axis (longitudinal) plane so that multiple slices per rotation may be acquired. Section thickness is determined by the thickness of each detector row on a MDCT scanner.[1] The number of data channels present in a specific CT scanner determines the actual number of slices that may be obtained.

MULTIDETECTOR COMPUTED TOMOGRAPHY

The use of MDCT is an advantage for CTC because the entire abdomen and pelvis may be scanned in a shorter amount of time using thinner slices. Shorter scan duration translates into a more tolerable breath hold for the patient and subsequently results in a decrease in respiratory and motion artifacts (see Figs. 3.1 to 3.3). Hara et al. performed a study comparing respiratory artifacts, colonic distention, and polyp detection at CTC by using single- and multidetector row helical CT systems.[2] Seventy-seven patients underwent CTC with single-detector CT and 160 patients were scanned on MDCT followed by optical colonoscopy. Mild respiratory artifacts were identified in 61% of patients who were scanned on single-detector CT compared with only 16% of patients who underwent MDCT. Similarly, there was a statistically significant larger number of patients with suboptimal colonic distention with single-detector CT involving at least one colonic segment in 52% of examinations versus only 16% of multidetector row CT examinations. There was no statistically significant difference in the sensitivity for detection of large polyps comparing single-detector CT versus MDCT at 89% (8/9) versus 80% (8/10) respectively although it was noted that there were a relatively small number of large polyps in each group.

SECTION THICKNESS

The acquisition of thin sections allows for less partial volume averaging and improved image quality of the multiplanar reformatted views and the three-dimensional (3D) endoluminal images. This has been evaluated in both phantom models and patient studies. An early study by Power et al. evaluated a phantom containing 10 spherical polyps between 1 mm and 10 mm in size using single-detector CT.[3] The phantom was scanned at slice thicknesses of 3 mm, 5 mm, and 7 mm and various pitches ranging between 1.0 and 2.0. It was found that a slice thickness of 3 mm with a pitch of 2 on single-detector CT provided optimal polyp conspicuity with a relatively low radiation dose. Laghi et al. used a colonic phantom containing 27 simulated polyps of various morphologies to evaluate the optimal scanning technique for CTC using a MDCT scanner.[4] Three different scanning protocols were tested—collimation and slice thickness of 1.0 mm, collimation of 2.5 mm with a slice thickness of 3.0 mm, and collimation of 2.5 mm with a slice thickness of 5.0 mm. Sensitivity for detection of lesions was 100% for protocol 1, 96% for protocol 2 and dropped to 85% for protocol 3. There was progressive blurring of polyp borders and worsening of image quality when slice thickness was increased. Increased stair-step and rippling artifacts were identified with increasing slice thickness. On the basis of these results it was recommended that CTC be performed with the use of a high-resolution CT protocol when using a MDCT scanner (1.0-mm effective slice thickness).

Lui et al. performed a study evaluating the effect of various section thicknesses at CTC and results showed improved specificity for thin sections.[5] Twenty-five patients

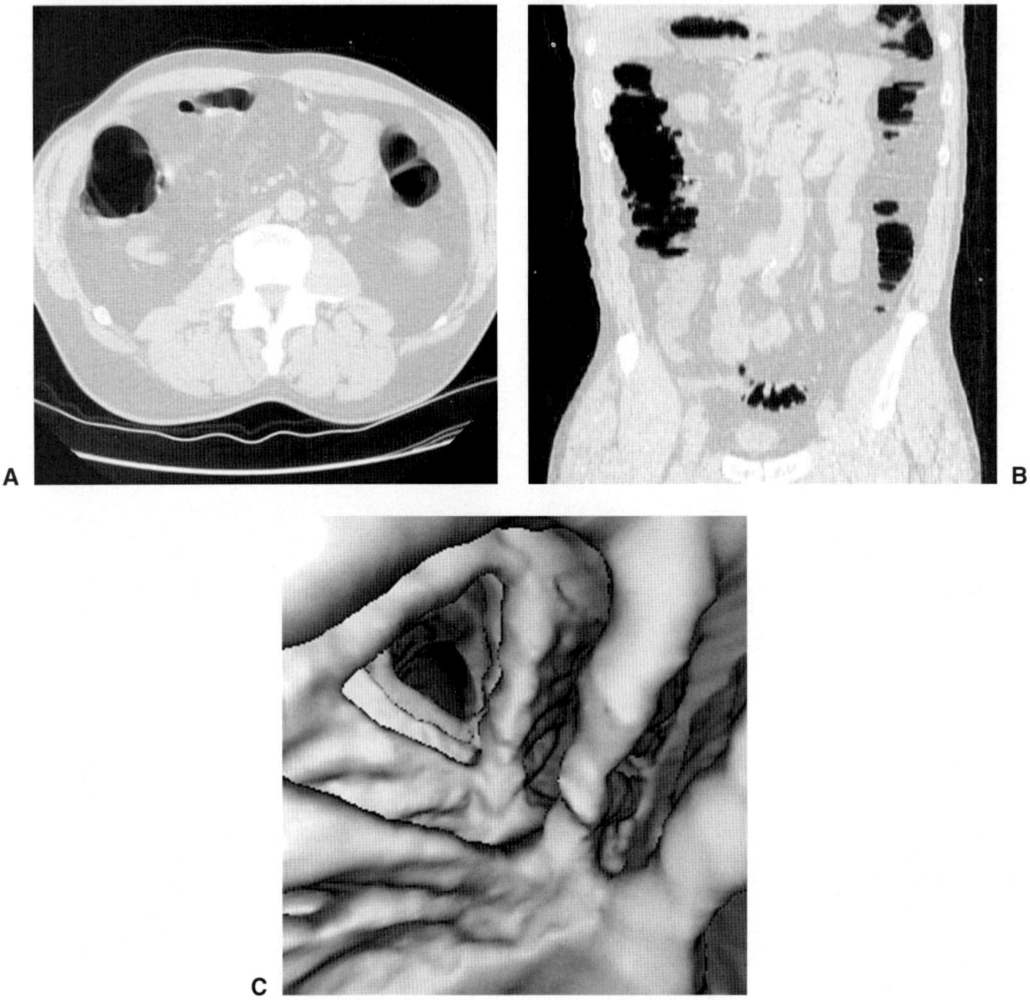

FIGURE 3.1 Mild motion artifact. Axial image **(A)** shows ill-defined edges of the colonic wall due to motion. Coronal multiplanar reformatted view **(B)** and 3D endoluminal image **(C)** demonstrates mild jagged appearance of the ascending colonic wall. This can make it more difficult to detect polyps.

underwent MDCT colonography and colonoscopy. The CT images were reconstructed using a "thin protocol" consisting of 1.25-mm sections reconstructed every 1.0 mm and a "thick method" consisting of 5.0-mm sections reconstructed every 2.0 mm. There was no statistically significant difference in sensitivity for polyp detection comparing thin and thick sections although there were only a total of 12 polyps in this study. However, it was found that the number of false-positive findings was significantly lower for thin sections compared with the thick sections for two readers. Specificity ranged between 80% and 93% for thin sections compared with 73% to 80% for thick sections. Mean interpretation time was significantly longer using thin sections for one reader and was 13 minutes for both thin and thick sections for the second reader.

With the evolution from single-detector to 4-, 8-, 16- and 64-detector row CT scanners, the collimation and the section thickness used for CTC has decreased. The typical collimation ranges between 3 and 5 mm for single-detector CT with a large percentage of overlap in the data acquisition. For 4- and 8-detector row CT, the collimation is approximately halved and ranges between 1 and 2.5 mm depending upon the specific CT scanner used. The collimation ranges between 0.625 and 1.25 mm for 16- and 64-detector CT (see Table 3.1). The American College of Radiology Practice Guidelines for the Performance of CTC in Adults recommend optimal slice collimation $\leq$3 mm with a reconstruction interval of $\leq$1.5 mm.[6] A breath hold of 25 seconds or less is suggested. A thicker slice collimation of up to 5 mm with a reconstruction interval of $\leq$2.5 mm is less preferable.[6]

RADIATION DOSE

One of the challenges facing CTC particularly as a screening examination is to maintain acceptable radiation

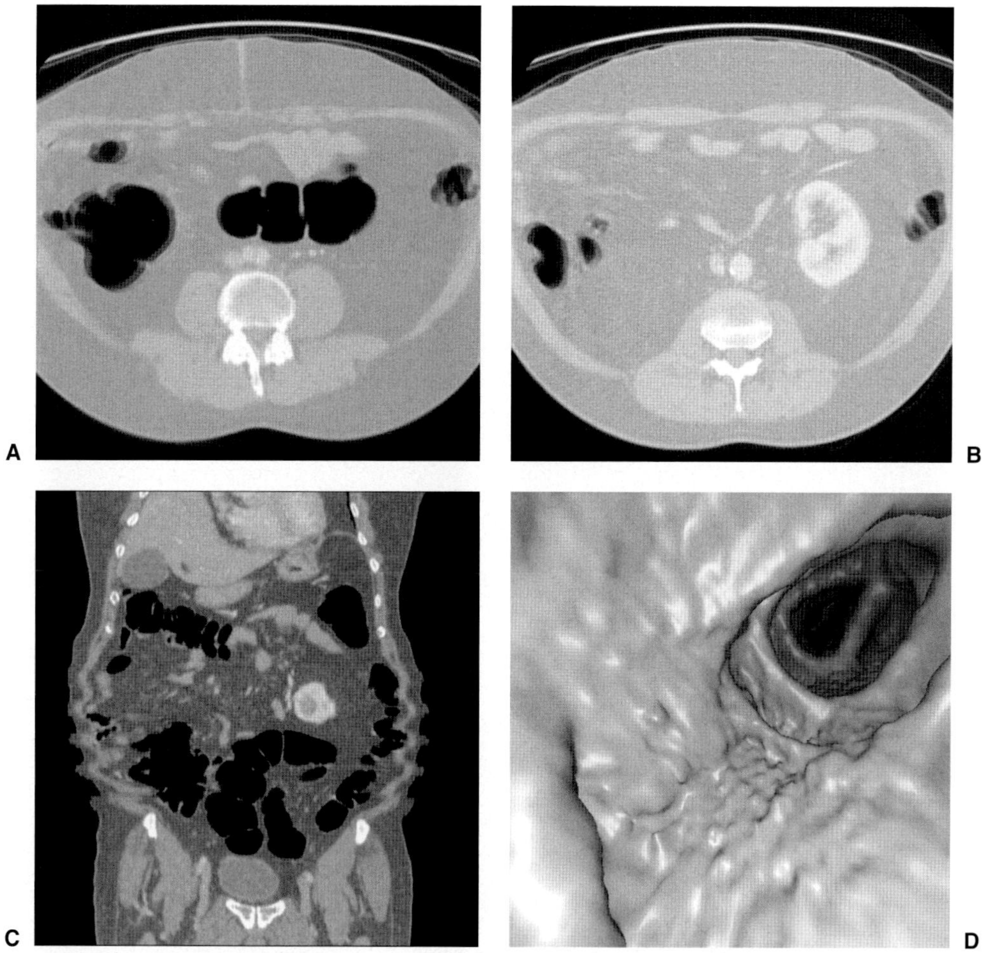

FIGURE 3.2 Moderate motion artifact is seen predominantly involving the ascending and descending colon segments on the axial **(A, B)** and coronal multiplanar reformatted **(C)** views. The 3D endoluminal view **(D)** demonstrates how motion that occurs during data acquisition can cause an irregular colonic wall with more focal protrusions that may potentially be misinterpreted as a polyp.

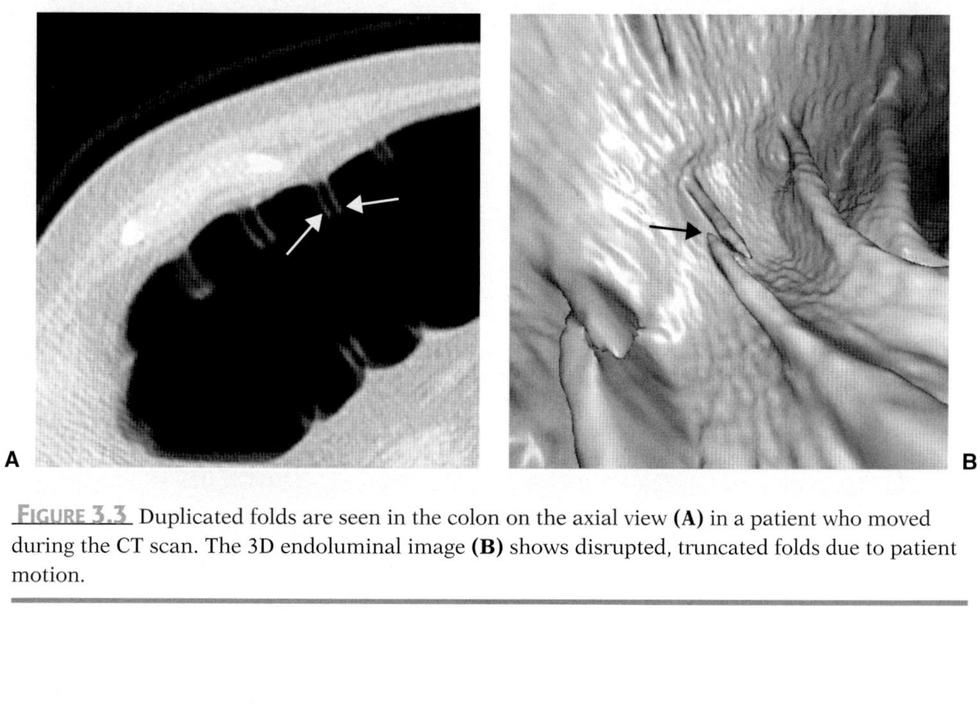

FIGURE 3.3 Duplicated folds are seen in the colon on the axial view **(A)** in a patient who moved during the CT scan. The 3D endoluminal image **(B)** shows disrupted, truncated folds due to patient motion.

TABLE 3.1 Sample Parameters for Computed Tomography Colonography

	Single Slice	4-Slice	8–16 Slice	64-Slice
Collimation (mm)	3–5	1.25–2.5	0.625–1.25	0.5–0.625
Pitch	1.5–2	1–1.5	1–1.5	0.98–1.4
Feed (mm/sec)	4.5	7.5–15	13–20	25–48
mAs	100–150	80–100	50–100	50–100
kVp	120	120	120	120
Rotation time (sec)	0.75–1	0.5–0.8	0.5	0.5
Reconstruction (mm)	1.5–2.5	1–1.25	1–1.25	1–1.25
Scan time (sec)	50–60	25–30	9–20	5–7

dose to the patient without compromising the diagnostic ability for lesions. The International Commission on Radiological Protection (ICRP) requires that radiation doses to patients are as low as reasonably achievable (ALARA).[7] There are multiple factors that affect radiation dose and the image quality of a CT scan. Better image quality is typically associated with increased radiation dose to the patient. Reducing radiation dose decreases the number of photons that reach the detectors and this consequently increases image noise (see Figs. 3.4 to 3.6).

DOSE PARAMETERS

Different parameters of dose include the weighted computed tomography dose index (CTDIw) and the dose

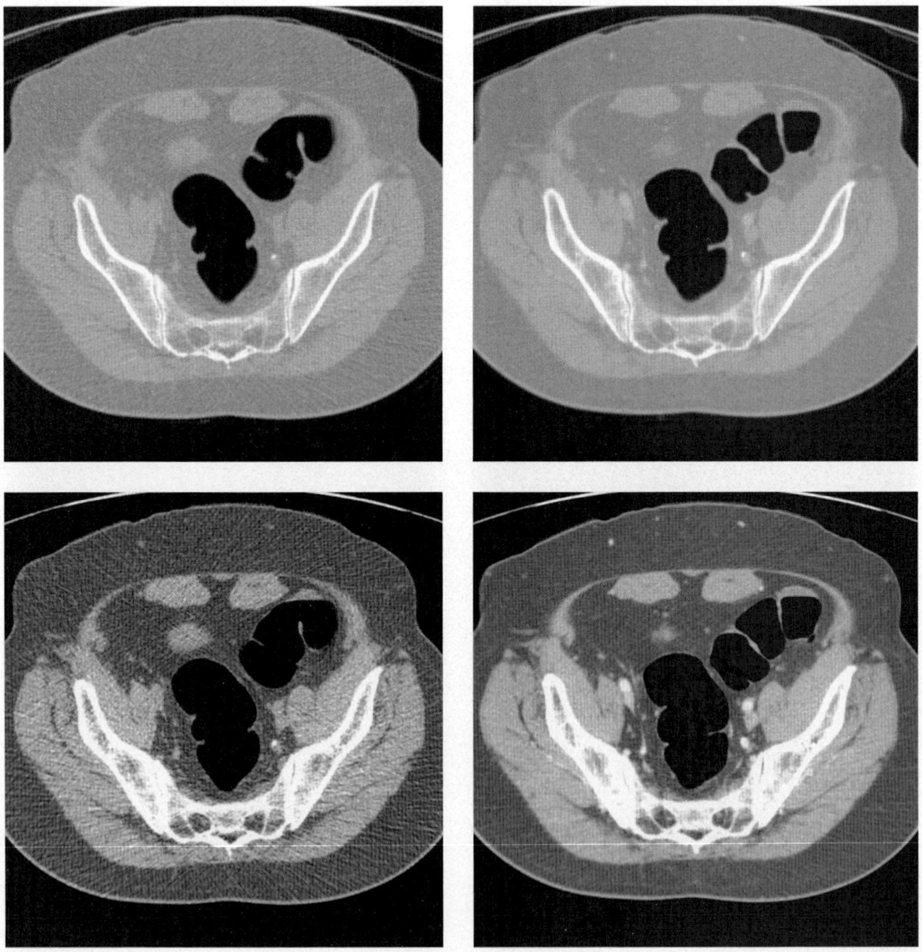

A B C D

FIGURE 3.4 Low mAs versus high mAs. Axial images using 50 mAs **(A, C)** have increased noise and appear more grainy than images acquired using 200 mAs **(B, D)**.

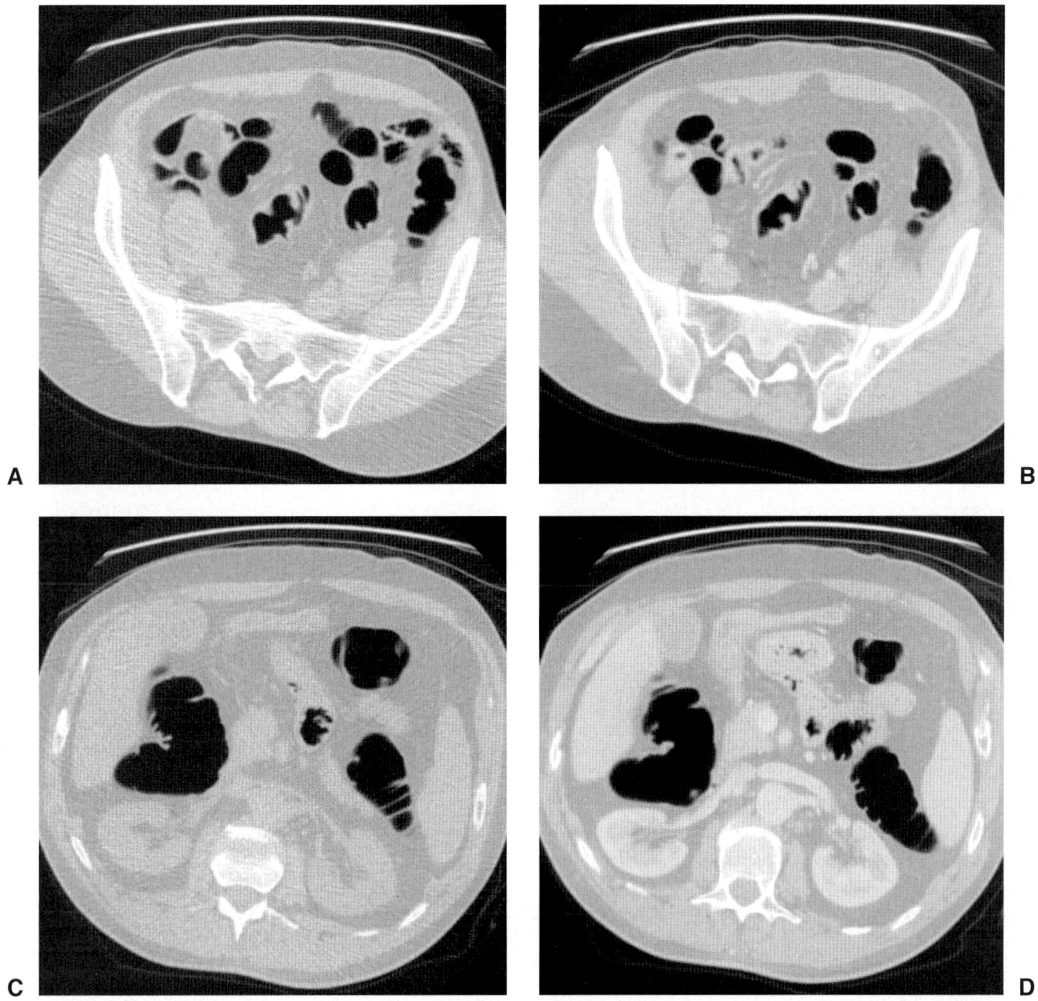

FIGURE 3.5 Axial images using low mAs **(A,C)** is of adequate quality for evaluation of the air–colon wall interface although overall image quality is noisier than the high mAs images **(B,D)**.

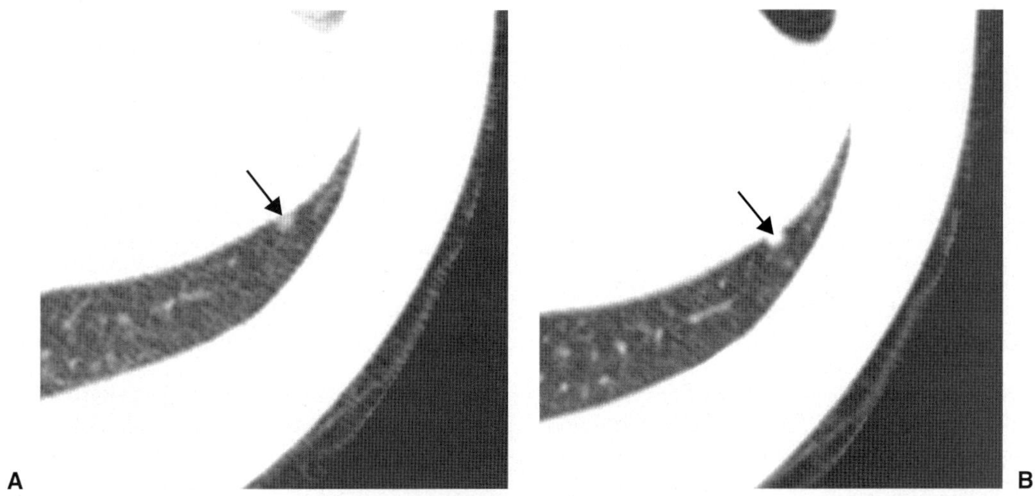

FIGURE 3.6 Decreasing the mAs will decrease the effective radiation dose to the patient. This may make it more difficult to detect or characterize extracolonic lesions. The left lower lobe lung nodule is less distinct on the 90 mAs image **(A)** than the 200 mAs image **(B)**.

length product (DLP).[8] The CTDIw takes into account acquisition parameters such as tube potential, tube current, and slice thickness. CTDIw is measured in milligray (mGy) and is used to calculate the DLP. The DLP is the product of the CTDIw and the length of the section scanned and is measured in milligray-centimeter (mGy-cm). The effective dose (ED) is derived from the DLP and also takes into account the radiation sensitivities of individual organs. ED is measured by the unit millisievert (mSv) and provides the best estimation of patient dose and its related biologic risk. Ware et al. examined the ED to patients undergoing routine abdominal CT examinations performed on single-detector CT scanners using 120 kVp with a section thickness of 7 mm and 287 + 67 mAs.[9] The mean ED for adults was 3.9 + 1.1 mSv for standard abdominal CT.

LOW-DOSE COMPUTED TOMOGRAPHY COLONOGRAPHY

Hara et al. initially demonstrated that tube current can be decreased to reduce radiation exposure without compromising polyp detection on CTC because of the high contrast between the air-filled colon and the soft tissue density of the colon wall.[10] Two single-detector CT protocols were compared with one group of eight patients with 31 polyps scanned using 140 mA, 5-mm collimation, pitch of 1.3 and 3-mm reconstruction interval. The other group of 10 patients with 30 polyps was scanned using the same parameters except for 70 mA, pitch of 1, and 1-mm reconstruction interval. The sensitivity for polyp detection was 100% for polyps 5 mm and larger for both groups. In this study, the radiation dose for CTC performed using supine and prone scans at 70 mA was 3.74 mGy for men and 5.70 mGy for women. These doses are 50% lower than the dose for a standard CT of the abdomen and pelvis and are equivalent to the radiation dose for a barium enema.

Phantom studies allow the evaluation of multiple different CT parameters simultaneously. Wessling et al. used a colon phantom containing nine simulated sessile polyps ranging in size between 2 and 12 mm to evaluate multidetector row CT with different combinations of detector collimation (4 × 1.0 mm and 4 × 2.5 mm), dose (10 to 140 mAs), and section thickness/reconstruction interval (1.25/0.6–5.0/2.0).[11] Polyps measuring 8 mm and larger were identified irrespective of the combination of parameters used. However, detection of polyps 6 mm and smaller was best using 4- × 1.0-mm detector collimation with a small section thickness of 1.25 mm even with a low-dose protocol using 10 mAs and 140 kV. The effective radiation dose for supine and prone CTC was calculated to be 1.8 mSv for men and 2.4 mSv for women using this low-dose protocol. Colon phantoms containing 240 synthetic polyps of different shapes and various sizes up to 10 mm were evaluated using 4-row MDCT in a study performed by Ozgun et al.[12] Twelve scanning sequences were performed with variable slice thickness between 1.25 and 3.75 mm, pitch of 0.75 or 1.5, and tube current between 20 and 200 mA. For a standard protocol using 2.5-mm slice thickness and pitch of 1.5, the detection rate of 5 mm and larger polyps was approximately 90% between 60 and 100 mA. If the radiation dose was kept constant, the highest detection rate of polyps >2 mm was obtained using the protocol with 1.25-mm slice thickness and the smaller pitch of 0.75.

Patient studies have helped to confirm some of the findings made using phantoms. Van Gelder et al. performed a feasibility study evaluating CTC at different radiation dose levels in 50 high-risk patients.[13] The CT scan parameters consisted of detector collimation 4 × 2.5 mm, 120 kV, and 100 mAs with two lower dose CT scans simulated at 50 mAs and 30 mAs. The per-patient sensitivity for detection of polyps measuring 5 mm and larger was 90% at all dose levels although it was noted that image quality decreased significantly at 30 mAs. Per-polyp sensitivity for detection of polyps measuring 5 mm and larger was also similar at all dose levels ranging between 85% and 92%. The specificity for patients without polyps 5 mm and larger was uniformly low at all dose levels and ranged between 53% and 60%. Also included in this study was a determination that the median ED for CTC in both supine and prone positions is 8.8 mSv which, using ICRP data, may result in a 0.02% risk for inducing cancer in a 50-year-old individual. This calculation involved the parameters for CTC at that time in 13 different research sites in the United States and Europe.

In a study by Macari et al., 105 symptomatic patients underwent same-day MDCT followed by conventional colonoscopy.[14] CT scan parameters included detector collimation 4 × 1.0 mm, 120 kV, 50 mAs, and 1.25-mm reconstructions at a 1.0-mm interval. Using this thin-section, low-dose protocol the per-lesion sensitivities for detection of polyps 5 mm and smaller, 6 to 9 mm, and 10 mm and larger were 12%, 70%, and 93% respectively. Overall specificity was excellent at 98%. The CTDIw for CTC combining supine and prone positions was 11.4 mGy. The EDs for combined CTC were 5.0 mSv for men and 7.8 mSv for women. It was concluded that low-dose MDCT colonography has excellent sensitivity and specificity for detection of large polyps.

ULTRA-LOW-DOSE COMPUTED TOMOGRAPHY-COLONOGRAPHY

Increasing attention has been focused on the evaluation of ultra low–dose CTC. An initial study by Iannaccone et al. reported the excellent preliminary experience with even lower dose CTC in 27 symptomatic patients.[15] The MDCT protocol consisted of 4 × 2.5-mm collimation, 3.0-mm slice thickness, 140 kVp, and 10 mAs. All nine cancers were identified and there was 100% sensitivity for polyps 10 mm and larger (3/3) as well as for medium-sized polyps between 6 and 9 mm (3/3). Total radiation dose for supine and prone sequences together was 1.7 mSv for men and 2.3 mSv for women, which was a 40% to 70% decrease in radiation dose compared with prior studies.

Iannaccone et al. followed this study up with a report of a larger experience using the same lower-dose CTC protocol in 158 patients.[16] Using 10 mAs, CTC had 100% sensitivity for carcinomas (22/22), 100% sensitivity for large polyps (13/13), and 83% sensitivity for medium-sized polyps (20/24). Specificity was 96.6% and the positive predictive value and negative predictive value were 94.1% and 97.7% respectively. The CTDIw considering both supine and prone acquisitions was 2.74 mGy. Iannaccone et al. also evaluated low-dose CTC (effective mAs of 10) in 88 patients who underwent two sequential colonoscopies that were performed within 2 weeks of each other.[17] Results of the second colonoscopy served as the reference standard for determination of the sensitivities of the CTC and the initial colonoscopy. The per-lesion sensitivities for polyps 6 mm and larger for CTC and the initial colonoscopy were 86% and 84% respectively. The initial colonoscopy failed to detect 16 polyps, 6 of which were detected by the CT. The per-patient sensitivities for polyps 6 mm and larger for CTC and the initial colonoscopy were 84% and 90% respectively with specificities of 82% and 100%.

The performance of ultra low–dose CTC was also studied in 137 symptomatic patients by Cohnen et al.[18] However, patients were scanned only in the supine position. CT scan parameters were detector collimation of 4×1 mm, 120 kVp, pitch of 2, 10 mAs (effective), and reconstruction width of 1.25 mm at an interval of 0.7 mm. The CTDIw for this protocol was calculated to be 1.14 mGy with an ED of 0.7 mSv for men and 1 mSv for women. The sensitivity for large polyps (>10 mm), medium polyps (5–9.9 mm) and small polyps (<5 mm) was 78.6%, 85.7%, and 57% respectively with the specificity for each size group at 100%, 92.8%, and 85.9% respectively. It was concluded that ultra low–dose CTC is feasible at a substantial radiation dose reduction, although in this study patients were scanned only in one position. Current standard practice consists of scanning patients in two opposing positions.[6]

In trying to determine whether radiation dose could be lowered even more, van Gelder et al. performed a study on 15 patients with variable mAs ranging between 0.4 and 100 mAs and doses ranging from 0.05 to 12 mSv.[19] Sensitivity was 80% to 100% for large polyps ($\geq$10 mm) across all mAs and dose levels. The mean sensitivity for detection of polyps 5 mm and larger remained at 74% across all mAs and dose levels except for the lowest level of 0.4 mAs. The number of false-positive results decreased as the mAs decreased for 5 mm and larger lesions and this was felt to be related to increased noise and smoothing algorithms applied to the lowest dose images.

In summary, there has been a shift to the use of low-dose CTC technique and even to ultra low–dose protocols at some sites. Other considerations include the size of the target lesion that should be detected by CTC and the desire and ability to detect extracolonic lesions. The CT protocol employed also varies depending upon the clinical indication for the test. If the patient is undergoing CTC as a screening examination, then intravenous contrast is not routinely used. Low-dose technique is recommended consisting of kVp = 120 and mAs $\leq$ 100.[6] The method of interpretation may require particular levels of mAs. When the reader uses a primary 2D interpretation method, then 10 mAs has been found in studies to be adequate. However, higher dosage of 50 to 100 mAs is needed for primary 3D interpretation.

REFERENCES

1. Saini S. Multi-detector row CT: principles and practice for abdominal applications. *Radiology*. 2004;233:323–327.
2. Hara AK, Johnson CD, MacCarty RL, et al. CT colonography: single- versus multi-detector row imaging. *Radiology*. 2001;219:461–465.
3. Power NP, Pryor MD, Martin A, et al. Optimization of scanning parameters for CT colonography. *Br J Radiol*. 2002;75:401–408.
4. Laghi A, Iannaccone R, Mangiapane F, et al. Experimental colonic phantom for the evaluation of the optimal scanning technique for CT colonography using multidetector spiral CT equipment. *Eur Radiol*. 2003;13:459–466.
5. Lui YW, Macari M, Israel G, et al. CT colonography data interpretation: effect of different section thicknesses preliminary observations. *Radiology*. 2003;229:791–797.
6. Glick SG, Johnson CD, Macari M, et al. *ACR Practice Guideline for the Performance of Computed Tomography (CT) Colonography in Adults. ACR Practice Guidelines and Technical Standards*. 2005–2006.
7. International Commission on Radiological Protection. *Summary of Recommendations ICRP 60. Report 60*. Bethesda, MD: International Commission on Radiological Protection; 1990.
8. Jessen KA, Shrimpton PC, Geleijins J, et al. Dosimetry for optimisation of patient protection in computed tomography. *Appl Radiat Isot*. 1999;50:165–172.
9. Ware DE, Huda W, Mergo PJ, et al. Radiation effective doses to patients undergoing abdominal CT examinations. *Radiology*. 1999;210:645–650.
10. Hara AK, Johnson CD, Reed JE, et al. Reducing data size and radiation dose for CT Colonography. *Am J Roentgenol*. 1997;168:1181–1184.
11. Wessling J, Fischbach R, Meier N, et al. CT colonography: protocol optimization with multi-detector row CT-study in an anthropomorphic colon phantom. *Radiology*. 2003;228:753–759.
12. Ozgun A, Rollven E, Blomqvist L, et al. Polyp detection with MDCT: a phantom-based evaluation of the impact of dose and spatial resolution. *Am J Roentgenol*. 2005;184:1181–1188.
13. van Gelder RE, Venema HW, Serlie IW, et al. CT colonography at different radiation dose levels: feasibility of dose reduction. *Radiology*. 2002;224:25–33.
14. Macari M, Bini EJ, Xue X, et al. Colorectal neoplasms: prospective comparison of thin-section low-dose multi-detector row CT colonography and conventional colonoscopy for detection. *Radiology*. 2002;224:383–392.
15. Iannaccone R, Laghi A, Catalano C, et al. Feasibility of ultra-low-dose multislice CT colonography for the detection of colorectal lesions: preliminary experience. *Eur Radiol*. 2003;13:1297–1302.
16. Iannaccone R, Laghi A, Catalano C, et al. Detection of colorectal lesions: lower-dose multi-detector row helical CT colonography compared with conventional colonoscopy. *Radiology*. 2003;229:775–781.

17. Iannaccone R, Catalano C, Mangiapane F, et al. Colorectal polyps: detection with low-dose multi-detector row helical CT colonography versus two sequential colonoscopies. *Radiology*. 2005;237:927–937.
18. Cohnen M, Vogt C, Beck A, et al. Feasibility of MDCT Colonography in ultra-low-dose technique in the detection of colorectal lesions: comparison with high-resolution video colonoscopy. *Am J Roentgenol*. 2004;183:1355–1359.
19. van Gelder RE, Venema HW, Florie J, et al. CT colonography: feasibility of substantial dose reduction- comparison of medium to very low doses in identical patients. *Radiology*. 2004;232:611–620.

CHAPTER 4 INTERPRETATION: NORMAL ANATOMY

Gregory M. Galdino and Judy Yee

The image displays used for the interpretation of computed tomography colonography (CTC) include standard two-dimensional (2D) axial images, multiplanar reformations (MPR) (coronal, sagittal, or oblique) and three-dimensional (3D) endoluminal views. Various options for the 3D view have been developed and include the "fly-through" navigational view, the subvolume cube view, as well as novel dissection and panoramic views. Various combinations of displays are commercially available, although one display technique (2D vs 3D) is typically chosen as the primary interpretation method, with the other used for problem solving. Debate exists as to the optimal reading strategy. There is evidence that supports the use of a primary 2D technique as well as published data that promotes a primary 3D reading approach. However, it is essential to recognize that both 2D and 3D displays are considered to be necessary and should be used as complementary reading tools for CTC.

DEVELOPING AN INTERPRETATION METHOD

Various factors should be considered when deciding which primary visualization method to use. Ease of use of the workstation and software, interpretation time, and the ability to rapidly generate and export a report are important considerations. Reader preference and training will also contribute to determining which interpretation method is used predominantly. If a computer workstation loaded with CTC software is already available on site, the reader will be more likely to adapt to a particular workstation and software which may be more amenable to one type of interpretation over another. Ultimately, the goal is accurate CTC interpretation irrespective of the primary reading method. Currently most radiologists still use primary 2D axial and MPR displays for interpretation with the use of 3D for problem solving.[1] Modification of reading preferences may occur with the development of newer software, allowing for improved and novel image displays, improved user interface, and increased automated ability.

The ease of use of the 2D and 3D display techniques is directly related to the features and the user interface of the computer workstation and CTC software (see Tables 4.1 and 4.2). The improved ergonomics of mouse controls compared with keyboard controls are often preferred by readers. User-friendly features that are easily accessible with a single mouse click support faster interpretation times and promote a more relaxed reading style. The CTC software should allow easy magnification (zooming) and panning (roaming) of the image within both 2D and 3D displays. The ability to bookmark a lesion on 2D and 3D with rapid and seamless transition between the two types of images is essential for accurate and efficient lesion identification. Easy linking or synchronization of supine and prone data sets is available on most workstations for axial image review and this feature helps to speed interpretation times.

The interpretation time for CTC consists of the time required to evaluate for both colonic and extracolonic lesions. Documenting colonic and extracolonic findings as well as generating a report are necessary components of the procedure and will contribute to the overall time for the procedure. Features related to data and image

TABLE 4.1 Key Workstation Features—Two-Dimensional

Supine and prone axial linking or synchronization
Magnification
Panning
Window width/level adjustment
Bookmarking
Measurement of lesion density
Size measurement tool
Easy correlation with MPRs and 3D views
Computer-aided detection/computer-assisted reader

MPR, multiplanar reformations.

storage, exporting images and movie clips, as well as documentation of findings vary widely between computer workstations.

Colon segments are evaluated for adequacy of distention, adequacy of cleansing as well as for the detection and characterization of colonic polyps and masses. When a polyp or mass is detected, the reader must also determine the segmental location of the lesion. The six colonic segments that are typically used include rectum, sigmoid, descending colon, transverse colon, ascending colon, and the cecum.[2] Automatic estimation of the distance of a lesion from the anorectal junction is a useful feature available with some computer software. Accuracy of this tool is dependent upon adequate and continuous distention of the entire colon.

Polyp Measurement

The ability to accurately and easily measure the size of lesions on both 2D and 3D views is an important feature for time-efficient interpretation. Errors in polyp measurement can directly impact on patient management by either causing lesions to drop below a significant threshold or by causing unnecessary referrals for optical colonoscopy. Large polyps measuring ≥10 mm will require a referral for optical colonoscopy and polypectomy

TABLE 4.2 Key Workstation Features—Three Dimensional

Automatic colonic segmentation
Automatic navigation
Speed control
Bookmarking
Size measurement tool
Easy correlation with 2D images
Electronic subtraction of tagged material
Distance from the anorectal junction
Computer-aided detection/computer-assisted reader

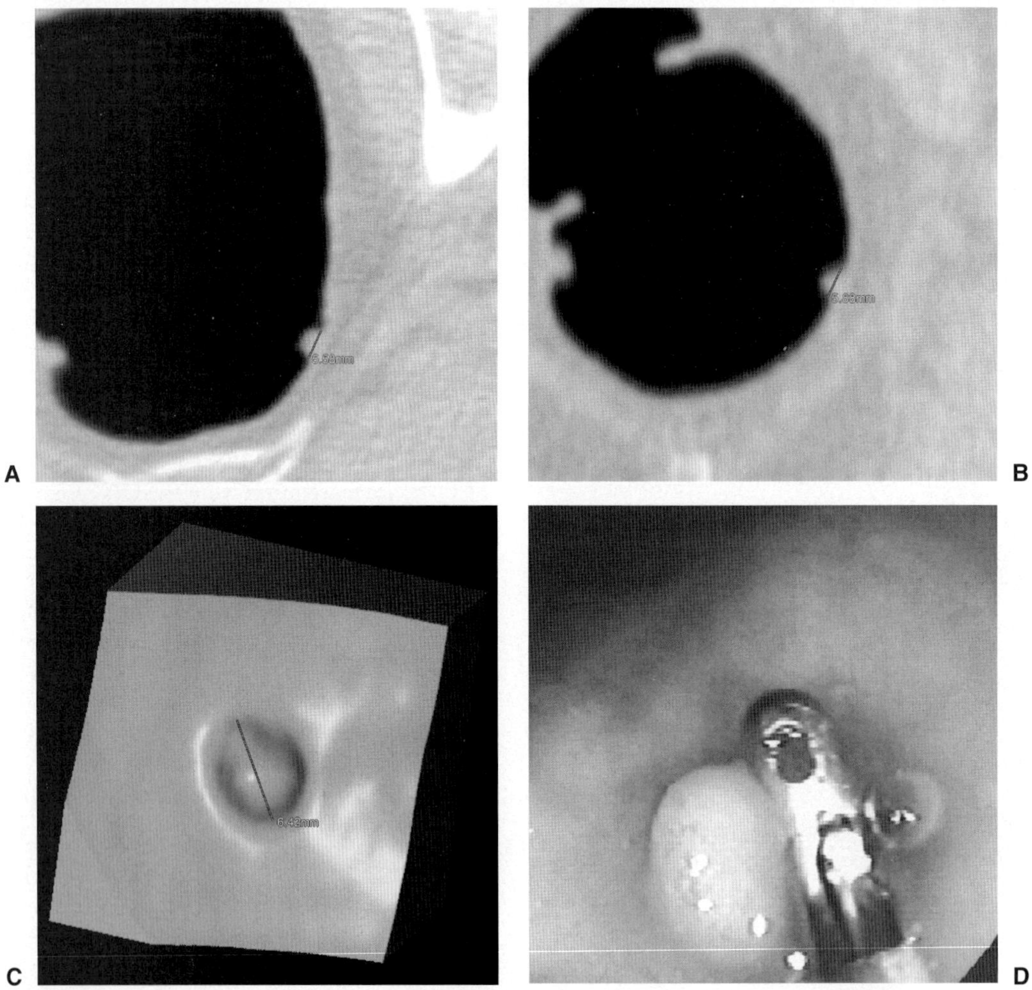

FIGURE 4.1 The axial image **(A)** shows a sessile rectal polyp measuring 5.6 mm. A coronal reformat **(B)** shows the same polyp measuring 5.9 mm. The 3D subvolume cube view **(C)** shows the polyp measuring 6.4 mm. Endoscopic view **(D)** demonstrates the technique of estimating polyp size by comparing to adjacent biopsy forceps. The endoscopic measurement was 7 mm.

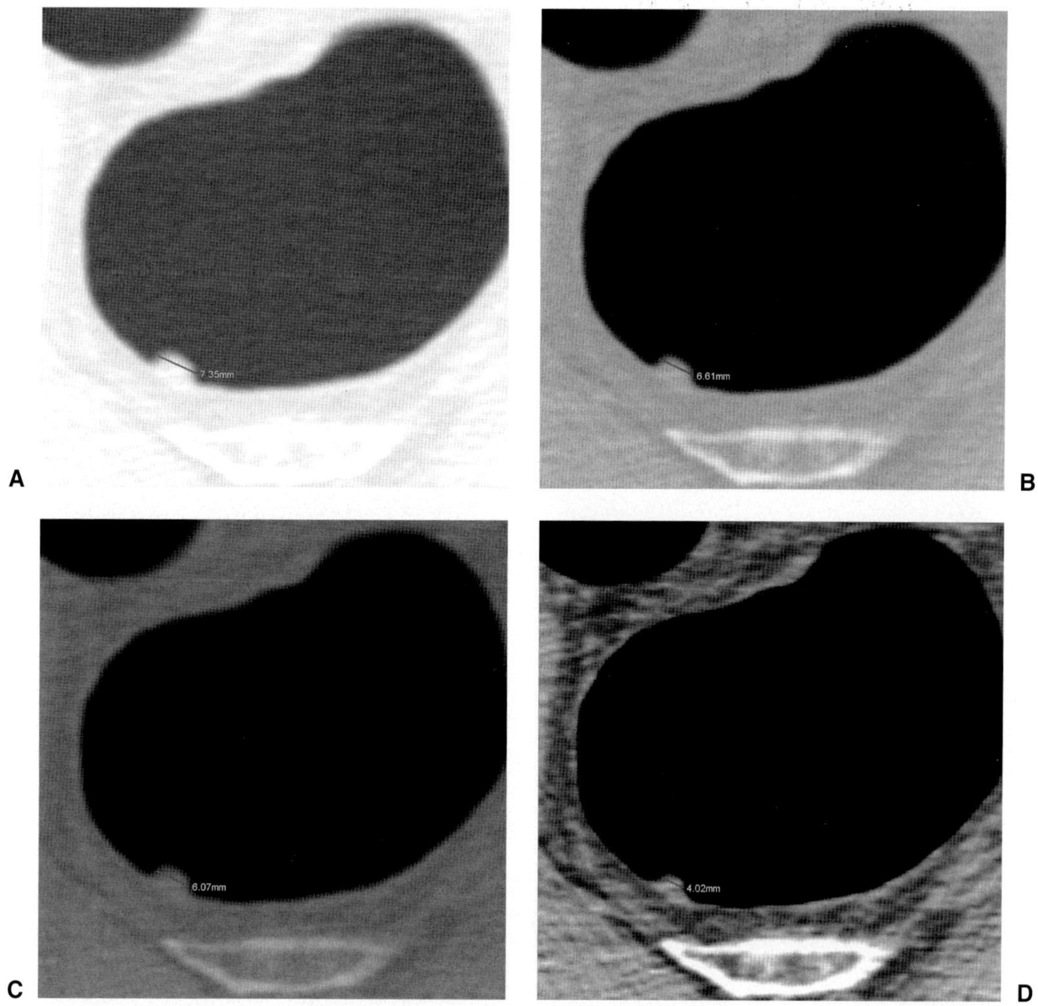

FIGURE 4.2 A high-contrast colon window width and level setting is recommended for viewing 2D images. Polyp size varies with different window settings: **(A)** lung window (W 700, L −600), **(B)** colon window (W 1,400, L −350), **(C)** bone window (W 1,500, L −700), **(D)** soft tissue window (W 400, L 40). A sessile rectal polyp measures 7.4 mm, 6.6 mm, 6.0 mm, and 4.2 mm in the respective window settings.

whereas small polyps measuring $\leq$5 mm are considered clinically insignificant and may be left in place and do not even need to be reported.[2,3]

Polyp size measurements obtained on CTC, particularly using the 3D endoluminal or subvolume cube views may be more accurate than the measurements determined by optical colonoscopy (see Fig. 4.1). Published studies have documented differences in the reliability between different endoscopic measurement methods. Direct measurement of polyps using a linear probe has been found to be the more accurate method whereas the use of an open biopsy forceps to estimate the size of an adjacent polyp is the less accurate method.[4]

Good intraobserver and interobserver agreement between measurements has been obtained on CTC using 2D views with a defined measurement protocol. This consists of a high-contrast window width and level with measurement of the largest diameter often found along the base of the polyp and cross-registration of the center of the lesion in three MPR images (axial, coronal, and sagittal) to determine the optimal plane for measurement[5] (see Fig. 4.2). Only the head of a pedunculated polyp is measured with exclusion of the stalk (see Fig. 4.3). The maximum diameter of 48 polyps measuring between 2 and 12 mm was measured by four observers using three different visualization displays: 2D colonography window, 2D abdominal window, and 3D surface rendering.[6] CT measurements, irrespective of the display used, were found to overestimate polyp diameters with the least amount of error found when using the 2D abdominal window setting. However, only two of the readers used a combination of the three multiplanar views for 2D measurements. Inter- and intraobserver agreement was poorest for the 3D display. Very large polyps and masses, particularly circumferential carcinomas are typically easier to measure using 2D multiplanar images.

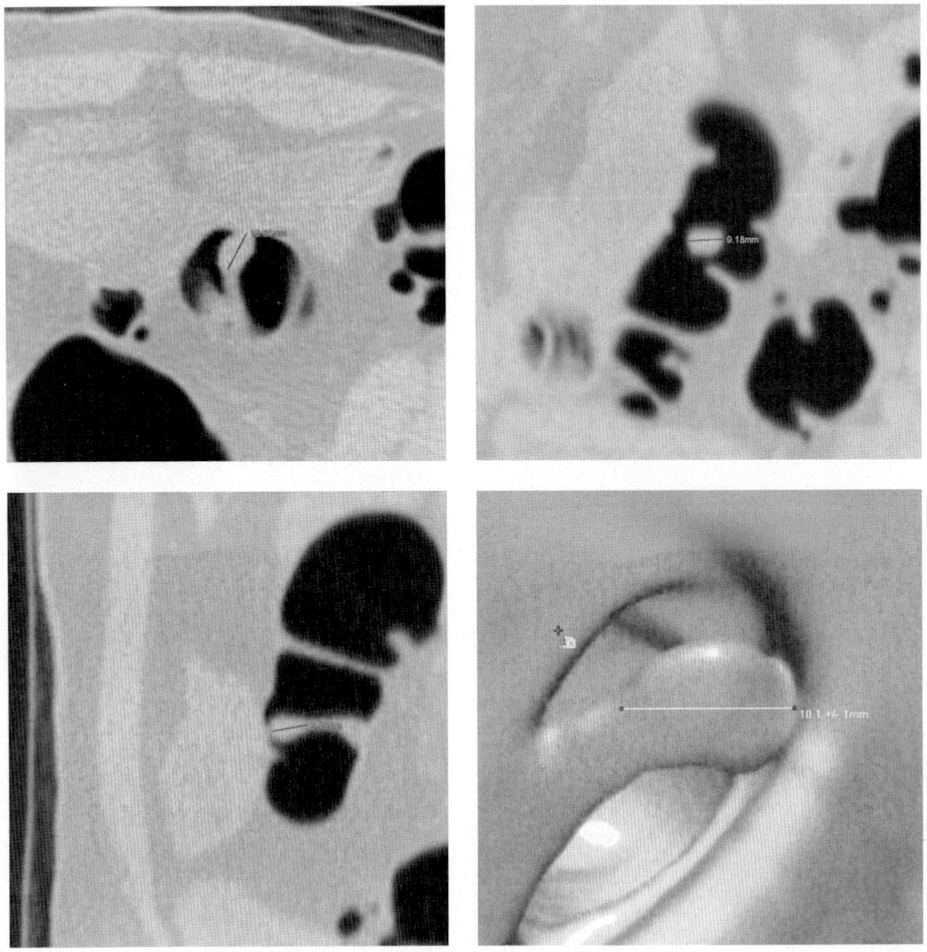

A B C D

FIGURE 4.3 Prone axial image **(A)** shows measurement of only the head of a pedunculated sigmoid polyp at 10.7 mm. The coronal **(B)** and sagittal **(C)** reformats show correlative measurements of 9.8 mm and 9.2 mm respectively. 3D endoluminal view **(D)** shows a polyp head measurement of 10.1 mm.

Additionally polyps located in a poorly distended segment are often more easily measured on 2D views.

In contrast, polyp measurement was found to be significantly more accurate on 3D endoluminal views than on 2D axial, coronal, or sagittal views in another study.[7] Four readers obtained measurements using 2D MPR and 3D endoluminal images on ten synthetic polyps (6–13 mm) in an *in vitro* phantom and on *in vivo* polyps in ten patients (10 polyps measuring 7–25 mm). It was also found that the 2D measurements underestimated polyp sizes in all cases. Shortening of polyps may be attributed to the fact that the long axis of polyps is often not aligned along a particular 2D view. The discrepancy between 2D and 3D measurements may be minimized by using an "optimized" 2D measurement, which is the largest diameter as determined from the three standard multiplanar views or by use of an oblique view, which is orthogonal to the axis of the colonic lumen (see Fig. 4.4).

Determination of maximum polyp diameter may be easier and faster on 3D endoluminal or subvolume cube images (see Fig. 4.5). The start and end points for a lesion on the 3D images may be difficult to ascertain unless the reader interactively manipulates the image to assure accurate point placement. Investigators are evaluating a method to automatically measure polyp size on CTC based on segmentation that grows a surface patch over the polyp surface starting from a seed.[8] The long axis of an ellipse that is fitted to a 2D point set determined from projection of patch points along the polyp axis determines the size of the polyp. The future development of automated polyp volume measurement may prove to be the most accurate method for detecting the relative change in the size of polyps that are followed noninvasively on CTC.[9]

PRIMARY TWO-DIMENSIONAL INTERPRETATION

The traditional approach to CTC interpretation is using a primary 2D technique, with the use of 3D views only

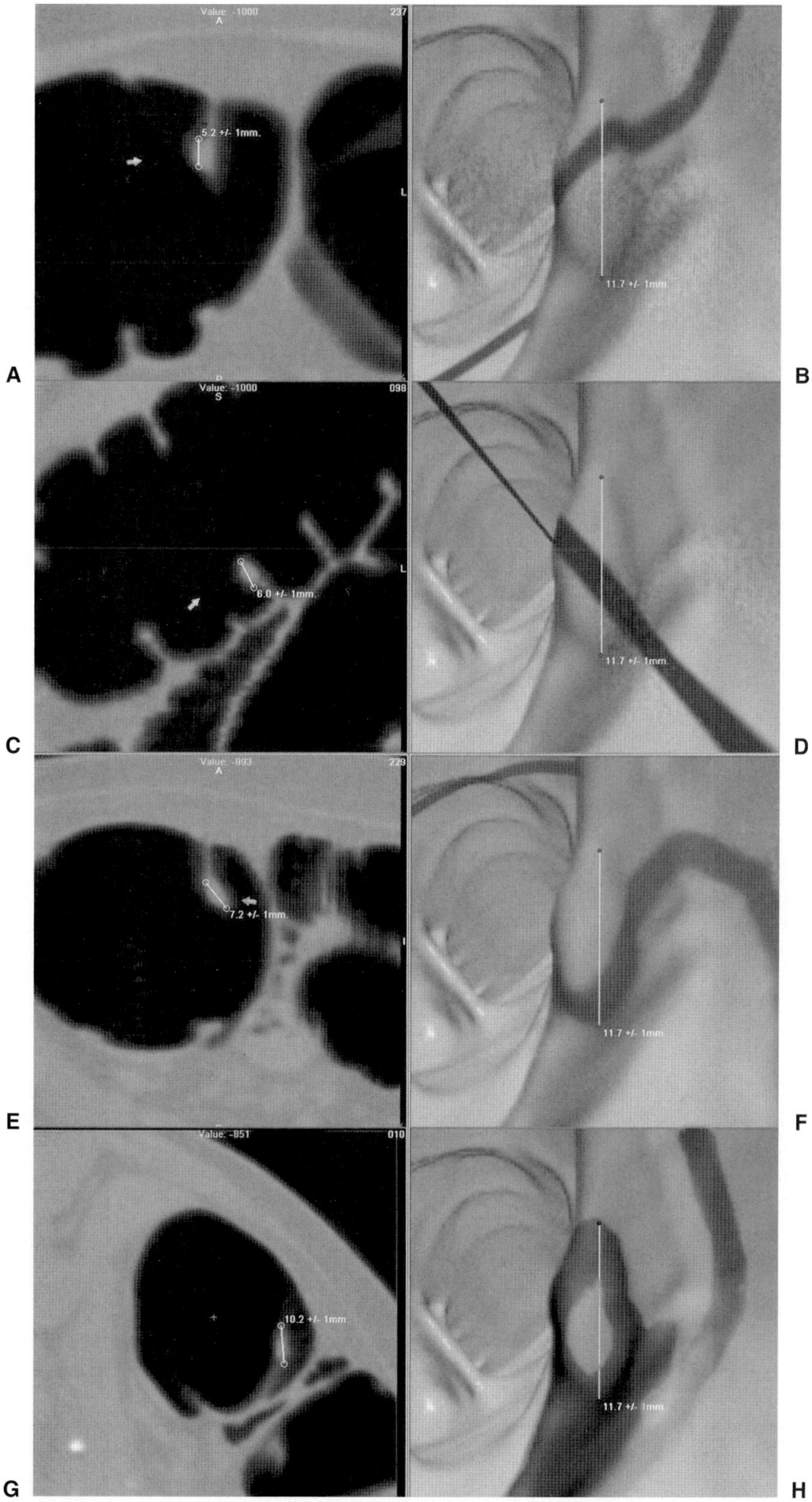

FIGURE 4.4 Axial **(A, B)**, coronal **(C, D)**, and sagittal **(E, F)** views underestimate true polyp size with measurements of 5.2 mm, 6.0 mm, and 7.2 mm respectively. Polyp measurement of 10.2 mm on an oblique view **(G, H)** most accurately approximates lesion size of 11.7 mm from the 3D view and endoscopic size of 12 mm.

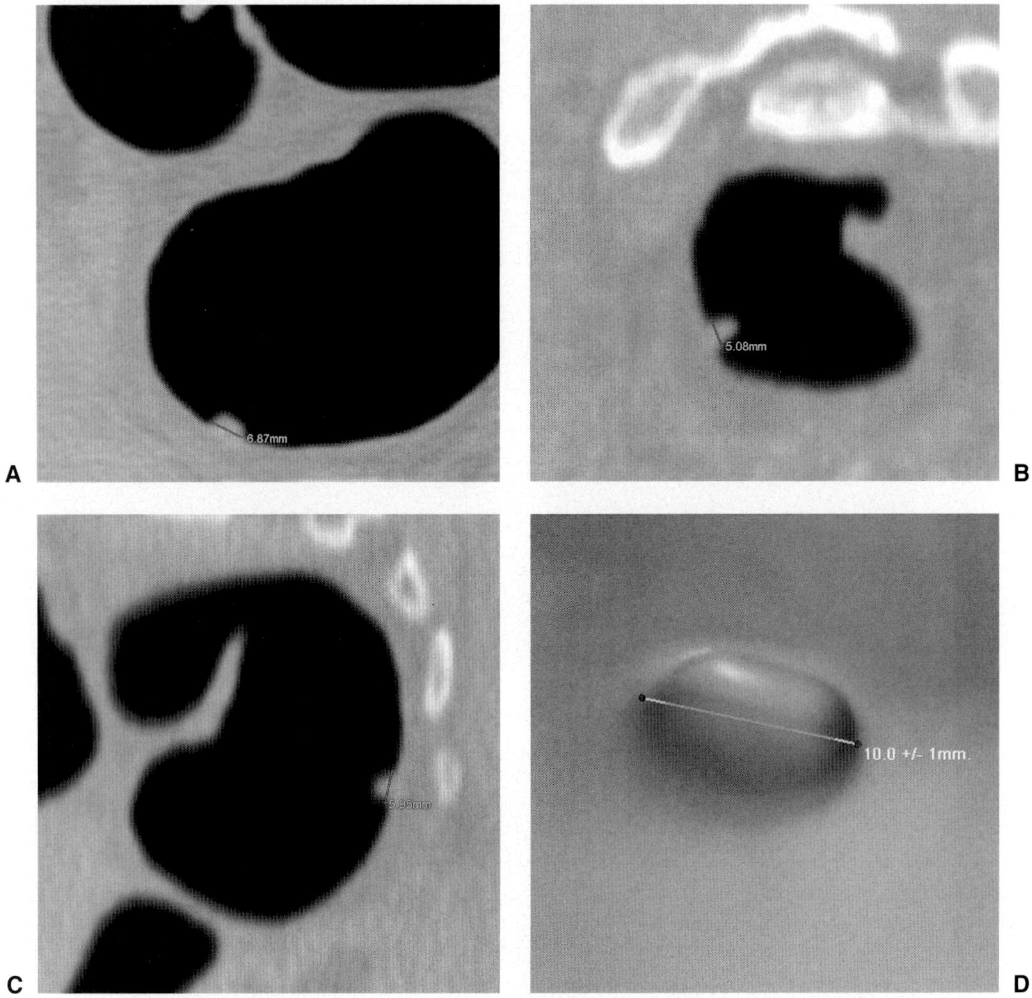

FIGURE 4.5 Supine axial image **(A)** shows a sessile rectal polyp measuring 6 mm. Coronal **(B)** and sagittal reformats **(C)** also underestimate polyp size at 5 mm and 6 mm respectively. The 3D endoluminal view **(D)** shows an elliptical polyp that measures 10 mm along the long axis. Note the different morphologic appearance of the polyp on coronal view as it is viewed along its short axis.

when necessary to problem-solve potential lesions. This 2D approach is similar to the typical approach to reading computed tomography (CT) scans that relies on the use of the axial images and may therefore be more familiar and comfortable for readers who are already experienced in interpreting CT data sets. Additionally, most computer workstations easily support a primary 2D interpretation method particularly early in the development of this technique. In a survey of experts in CTC, it was found that most respondents (80%, 20/25) believed that a primary 2D approach with 3D reserved for problem solving was the optimum method for CTC interpretation.[1]

The primary 2D approach requires evaluation of the colon in a systematic manner typically from the anorectum to the cecum using the 2D axial supine and prone images with the use of the MPR and 3D endoluminal images to aid in differentiating polyps from other structures such as bulbous folds and stool. CTC software should allow the ability to display the supine and prone axial data sets side by side (see Figs. 4.6 and 4.7). It is also useful to have the MPR and 3D views easily accessible, which may be available in the same display as the axial images.

The reader begins by scrolling to approximately the same level on both the supine and prone axial views. When starting at the level of the anorectal junction, the bony landmarks in the pelvis may be used for initial orientation and registration of similar levels on the supine and prone images. Intracolonic landmarks such as the inferior valve of Houston in the rectum, or specific folds or diverticulae in other parts of the colon may also be used. The supine and prone axial data sets are then linked or synchronized as the reader evaluates each colonic segment systematically (segmental lumen tracking) being sure to scroll through the top and bottom of each portion of the colon. The colon should be magnified so that the gas-filled colonic segment occupies most of the display in each position. The reader will have to link and unlink

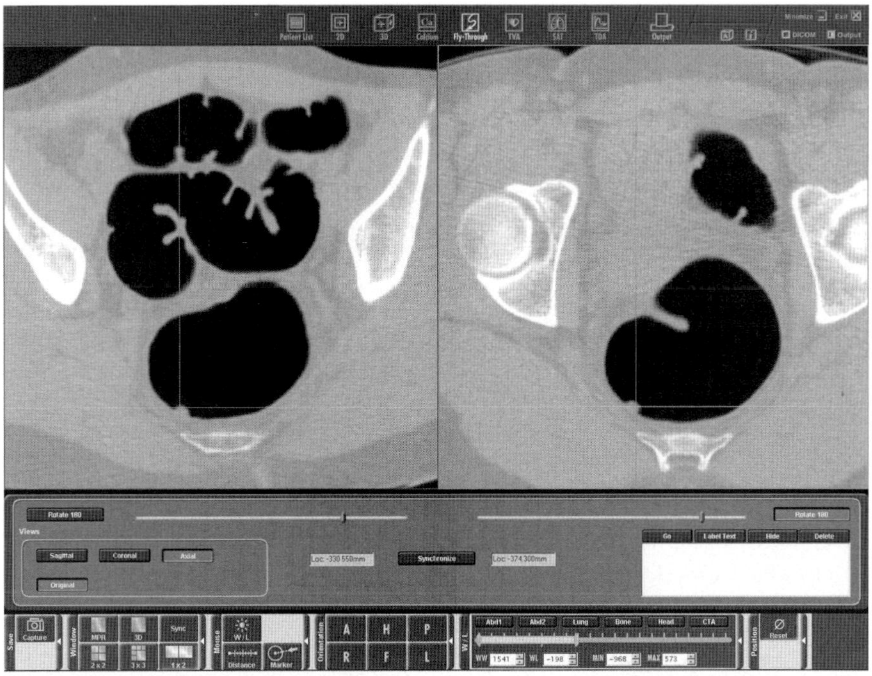

FIGURE 4.6 Display format for primary 2D interpretation shows adjacent magnified supine and prone axial images with a crosshair placed on a rectal polyp. There are easily accessible buttons for image synchronization and alternative layout windows allowing time-efficient correlation with MPRs and 3D views. Functions such as measurement, bookmarking, image capture, windowing, and reporting are also accessible. MPRs, multiformat reformations.

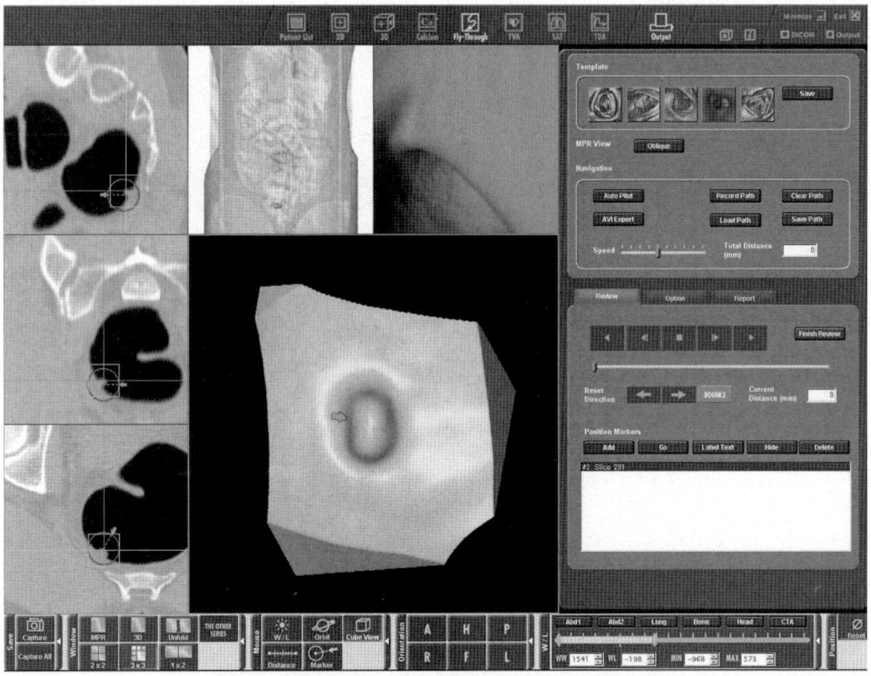

FIGURE 4.7 Display format which may be used for further evaluation of a potential lesion initially identified on axial views. A single data set is evaluated with multiple windows typically including MPRs, 3D endoluminal or subvolume cube views, and an overview image showing the position within the entire colon. An endoluminal view at 180 degrees is available. A particular view can be maximized or brought to the dominant window typically by selection. MPRs, multiformat reformations.

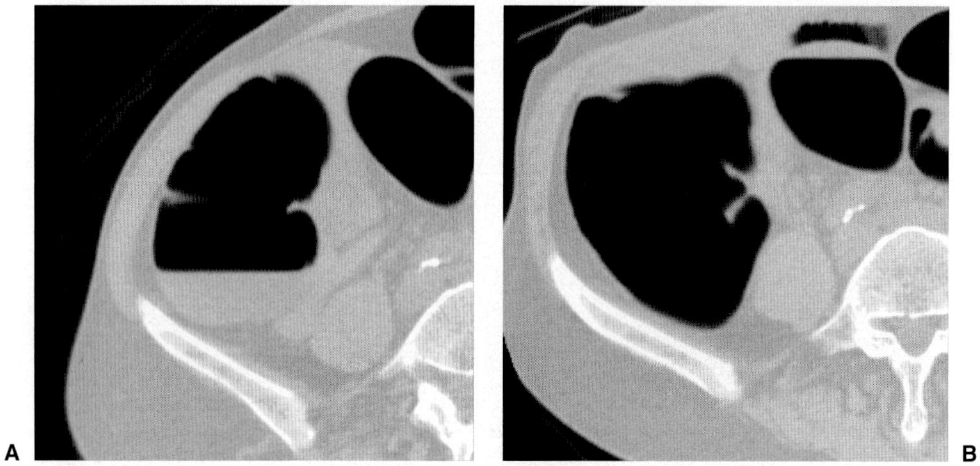

FIGURE 4.8 Axial supine **(A)** and prone **(B)** images show shifting of the remaining fluid in the opposing position to reveal the previously hidden colonic surface for evaluation.

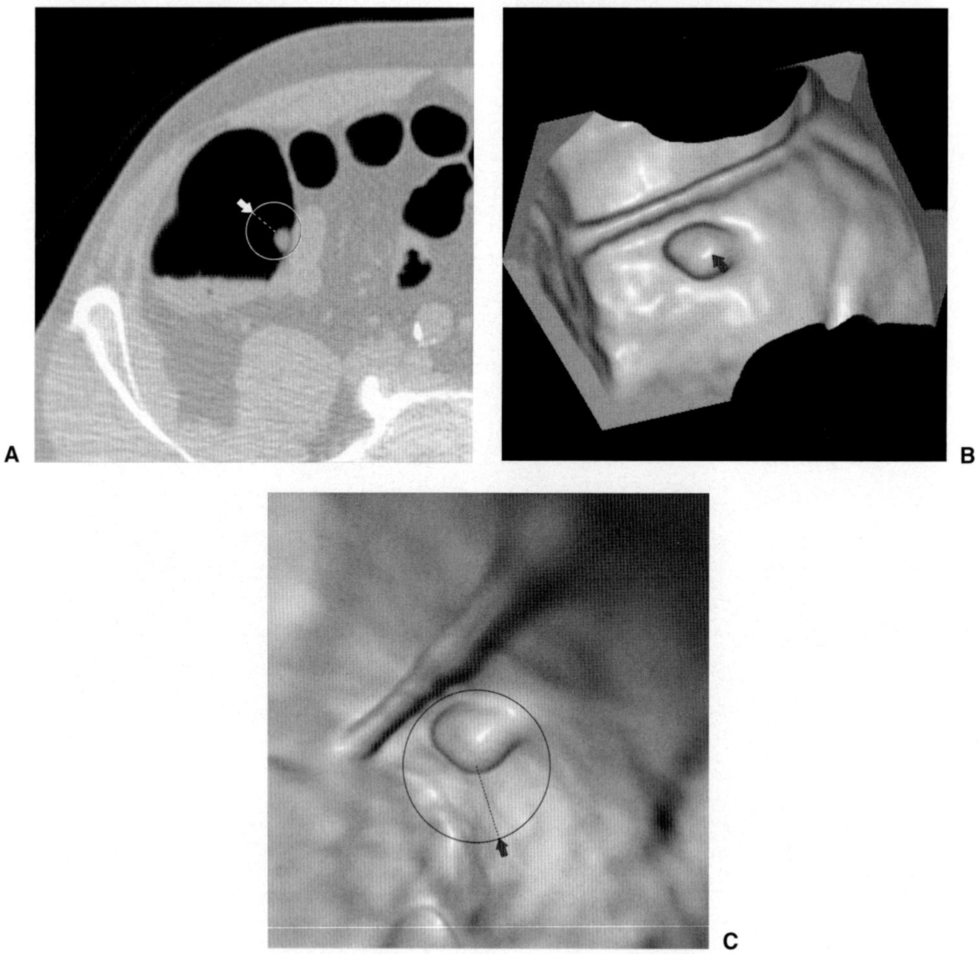

FIGURE 4.9 Cecal polyp identified on the supine axial image is bookmarked **(A)** and may be correlated with the prone axial image and MPRs. If needed the 3D cube view **(B)** or the endoluminal view **(C)** may be used to help differentiate a polyp from a haustral fold.

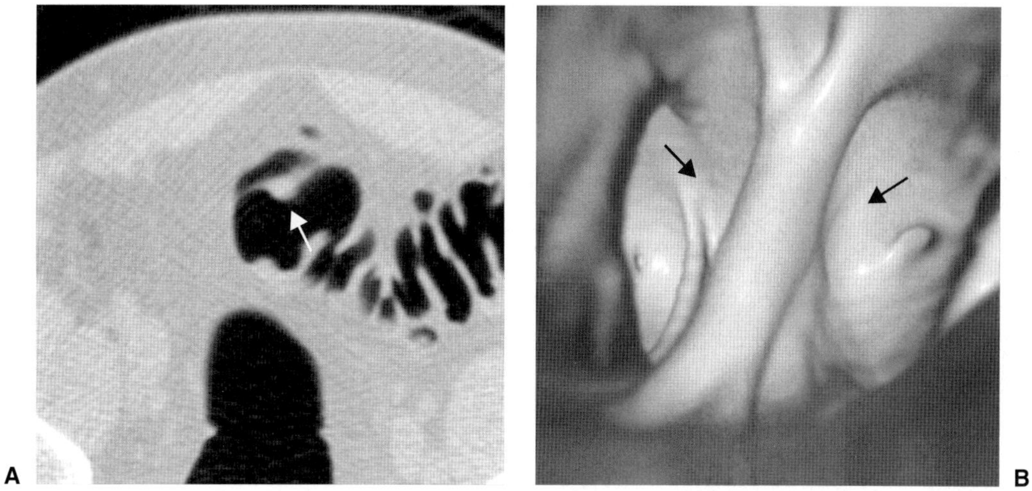

FIGURE 4.10 Axial image **(A)** shows a polypoid lesion in the sigmoid colon. The 3D endoluminal view **(B)** shows the lesion to represent a bulbous fold.

the supine and prone data sets multiple times to maintain similar orientation of a particular colonic segment in both positions during the evaluation. Additionally, supine and prone axial images will require panning or roaming to keep the gas-filled lumen in the center of the display field. This method allows direct comparison of segments that cannot be fully evaluated in one position either due to residual layering fluid or stool obscuring the dependent colonic surface or due to suboptimal distention (see Fig. 4.8).

If a suspicious lesion is detected on 2D axial images, it is bookmarked so that it can be quickly located and reviewed using 3D views (see Figs. 4.9 and 4.10). Depending on reader preference, potential lesions identified on 2D images may be evaluated immediately with 3D views, or they can all be evaluated at the end of the 2D interrogation of the colon. Most CTC software provides a crosshair visible on axial, multiplanar, and 3D views to show the particular location of a lesion on all views.

A high-contrast colon display window (width 1,400, level −350) is recommended to maximize visualization of polyps at the air–soft tissue interface and to help display air or heterogeneous density within stool. A standard soft tissue or abdominal window (width 400, level 40) is used to evaluate for mural thickening due to involvement by cancers. The abdominal window is also used to distinguish the fat density of colonic lipomas as well as the high density of pills and contrast material. In addition, this window is sometimes helpful in tracking the colonic lumen in very tortuous colonic segments. Flat lesions may be easier to visualize using a soft tissue window. Following complete colonic evaluation, the abdominal window is used to review the entire 2D axial data set for extracolonic lesions.

Multiplanar reformations must often be referred to when evaluating very tortuous segments or segments of collapse and should be easily available. The display layout can often be customized and listed as a specific user preference. Multiple types of images may be displayed at one time including 2D axial images in combination with sagittal, coronal, and/or oblique MPRs, and/or 3D views such as either the cube view, fly-through or dissection view for problem solving. A 3D overview of the colon that simulates an air-contrast barium enema may be included and is useful for showing the location of the viewing point or a potential lesion (see Fig. 4.11). This view also allows easy review of the anatomy of the colon and the detection of variants. 3D thick-slab MPR is also available on some workstations, and has the advantage of the extraluminal

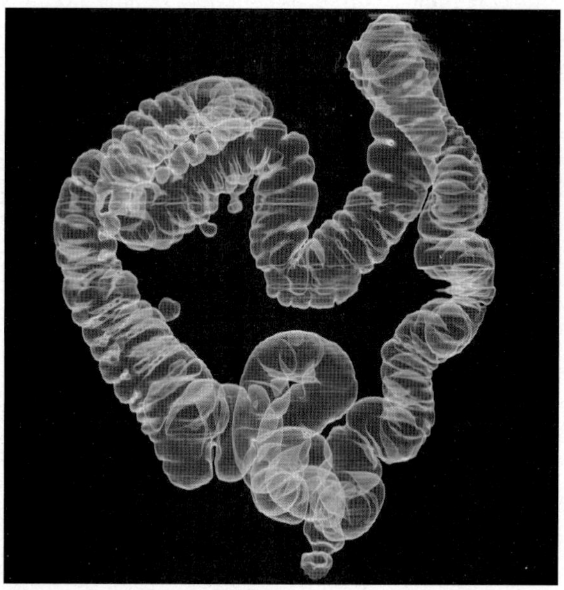

FIGURE 4.11 Colon overview resembles the appearance of a double contrast barium enema and is helpful in demonstrating colon tortuosity and mobility. Note diverticulosis involving the ascending colon and transverse colon.

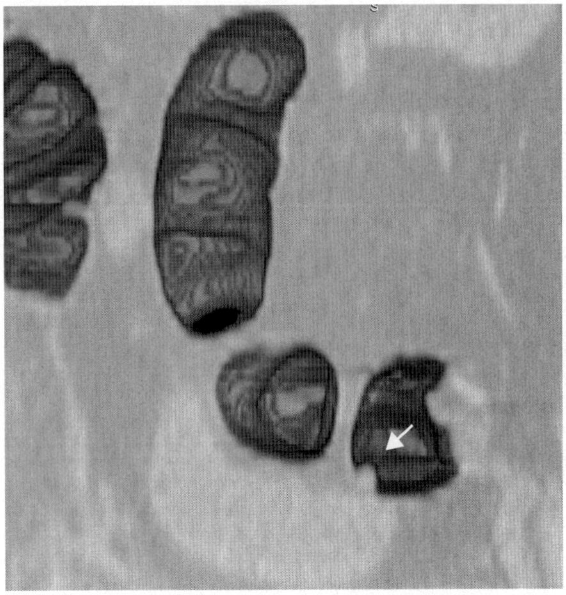

FIGURE 4.12 Thick slab view in the coronal plane provides a 3D perspective to the MPR view. A small polyp is demonstrated protruding into the sigmoid colon lumen with visualization of adjacent structures. MPR, multiformat reformation.

orientation of 2D MPR and the ability to display a finite volume beyond a single slice (see Fig. 4.12).

Advantages of 2D interpretation include the ability to directly visualize the texture and density of potential lesions (heterogeneous stool-containing air, fat density of lipomas, high density of contrast material or pill fragments) (see Table 4.3 and Figs. 4.13 and 4.14). The mobility of stool and pedunculated polyps are easily assessed, and structures causing external compression of the colon are quickly identified. 2D views allow the reader to easily avoid the potential pitfalls that occur with primary 3D interpretation such as diverticulae. The entire wall of the colon may be visualized on 2D if there is optimal cleansing and distention. Interpretation times using primary 2D are typically faster than for primary 3D interpretation, ranging between 5 and 20 minutes, and often 10 minutes or less particularly in normal studies. As a reader becomes more experienced in distinguishing true polyps from false positives on 2D images, interpretation times can decrease and 3D problem solving is used less frequently.

Disadvantages of using 2D as a primary method include the difficulty of tracking the colon when there are redundant segments, aberrant anatomy (i.e., cecal bascule), or if multiple collapsed segments are present. Although there have been many single-center studies that have shown excellent sensitivity of CTC for the detection of clinically significant polyps using a primary 2D interpretation approach, results from multicenter trials to date performed in low-prevalence populations have been disappointing.[10,11] Poorly cleansed colons containing large amounts of residual fluid or solid stool can pose a problem for both 2D and 3D interpretation methods.

PRIMARY THREE-DIMENSIONAL INTERPRETATION

Advances in computer processing power, graphics cards, and the user interface of CTC software have improved the resolution of the 3D view as well as the ability to easily navigate through the endoluminal view. The user should ensure the availability of high quality 3D viewing and usability before attempting a primary 3D interpretation method. Most 3D display techniques currently employ volume rendering for postprocessing of the CT data sets

TABLE 4.3 Comparison of Advantages of Primary Two-Dimensional vs. Primary Three-Dimensional Interpretation Methods

Primary 2D	Primary 3D
1. Shorter interpretation time 2. Easy assessment of lesion density—differentiation of stool from true lesion, lipomas, can measure attenuation 3. Easier registration of colon segments in supine and prone positions 4. Easier differentiation of annular tumor/strictures from collapsed/poorly distended segments 5. Visualize entire wall as you scroll 6. Visualize wall thickening and extracolonic extension of colonic lesions 7. Avoid 3D pitfalls such as diverticulae	1. Potential higher sensitivity for small lesions 2. Less eye strain—more relaxed reading style 3. Easier to learn for the novice reader (although some radiologists are more familiar with 2D and 3D is harder to learn) 4. Easier to identify polyps on or adjacent to folds 5. Ability to quickly screen large areas of colon—virtual dissection view 6. Avoid 2D pitfalls such as bulbous or converging folds

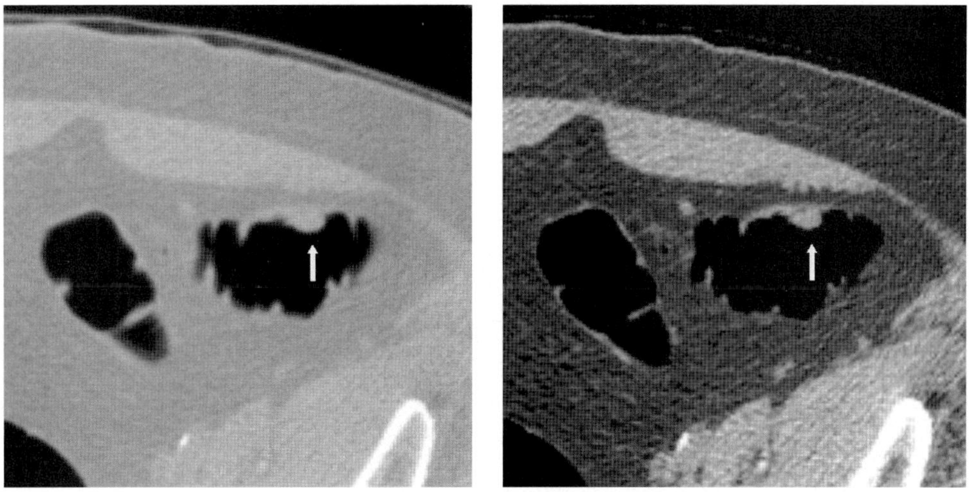

FIGURE 4.13 The abdominal window is useful for evaluating the density of a lesion. Axial image of the sigmoid viewed using a colon window **(A)** shows a homogeneous, ovoid lesion typical of a polyp. The abdominal window **(B)** confirms the homogeneous soft tissue density of the lesion characteristic of a polyp.

although surface rendering has been used in the past (see Fig. 4.15). 3D data can be visualized using monochromatic or color shaded displays which simulate the appearance of colonic mucosa. Perspective lighting can also be adjusted to provide near-field and far-field differentiation. Current CTC software offers real-time interactive 3D viewing and navigation, and offers either a partially or completely automated centerline flight path. Older software only allowed manual adjustment of the centerline flight path for 3D endoluminal navigation.

Several features have been developed to assist interpretation using a primary 3D method. Rapid, automatic segmentation of the gas-distended colon with automatic centerline generation are now available. Automated seed placement for colonic segmentation is available that effectively excludes extracolonic air.[12–14] Computation methods for the colonic centerline include decimation and topological thinning.[15–17] Some software algorithms use the colonic lumen or wall as a basis for computation of the centerline, although other methods have been developed that do not rely on identification of complete colon segments and this has decreased centerline computation times from 17 seconds down to approximately 10 seconds.[18] Other gas-filled structures such as the stomach or small bowel are initially segmented and identified by different colors and can be manually excluded from evaluation (see Fig. 4.16).

The display format used for primary 3D interpretation should feature central placement of an enlarged endoluminal 3D view (see Fig. 4.17). 3D interpretation

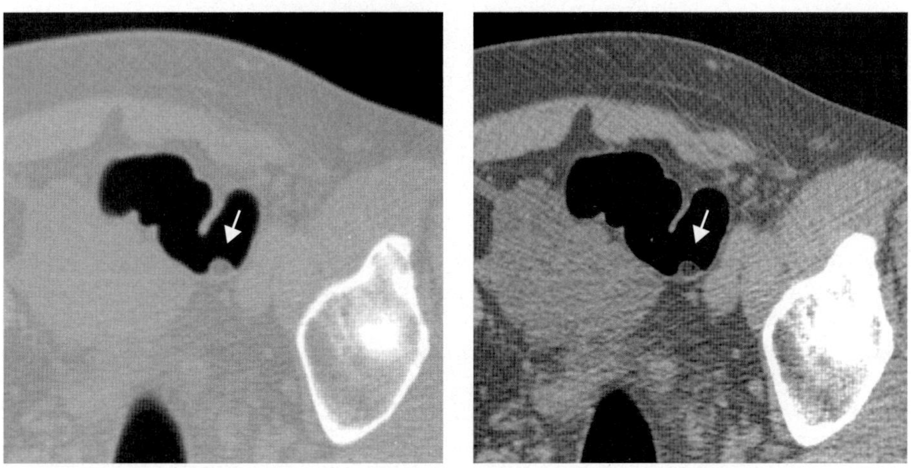

FIGURE 4.14 Axial image using a colon window **(A)** shows a lesion in the sigmoid colon with internal heterogeneity and low density, more apparent on the abdominal window image **(B)**, and characteristic of stool.

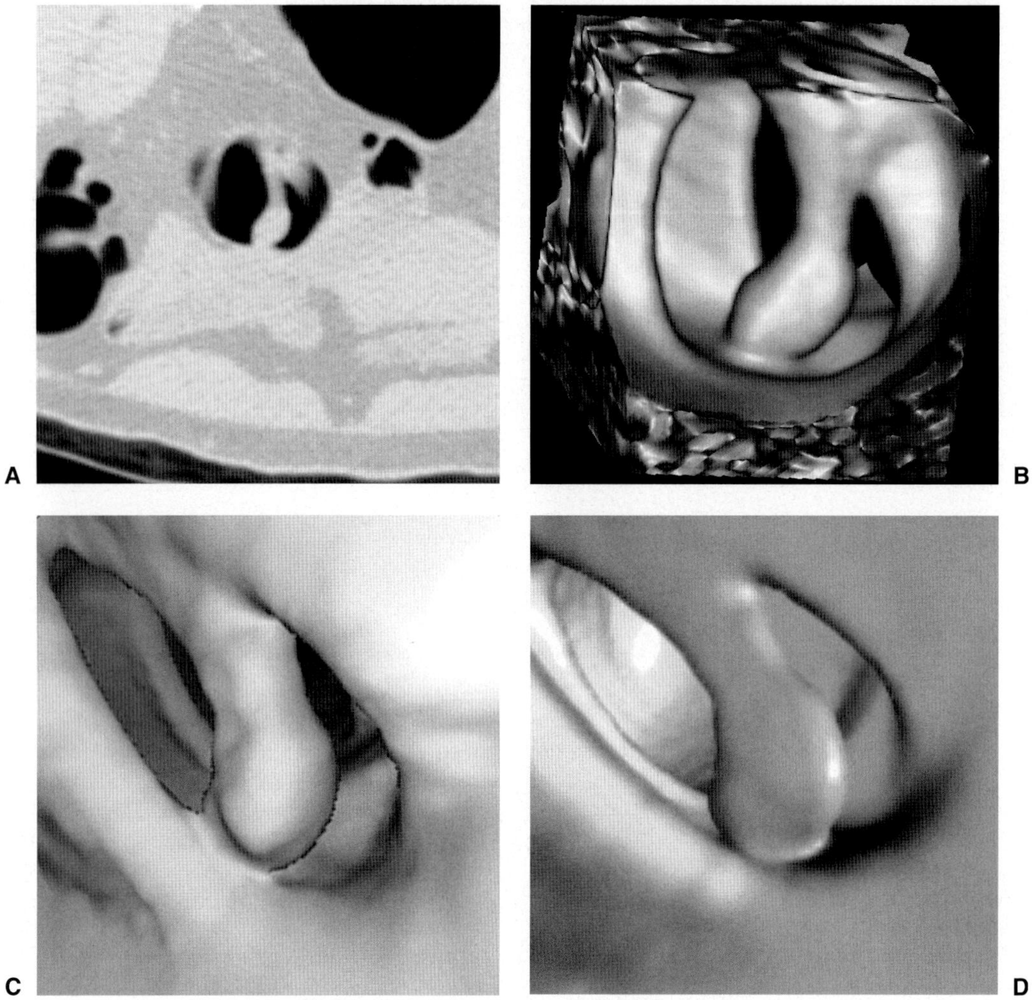

FIGURE 4.15 Volume rendering is the preferred postprocessing technique for 3D views. Surface-rendered images have more artifacts at the air–soft tissue interface, appear less smooth, and are higher contrast than volume-rendered images. The axial image **(A)** and 3D volume rendered cube view **(B)** shows a pedunculated polyp in the sigmoid colon. The surface rendered 3D endoluminal image **(C)** appears less smooth, with more contrast compared to the volume rendered image **(D)**.

begins by flying although the colon segments along the centerline, first in a retrograde direction (anorectum to cecum) and then in an anterograde direction (cecum to anorectum). A total of four "fly-throughs" are performed: once in each of the two directions in both supine and prone positions. In a study of 50 patients undergoing both CTC and colonoscopy, the value of two-way 3D interpretation was compared to one-way 3D interpretation.[19] It was found that using three readers, the mean sensitivity of CTC for polyp detection with two-way navigation was significantly higher (88.4%, 411/465) than for one-way navigation (78.1%, 363/465). An increased number of false-positive findings were present when using two-way interpretation as well.

Navigation through the colon is real time (variable renderings ranging between 5–30 frames per second) so that the reader may deviate off of the flight path at any time to further evaluate a suspicious lesion. The user should have the ability to modify navigation speed as needed. If a potential lesion is identified, it should be bookmarked and then interrogated on 2D views to determine its density and mobility (see Figs. 4.18 and 4.19). Bookmarking of potential lesions performed on 3D views should automatically transfer onto the 2D views and there should be ready accessibility of the axial and MPR images for correlation of findings. Once a polyp is confirmed, there should be easy ability to measure the largest diameter.

Software is available to track the walls of the colon that have been visualized and can paint the surface a different color to indicate that it has been evaluated. After anterograde and retrograde evaluation, skipped areas or "missing patches" (often located behind haustral folds) may be reviewed automatically. In a study of 223 patients undergoing CTC, the mean surface coverage after one-way retrograde 3D navigation was 76.6%, which increased to

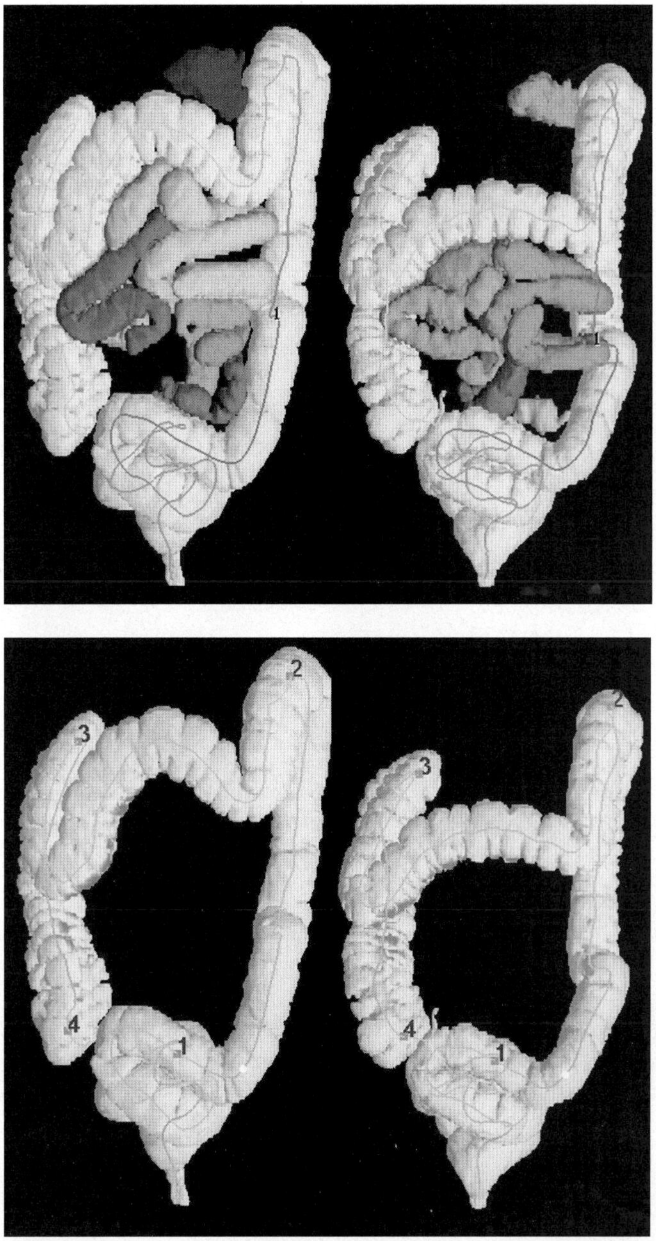

FIGURE 4.16 Primary 3D interpretation requires initial segmentation of the colon from surrounding structures. Supine segmentation view **(A)** and prone segmentation view **(B)** shows inclusion of the stomach and small bowel. The colonic centerline is automatically generated and visible. Only the colon is selected for evaluation by the user and the stomach and small bowel segments are removed. **(C, D)**.

94.1% when anterograde navigation was added.[20] A review of missed areas measuring 300 mm or larger increased coverage to 97.9% and added an average of 21.4 seconds to the interpretation time. If residual stool and fluid has been tagged, software is available to digitally subtract the tagged material from the data set. A 3D translucency view consisting of a color map based on density is helpful for quickly determining the internal attenuation of lesions and can aid in differentiating tagged stool from a true polyp or mass.[21]

Advantages of using 3D as a primary reading method include a fairly relaxed reading style with the use of automatic navigation through the colon (see Table 4.3). 3D navigation may be easier for some novice readers to learn and experienced readers using this approach can have high accuracy for polyp detection. Polyps on or adjacent to folds are often easier to discern on 3D images and complex, truncated, or bulbous folds are quickly identified. Some lesions, particularly small polyps measuring 5 mm or less may be more conspicuous on 3D images.

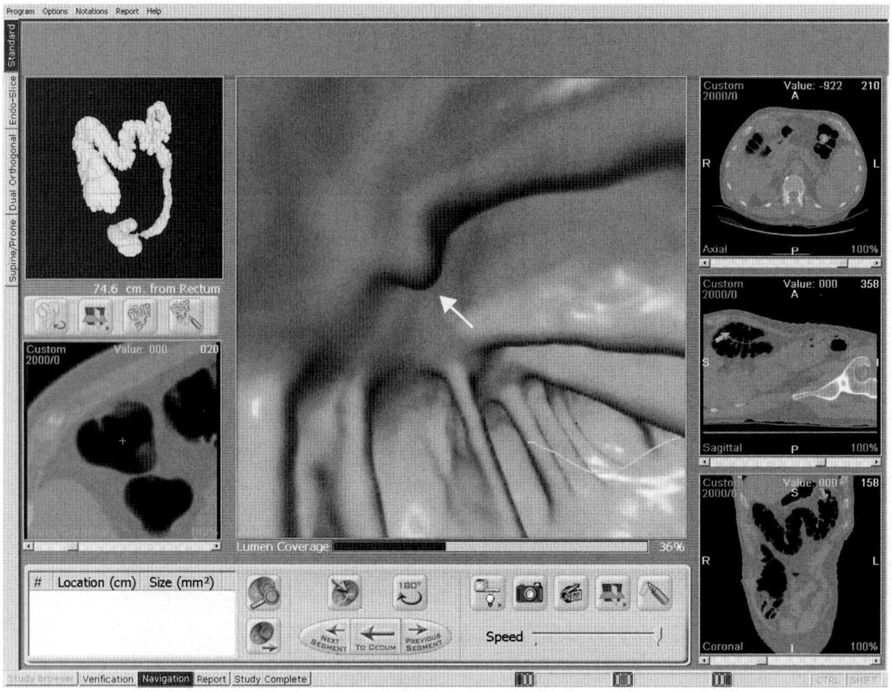

FIGURE 4.17 Primary 3D interpretation features a display format with a dominant window for the 3D endoluminal view. The endoluminal 3D view shows a polyp on a fold in the transverse colon. MPR views are to the right and include axial (**top**), sagittal (**middle**), and coronal (**bottom**) planes. A colon overview (**top**) and oblique reformat (**bottom**) are included on the left. Useful functions for 3D interpretation are easily accessible: navigation speed, direction and position change, measurement, image capture, and painting of visualized surfaces. Distance from the anorectal junction is provided. MPR, multiformat reformation.

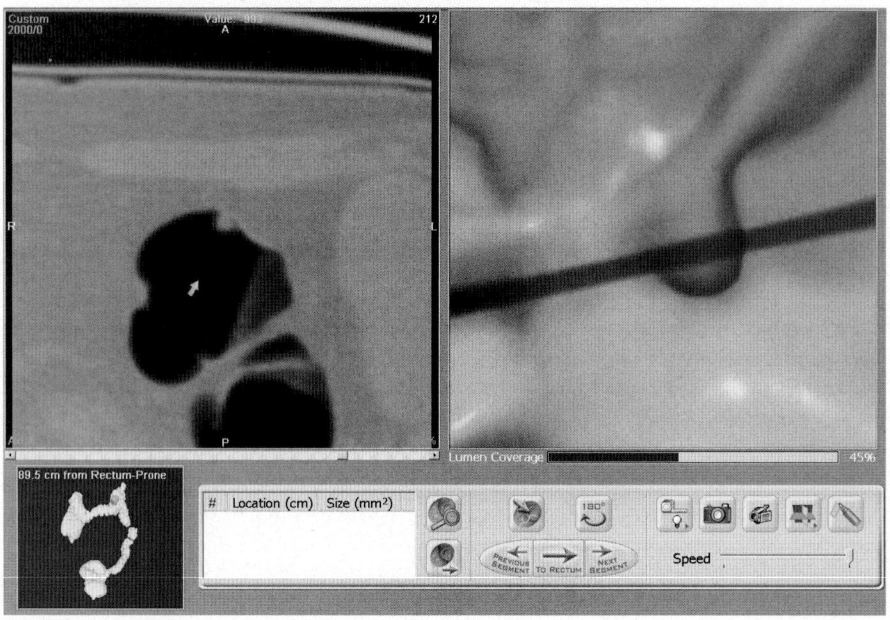

FIGURE 4.18 Polypoid lesion on a fold initially identified on 3D endoluminal view (**right**) is correlated with the prone 2D axial image (**left**). The exact axial location is indicated by a stripe that is displayed on the 3D endoluminal view. The location of the bookmarked polyp is indicated on the colon overview image.

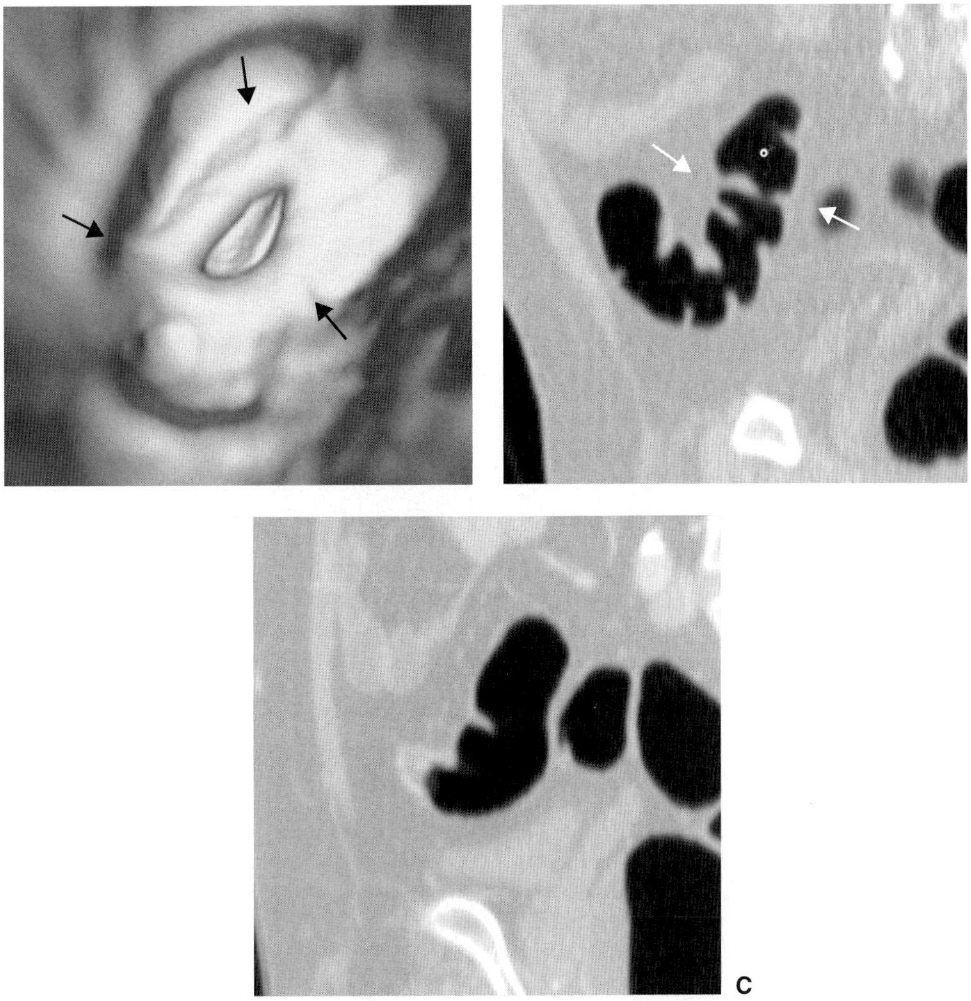

FIGURE 4.19 Endoluminal image **(A)** shows an annular type lesion, suspicious for a carcinoma. On the 2D supine sagittal image **(B)**, it is clear that the sigmoid colon is not well distended, allowing two prominent folds to mimic this annular lesion. The 2D prone sagittal image **(C)** in the same location is better distended.

Disadvantages of primary 3D interpretation include the detection of pitfalls specific to the 3D view, the inability to assess for wall thickening, the possibility of identifying more false-positive lesions, and difficulty assessing lesion density except on specific workstations. Additionally, if fluid and/or fecal tagging is being performed, it is important to have software available that can electronically subtract out the tagged material for easy and accurate primary 3D interpretation. Another drawback of primary 3D interpretation is the relatively longer interpretation time depending upon the hardware and software available. The mean time for 3D interpretation has been found to range between 12 and 39 minutes.[20,22,23] With automated 3D navigation, reading times may be comparable to the 2D navigation approach. However, with the use of semiautomated navigation, the time for 3D interpretation is significantly longer than for 2D interpretation.

TWO-DIMENSIONAL VERSUS THREE-DIMENSIONAL: THE EVIDENCE

Early in the investigation of CTC as a diagnostic tool, Royster et al. compared 2D CTC with 3D antegrade and retrograde navigations in 20 patients with colonoscopic findings suggestive of colorectal carcinoma.[24] Axial 2D interpretation alone revealed all 20 masses and 14 of 15 polyps. 3D navigations alone detected 19 of 20 masses and 13 of 15 polyps. It was concluded that both methods of interpretation are effective techniques.

Hara et al. compared 2D display only, 3D display only, and a combination of both displays for the detection of simulated polyps in five identical normal colonic data sets (15 total).[25] Two radiologists independently evaluated all data sets. The use of a combination of 2D and 3D views resulted in polyp detection rates that were higher or similar to those of 2D or 3D alone. This initial study recommended complete 2D and 3D interpretation for CTC.

Yee et al. evaluated the performance of CTC in a large single-center study of 300 patients using the combination of both complete 2D and 3D interpretations (anterograde and retrograde evaluation) in both the supine and prone positions.[26] Excellent results were achieved although interpretation times were relatively long. The mean interpretation time for two different radiologists was 27 minutes (range 15–40) and 31 minutes (range 15–45 minutes).

Beaulieu et al. compared the 2D axial display, a novel panoramic endoscopic volume-rendered display, and 3D endoluminal display.[27] Forty digitally synthesized polyps ranging between 3.5 and 10 mm in size were evaluated by two radiologists. Considering visible lesions only the sensitivities were 60%, 81%, and 85% for one reader and 28%, 62%, and 65% for the other reader for axial CT, panoramic views, and 3D endoluminal display respectively. The two radiologists differed significantly in sensitivity using 2D interpretation, which was attributed to differences in the search patterns used by each reviewer. The radiologist with the higher sensitivity using 2D interpretation systematically examined the colon from the rectum to the cecum by following the colonic lumen. The reader with lower sensitivity using 2D interpretation used a section-by-section approach, attempting to detect lesions in all parts of the visible colon on a particular axial slice. Three-dimensional displays were found to be more sensitive than 2D displays. The authors suggested that 3D views might contain visual cues that make lesion detection easier.

Primary 2D interpretation with 3D problem solving was used to evaluate 44 patients who underwent CTC in a study by Dachman et al.[28] The per-polyp sensitivity was 83% (5/6) for lesions 8 mm or larger. 3D problem solving was required in 23 (52%) of 44 patients. Interpretation times decreased from 29 to 22 minutes in one reader and 35 to 26 minutes in another reader without the use of 3D endoluminal views. The authors concluded that CTC may be interpreted using the axial images and that the endoluminal views should be used only when necessary to help distinguish folds from polyps.

Another study was performed with results supporting the use of primary 2D interpretation with the use of 3D endoluminal views for problem solving. Macari et al. performed CTC on 42 patients.[29] The CT data sets were examined by two radiologists using one of two methods of interpretation. Method 1 consisted of use of the 2D axial images for interpretation and referral to the 3D surface-rendered endoluminal display only if findings were suggestive of an abnormality. Method 2 consisted of complete review of the CT data sets using the 2D axial images and complete 3D "fly-throughs" in anterograde and retrograde manner. Both reading methods found the same number of polyps and no additional polyps were identified with 3D analysis. Interpretation time with Method 1 averaged 16 minutes (range 10–23 minutes), although the reading time for Method 2 averaged 41 minutes (range 28–62 minutes). A more recent study by the same group reported a mean interpretation time of 11 minutes using primary 2D reading with the use of 3D views for problem solving although maintaining a high sensitivity for large polyps.[30]

Diagnostic performance and reader agreement comparing 2D and 3D display techniques were evaluated by McFarland et al.[31] Three experienced abdominal radiologists independently evaluated 30 test segments and were then retested 6 weeks after the initial interpretation. The authors concluded that similar diagnostic performance in polyp detection was found when comparing 2D and 3D display techniques among experienced abdominal radiologists. Results showed good intraobserver reader agreement and variable interobserver agreement.

In a study by Bruzzi et al, CTC was performed in 82 patients at increased risk for colon cancer.[32] Using 2D axial views only with no review of multiplanar or 3D views, the sensitivity for detection of polyps measuring 9 mm, 6 to 9 mm, and <6 mm was 100%, 33%, and 19% respectively with specificities of 99%, 96%, and 82%.

In contrast to most other studies that had been performed to date, Pickhardt et al. performed a study in 1,233 asymptomatic patients where the readers employed a primary 3D interpretation method with 2D views used for problem solving.[23] Patients underwent a relatively rigorous colonic preparation method as well as the ingestion of barium for solid stool tagging and iodinated contrast for fluid tagging. The specific workstation and software employed allowed automatic subtraction of tagged material. Excellent results for adenomatous polyp detection were achieved with per polyp sensitivity for ≥10 mm, ≥8 mm, ≥6 mm polyp size categories of 92%, 93%, and 86% respectively.

Many of the earlier studies in the CTC literature performed both complete 2D and 3D interpretations. Since the publication of many of these earlier studies, computer processing power for 3D navigation and display has increased dramatically, and real-time 3D navigation with automated flight path is now widely available. Additional studies are being performed evaluating current software for the use of primary 2D versus primary 3D interpretation methods. There will likely be continued advocates for the various types of interpretation methods. The development of computer-aided detection and computer-assisted reading may make the specific type of primary interpretation method less relevant.

ALTERNATIVE VIEWS

The typical 3D endoluminal view used for CTC is similar to what is visualized on optical colonoscopy. Antegrade and retrograde navigations through the lumen of the colon visualized as a tubular structure are generated and viewed dynamically and interactively. Alternative 3D displays including the unfolded cube display, map projections, planar virtual pathology, and dissection view have been developed to help optimize visualization of the entire colon surface and to decrease interpretation times.

Vos et al. compared two-directional (antegrade and retrograde) 3D display versus an unfolded cube display in 30 patients.[33] The unfolded cube display renders six planar projections at 90-degree viewing angles from points along the central path. This allows visualization of the complete field of view at a particular path position. Sensitivity for the detection of large polyps was 89% and 100% for each of two readers and there no statistically significant difference between the two display methods was found. Mean interpretation times using the typical 3D endoluminal display (35–36 minutes) were significantly longer than for the unfolded cube display (19–20 minutes). Approximately 93.8% of the colon surface was viewed with the 3D endoluminal view. Colon surface visibility was higher at 99.5% using the unfolded cube view.

Map projection CTC using Mercator projection and stereographic projection were evaluated for polyp detection sensitivity in a study by Paik et al.[34] Forty digitally synthesized polyps of different sizes were inserted into copies of a CT data set. For two readers and polyp sizes of 7 mm or larger, the sensitivity for the Mercator projection (87.5%) and for stereographic projection (82.5%) was significantly higher than for viewing the axial slices (62.5%). Positive predictive value for the Mercator and stereographic projections was 75.4% and 78.9% respectively. It was determined that in order for the amount of mucosal surface visualization to approach that of map projection (98.8%) significant distortion occurred in other views. Therefore, map projection was determined to have higher sensitivity for polyp detection because a greater percentage of the mucosal surface was visualized.

Planar virtual pathology (PVP) generates volume-rendered images of segments of the colon. Cut planes are used to display the lumen of the colon and surrounding tissue. Isometric images are produced that do not cause distortion of the colon. Fletcher et al. compared traditional 2D axial images, multiplanar reformatted images, 3D endoluminal views and PVP images in 10 patients with 36 polyps.[35] PVP performed better than the other methods and detected 13 of 17 (76%) of large polyps, whereas 11 of 17 (65%) were identified using the other viewing methods.

The virtual dissection method bisects the colon along its longitudinal axis and unfolds it for display (see Figs. 4.20–4.23). Hoppe et al. performed an early study evaluating the polyp detection sensitivity and time for reconstruction of the dissection view compared with 2D axial interpretation in 20 patients with 31 lesions.[36] The software employed first defined the centerline of the colon using a semiautomatic technique. One fourth of the circumference of the colon was captured with a 90-degree

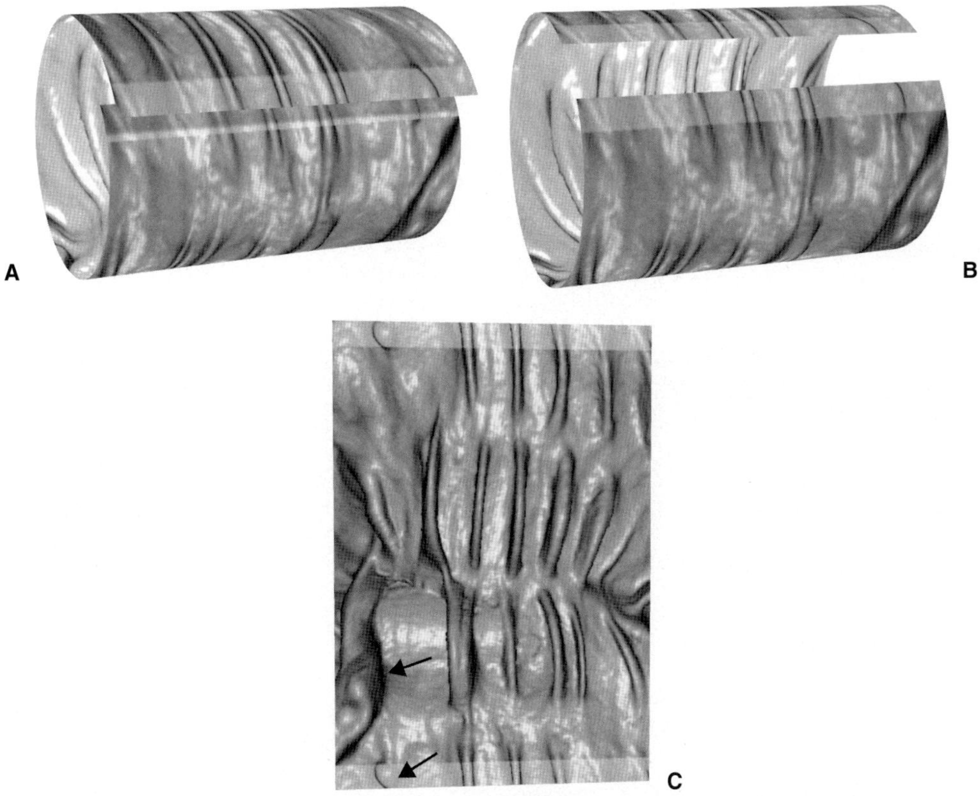

FIGURE 4.20 The virtual dissection view bisects the colon along its longitudinal axis and unfolds it for display **(A, B)**. A larger area of the colonic wall is available for viewing at one time. Stripes on both sides of the display indicate an area of wall overlap. Note the ileocecal valve in the lower left and a small diverticulum in a portion of the wall that is overlapped **(C)**.

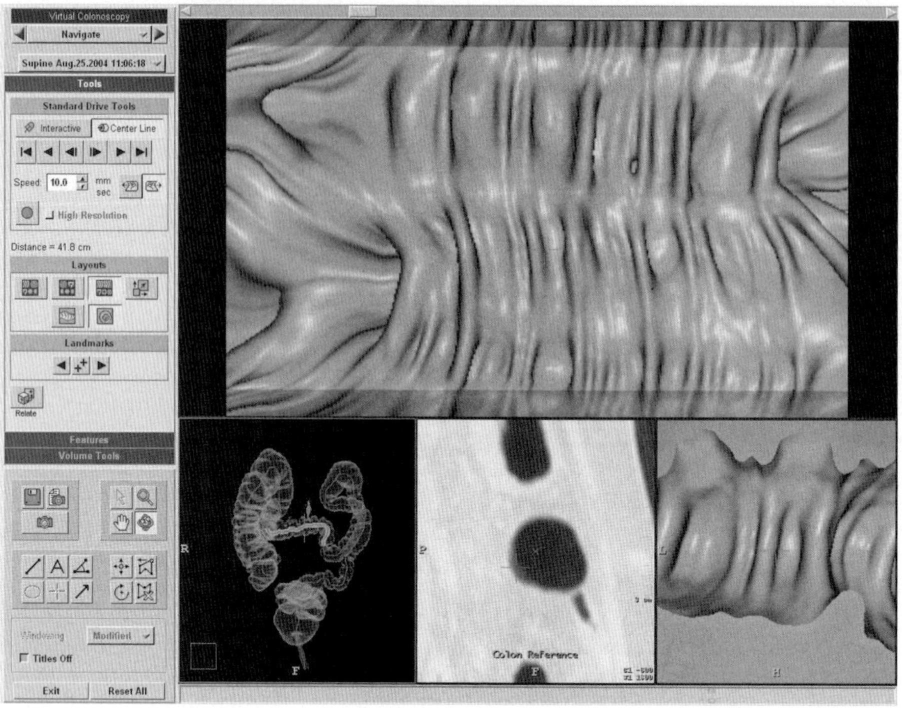

FIGURE 4.21 Display format that includes the dissection view as the largest window with smaller windows on the bottom for a colon overview (**left**), 2D axial view (**middle**), and 3D view (**right**). Distortion of folds and lesions may occur particularly in areas of acute curvature. (See also color plate.)

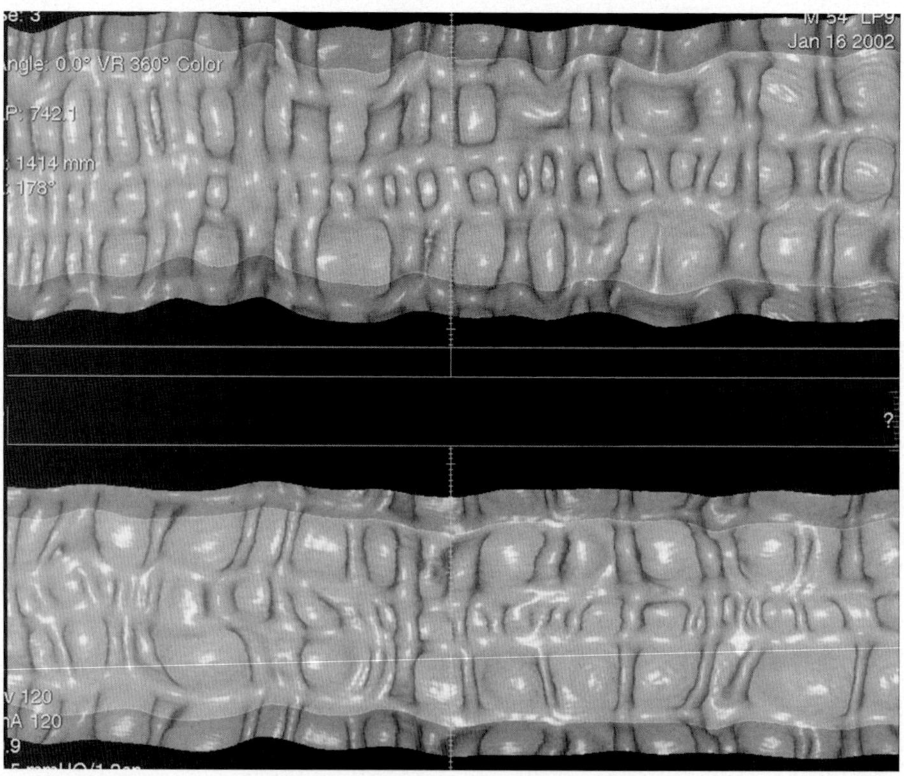

FIGURE 4.22 Excellent demonstration of normal haustral folds on this 360-degree dissection view using volume rendering. (See also color plate.)

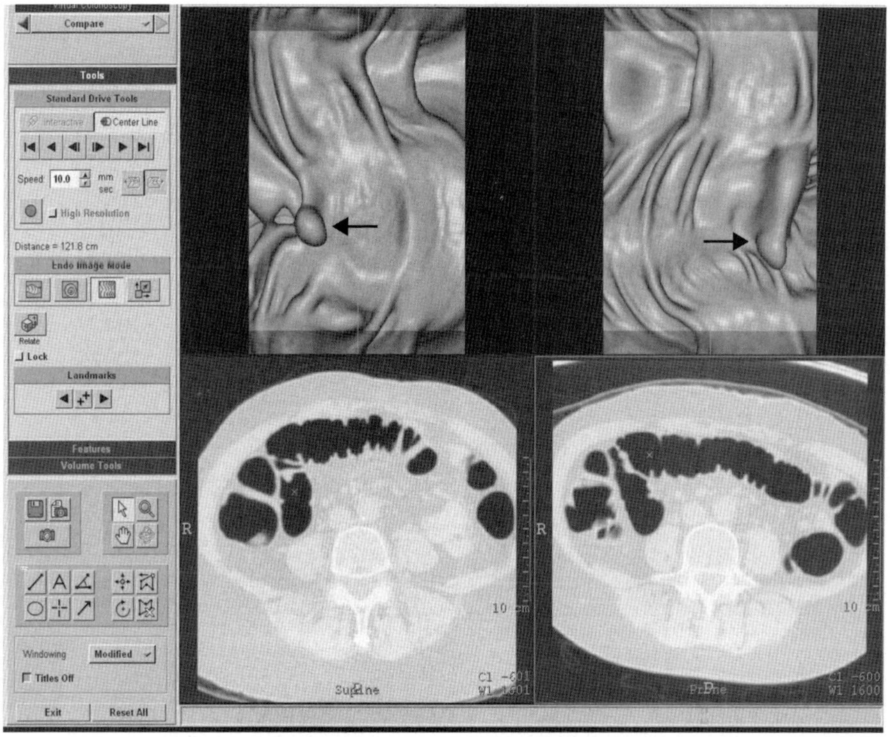

FIGURE 4.23 Supine and prone CTC data sets may be viewed together with the dissection views on top and the corresponding 2D axial images below. Note a small polyp more easily identifiable on the dissection views. (See also color plate.)

camera field of view that could be rotated in 45-degree increments. Eight connected panels of the colonic surface were generated when the camera was rotated in 45-degree increments. The sensitivities of two readers for detecting 10 mm and larger polyps using the dissection view were 67% and 87% compared with 89% and 100% using 2D axial interpretation. Results using this early version of the dissection software produced were suboptimal when compared with 2D axial interpretation.

Johnson et al. performed a feasibility study evaluating CTC using 360-degree virtual dissection.[37] Assuming a 5% incidence of 1-cm polyps in a screening population and the acquisition of 700 images per CTC data set, it was calculated that a radiologist would have to review >4,000 images to detect 1 large polyp. It was postulated that by decreasing the number of images to interpret there might be a reduction in reader fatigue and improved polyp detection. The sensitivities and specificities for large polyp detection in 20 patients for three observers were 94% (16/17), 82% (14/17), and 88% (15/17) respectively and 100% (5/5), 100% (5/5) and 80% (4/5) respectively. Evaluation of the virtual dissection view using a phantom containing 144 polyps of different sizes and shapes, it was determined that although there is distortion of structures it occurs in patterns that may be recognized so that detection of polyps is not compromised.

Forty-eight patients underwent CTC and analysis of the CT data sets was performed using various types of image display in a study by Rottgen et al.[38] Sensitivity and specificity for polyps detection for the virtual dissection view, the 3D endoluminal view, and the 2D axial images were 94% and 94%, 89% and 94%, and 62% and 100% respectively. The virtual dissection view outperformed the other two types of display for detection of polyps smaller than 5 mm. Juchems et al. performed a study in 21 patients and compared polyp detection using the dissection view and the 3D endoluminal view.[39] The per lesion sensitivity for polyps smaller than 5 mm, 5 to 10 mm, and larger than 10 mm were 47%, 56%, and 75% respectively for the dissection view versus 35%, 82%, and 100% respectively for the 3D endoluminal view. The average interpretation time for the dissection view was 10 and 38 minutes for the endoluminal view. It was concluded that the dissection view was superior for the detection of polyps smaller than 5 mm similar to the study by Rottgen et al.

NORMAL ANATOMY

Normal anatomy of the colon has been well described in the surgery and gastroenterology literature.[40–43] The colon is typically 150 to 180 cm in length, with the greatest segmental variability in the sigmoid and transverse colons.[40,41] Traditionally the colon is divided into the following six segments which is also most useful for describing the colon on CTC—rectum, sigmoid, descending colon, transverse colon, ascending colon, and cecum[44]

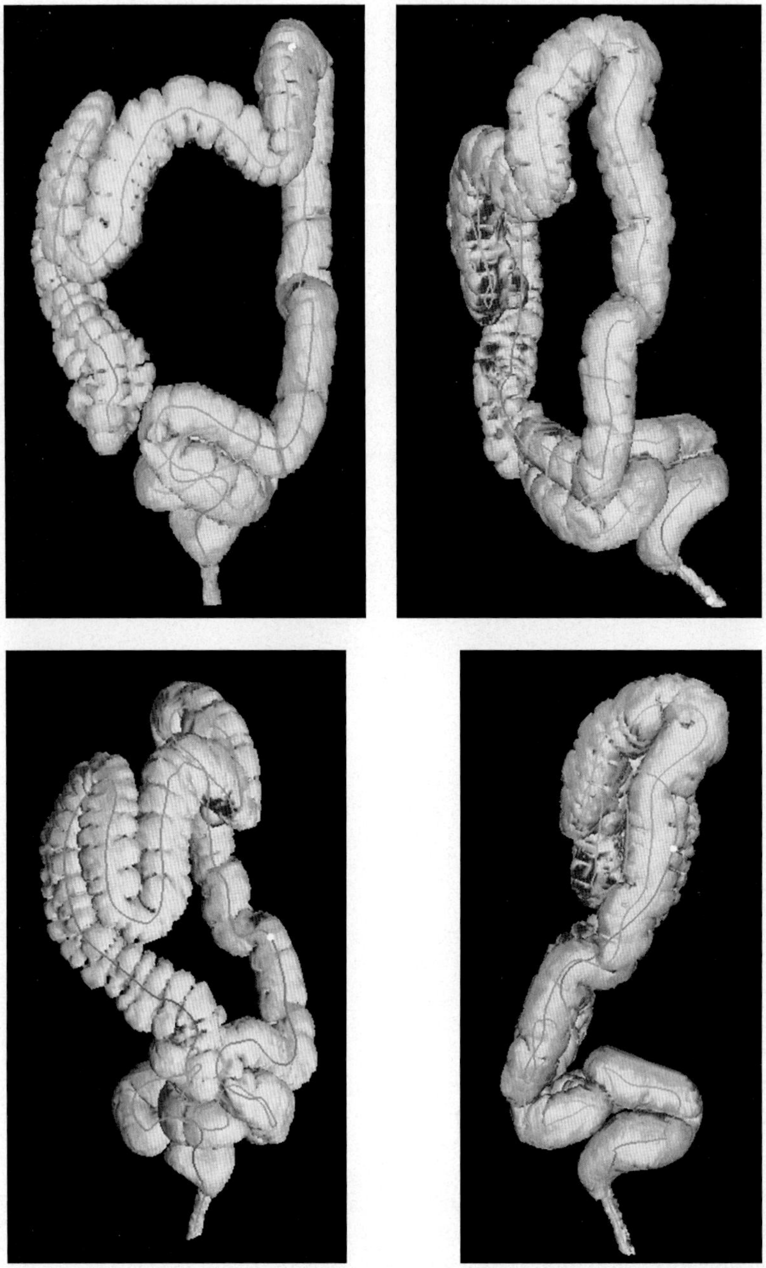

A B C D

FIGURE 4.24 An overview of the colon may be rotated in multiple projections after CT data acquisition without the need for additional radiation: Anterior-posterior **(A)**, left anterior oblique **(B)**, right anterior oblique **(C)**, and lateral **(D)** views.

(see Fig. 4.24). Although the hepatic and splenic flexures may also be included as colonic segments, they are less useful for CTC when compared with optical colonoscopy given the difficulty in identification of the flexures on endoscopy.

Evaluation of the distal colon on CT should begin with the anal verge and proceed into the rectum (see Fig. 4.25). It is imperative to include the anal verge within the field of view as this area should be evaluated for the presence of polyps, internal hemorrhoids, and hypertrophied anal papillae. Typically, there are radiating folds around the anal verge caused by the action of the anal sphincter. The dentate line, hypertrophied anal papillae, and prominent vertical folds at the anal verge may occasionally simulate a polyp. Additionally, there should be careful examination of the area around the rectal tube to avoid missing low rectal lesions. The sagittal and coronal views of the anorectal verge are often helpful as a problem-solving tool when trying to distinguish folds or hemorrhoids from polyps.

The rectum is 12 to 15 cm in length and is devoid of haustra because the longitudinal taeniae coli end at the rectosigmoid junction and continue only as

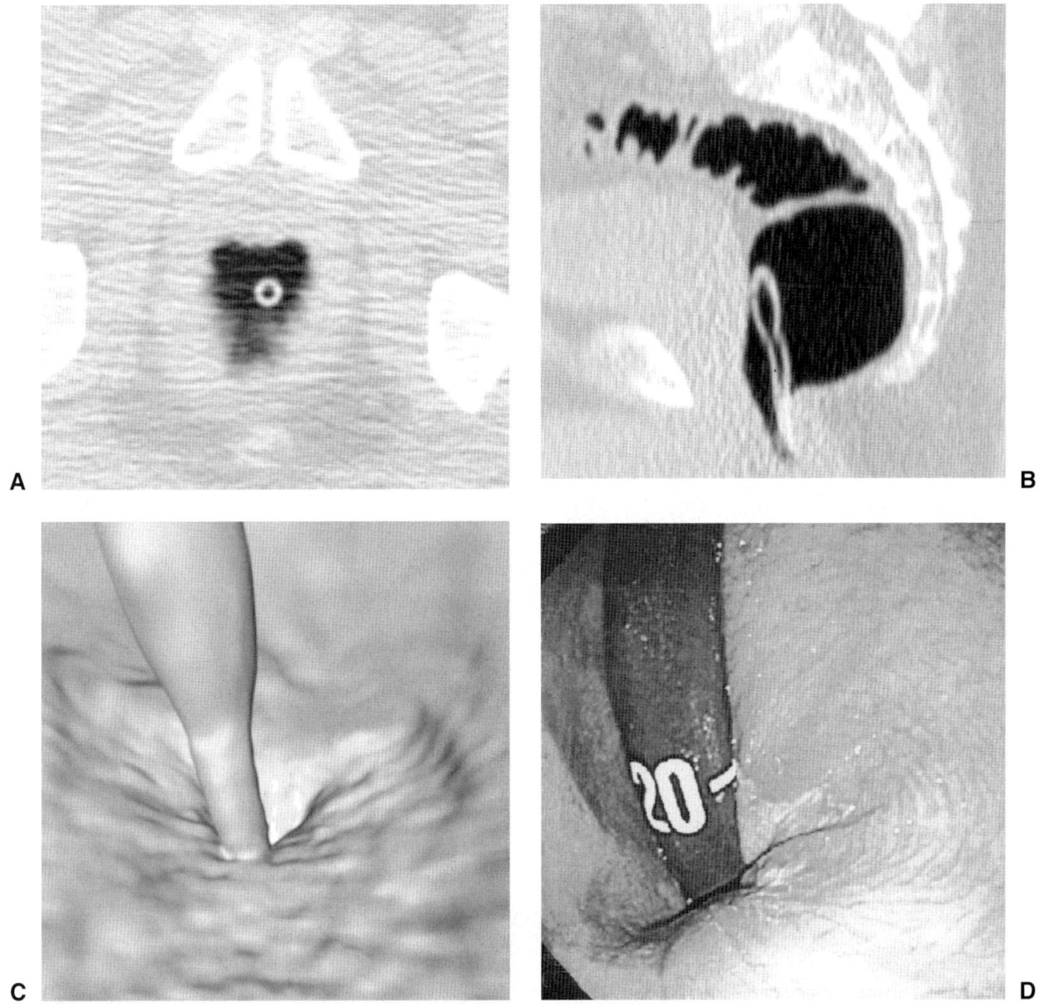

FIGURE 4.25 Normal appearance of the anorectum with a tube in place on the axial image using a colon window **(A)**, in sagittal reformat **(B)**, 3D endoluminal **(C)** and endoscopic **(D)** views. Careful inspection is necessary to avoid missing polyps that may be obscured by the rectal tube.

a circumferential smooth muscle layer in the rectum.[44] The posterior and lower third of the anterior rectum is extraperitoneal. In most patients, three prominent semilunar folds called the valves of Houston are commonly observed within the rectum in a spiral arrangement, convex in shape at the rectal wall and concave in shape at the free edge.[45,46] In approximately half the number of individuals, the inferior and superior valves are located on the left side of the rectum and the more prominent middle valve is located on the right[44,45] (see Fig. 4.26). However, variation in the number (0–4), location, and size of these valves has been described.[45] In approximately a third of individuals the configuration is reversed (see Fig. 4.27). Remaining individuals demonstrate a more variable configuration.[45] These valves may serve as landmarks for the location of lesions in the rectum (see Fig. 4.28). The middle valve indicates the level of the abdominal–peritoneal reflection anteriorly. It is typically located 8 cm from the anal verge and demarcates the lower and middle third of the rectum.[42] It is important to evaluate for lesions on both sides of these folds particularly when using primary 3D interpretation.

The rectosigmoid junction is an important anatomic landmark for surgical treatment of rectosigmoid tumors. The rectosigmoid junction is a 4-cm transition zone located ventral to the sacral promontory.[47] It can be easily identified on coronal and sagittal MPR images by the change in course of the rectosigmoid colon from upward and posterior to upward and anterior (moving toward the cecum) (see Fig. 4.29A, B). For rectal tumors in the lower third of the rectum (located between the anorectal ring and 7–8 cm from the anal verge), abdominal–peritoneal resection (APR) is typically the surgical treatment of choice, provided no intraperitoneal spread has occurred. For tumors located in the middle (8–12 cm from anal verge) and upper third of the rectum, anal sphincter sparing surgery such as low anterior resection (LAR) is performed. This technique generally requires at least 2 to 3 cm of preserved rectal stump for anastomosis and to preserve bowel continuity.[43]

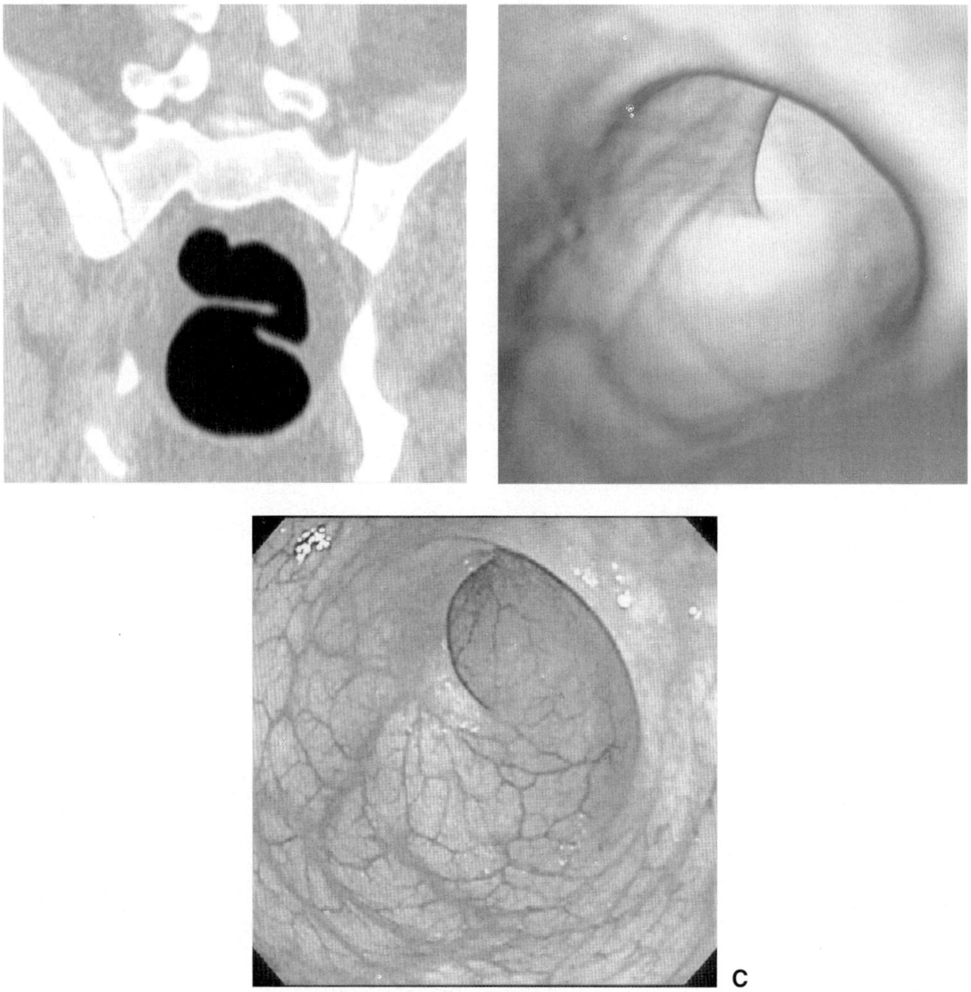

A B C

FIGURE 4.26 The inferior and middle rectal valves of Houston are shown on the coronal reformat **(A)** and correlated with the 3D endoluminal **(B)** and endoscopic images **(C)**.

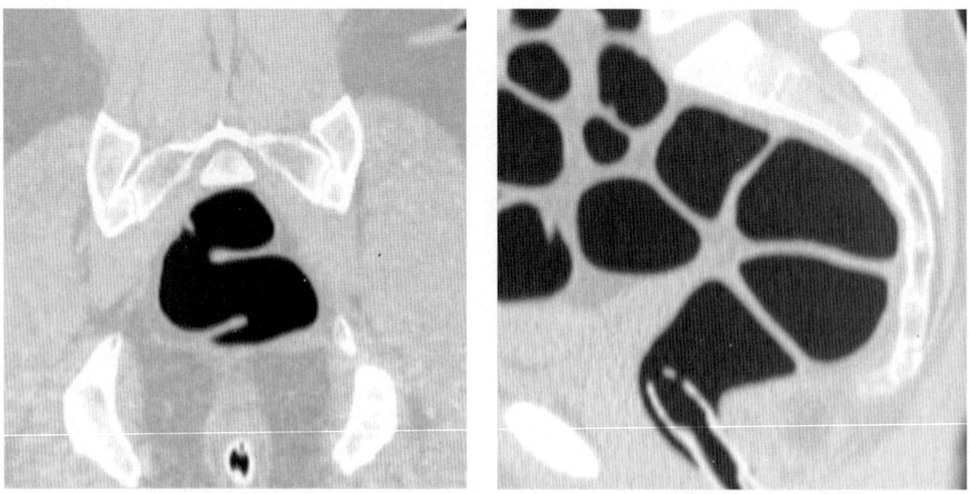

A B

FIGURE 4.27 Variation may be seen in the number, location, and size of the valves of Houston. The coronal reformat **(A)** shows the inferior and superior valves located on the right rectal wall, and the middle valve located on the left rectal wall. The sagittal reformat **(B)** shows all three valves.

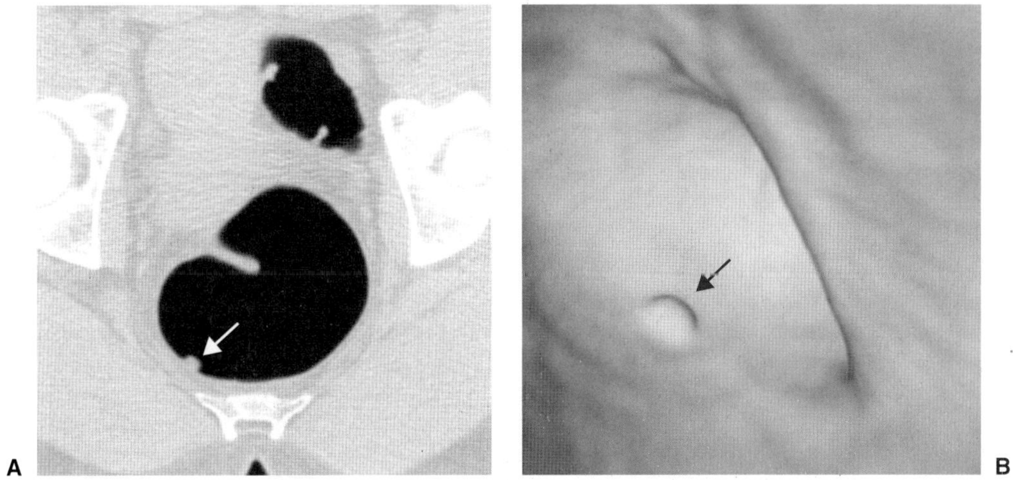

FIGURE 4.28 The axial image **(A)** shows a small polyp located on the posterior wall below the level of the inferior rectal valve and correlated with the 3D endoluminal image **(B)**.

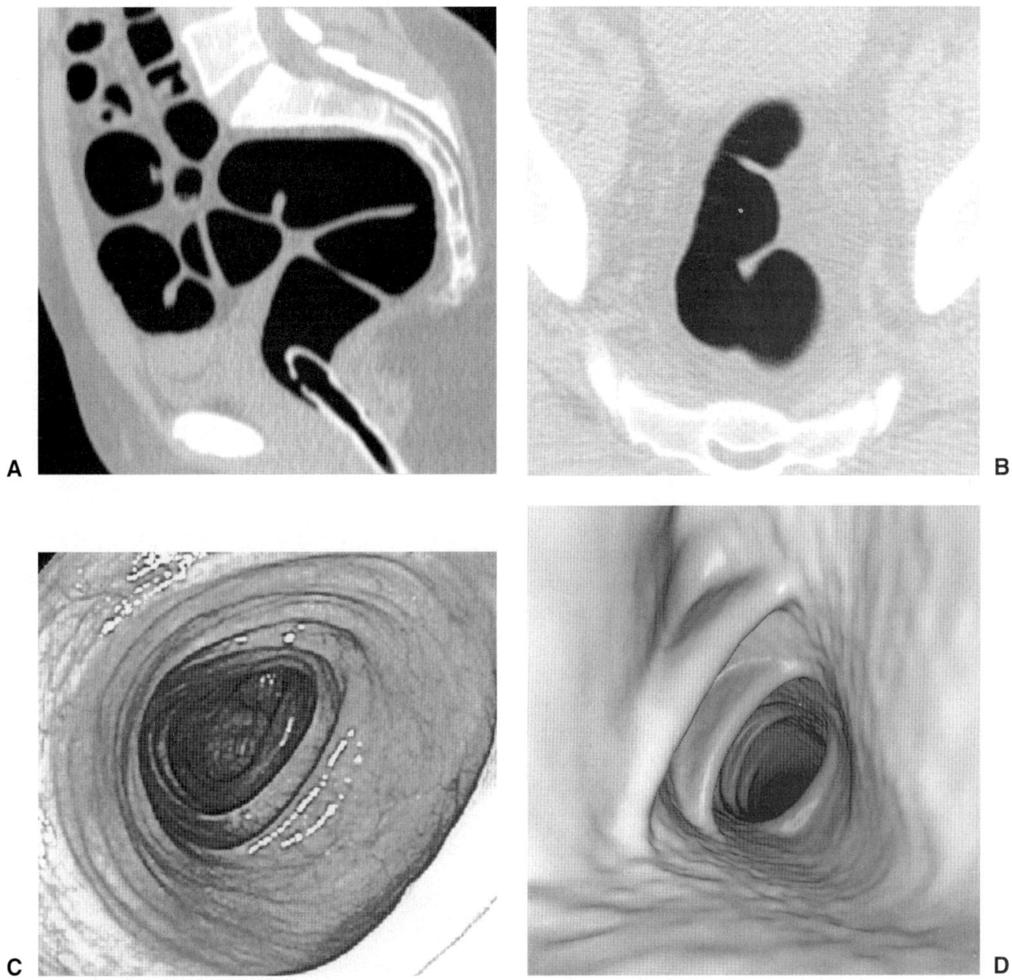

FIGURE 4.29 The sigmoid colon may be tortuous and redundant but typically has an anterior–posterior course as it transitions into the rectum as seen on the sagittal reformat **(A)** and axial **(B)** views. The endoscopic view **(C)** and 3D view **(D)** shows that the lumen of the normal sigmoid is typically rounded or ovoid. (View C: See also color plate.)

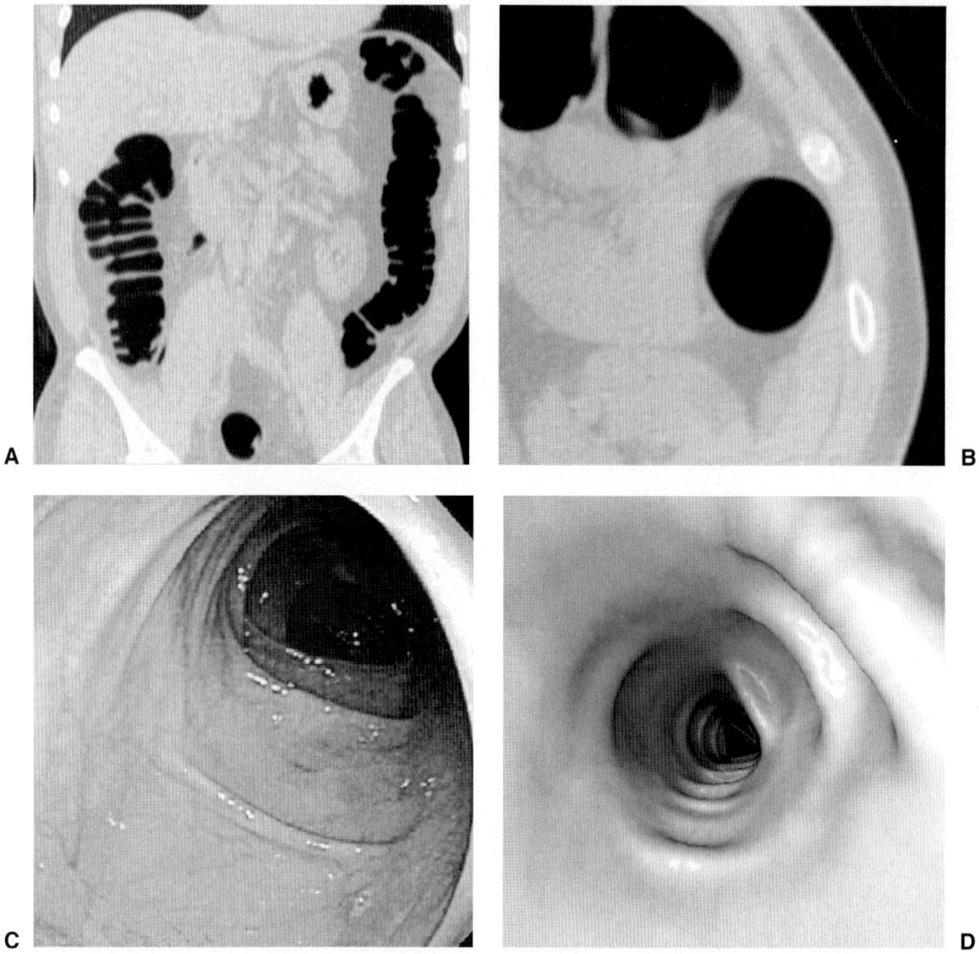

FIGURE 4.30 The descending colon has a straight course that is well demonstrated on the coronal reformat **(A)**. A round lumen with an imperceptible wall is seen on the axial image **(B)**. Colonoscopy **(C)** and the 3D endoluminal view **(D)** show haustral folds in the descending colon that are typically at more regular intervals than in the sigmoid colon.

The sigmoid colon has a loosely attached mesentery, allowing for mobility, and may be particularly redundant and tortuous. The mobility and redundancy of a segment may make tracking the colonic lumen difficult when performing 2D interpretation using the dual-linked axial data sets. It may be necessary to use MPR views to evaluate the segment in supine and prone positions independently. The 3D endoluminal "fly-through" may also be useful for evaluation of redundant and tortuous segments. The sigmoid colon is typically smaller in diameter than the remainder of the colon especially if there is muscular hypertrophy and associated diverticulosis. It contains rounded haustral folds that often incompletely encircle the colonic lumen and this is best seen on endoluminal view[40,41] (see Fig. 4.29C, D).

The junction of the sigmoid and descending colon occurs as the colonic lumen assumes an immediate upward course and the colon may demonstrate acute angulation in the area of transition[34] (see Fig. 4.30A, B). The descending colon is retroperitoneal and relatively fixed in position throughout most of its course. Appearance of the descending colon on axial images typically shows a straight course of the lumen with a variable degree of tortuosity before the splenic flexure. The haustral folds demonstrate a more regular appearance compared with the sigmoid colon and this segment maintains a tubular, rounded shape (see Fig. 4.30C, D).[40,41]

The splenic flexure is identified radiographically as the highest segment of the left colon (see Fig. 4.31A, B). Diaphragmatic ligaments help fixate this segment. The splenic flexure may be recognized on endoscopic and 3D endoluminal views as an acute change in the course of the colonic lumen, turning posteriorly and downward[44] (see Fig. 4.31C, D). Anatomically, the splenic flexure is defined as the transition point from the intraperitoneal transverse colon to the retroperitoneal descending colon. The anatomic splenic flexure is often inferior to the radiographic splenic flexure and the transition point may be difficult to identify on endoscopy. Use of this segment in defining colonic anatomy on CTC is often avoided.[48]

The lumen of the transverse colon has a characteristic triangular appearance of the haustral folds due to the

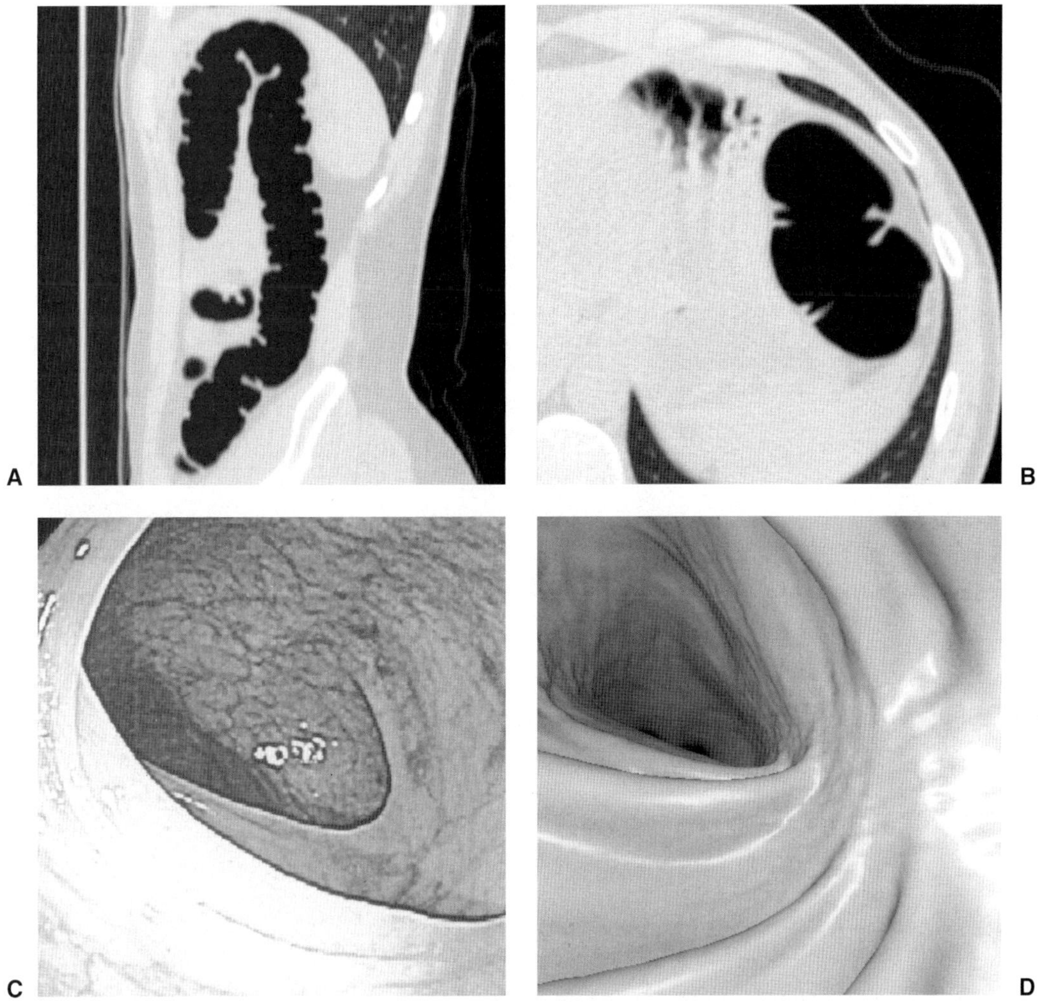

FIGURE 4.31 The radiographic splenic flexure is identified as the highest point of the left colon and is shown on the sagittal reformat **(A)** and axial image **(B)**. Colonoscopy **(C)** and the 3D view **(D)** show acute angulation at the flexure. Use of this segment in defining colonic anatomy on CTC is avoided because there is often difficulty identifying this segment on endoscopy. CTC, computed tomography colonography.

arrangement of the taeniae coli[40,41] (see Fig. 4.32). The transverse colon has a loose mesenteric attachment and often demonstrates a shift in location from the supine to the prone position. The transverse colon tends to have better distention in the supine position.[49] The hepatic flexure is the highest point of the right colon and has a characteristic sharp angle although it is often less pronounced than the splenic flexure.[40,41] On the endoluminal view, the lumen demonstrates acute alteration in course inferiorly. The haustral folds within the ascending colon are typically thicker than in the transverse colon and may not completely encircle the lumen. A triangular configuration may also be observed.[41] The ascending colon is typically larger in diameter than the distal colon and often distends well on both supine and prone positions (see Fig. 4.33).

The ileocecal valve (ICV) demarcates the cecum from the ascending colon and is usually located medially at the junction where the terminal ileum enters the cecum. Its position can change with rotation of the cecum. The ICV can serve as an anatomic landmark to help define cecal mobility when comparing the supine and prone images. Three types (papillary, labial, intermediate) of ICV have been described based on the morphologic appearance.[41,50] The papillary or polypoid type is the most common and appears as a prominent ovoid mass with a characteristic central depression that is typically easily identifiable on 3D endoluminal views (see Figs. 4.34 and 4.35). The labial type assumes a slit-like appearance and can be inconspicuous, especially compared with the papillary type (see Fig. 4.36). The intermediate or semilabial type has characteristics of both the papillary and labial types (see Fig. 4.37). The ICV may contain fat and exhibit a mass-like appearance. The intrinsic fat density can be easily identified on 2D views by using an abdominal window. The attenuation and appearance of the normal ICV were

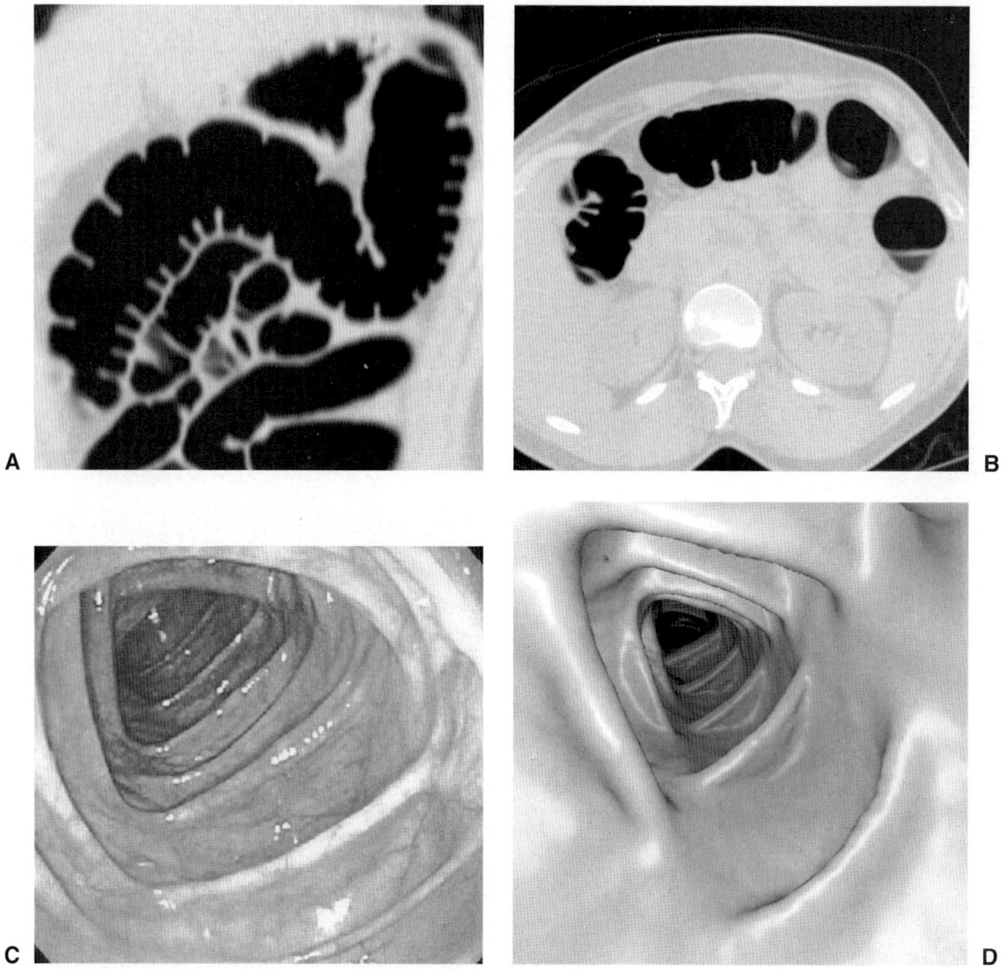

FIGURE 4.32 The transverse colon tends to be better distended in the supine position. A well-distended transverse colon is seen on the coronal reformat **(A)** and on the axial image **(B)**. The endoscopic **(C)** and 3D **(D)** images demonstrate the typical triangular appearance of the haustral folds in the transverse colon due to arrangement of the taeniae coli. (View C: See also color plate.)

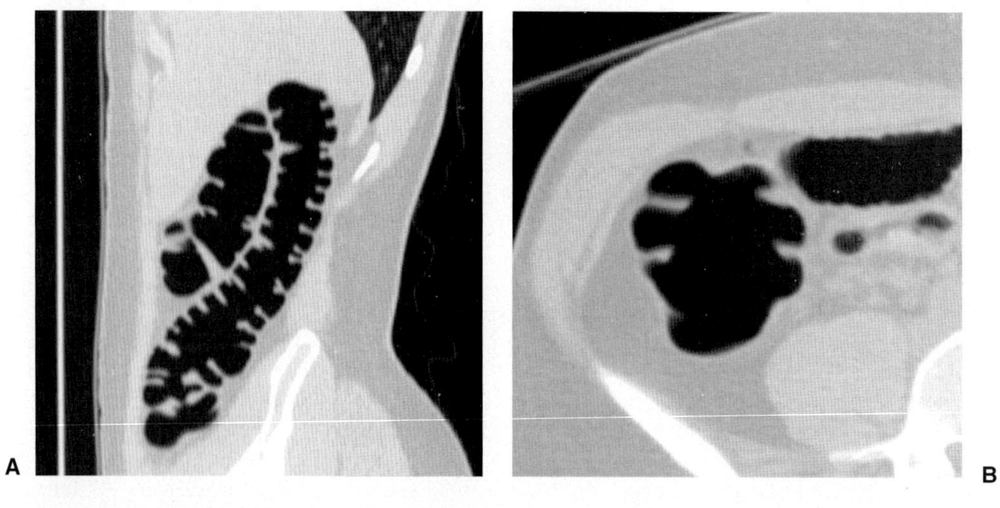

FIGURE 4.33 The hepatic flexure and straight course of the ascending colon are demonstrated on the sagittal reformat **(A)**. The lumen of the ascending colon is rounded or ovoid on the 2D axial image **(B)** and correlates well with the endoscopic appearance **(C)** and the 3D endoluminal view **(D)**.

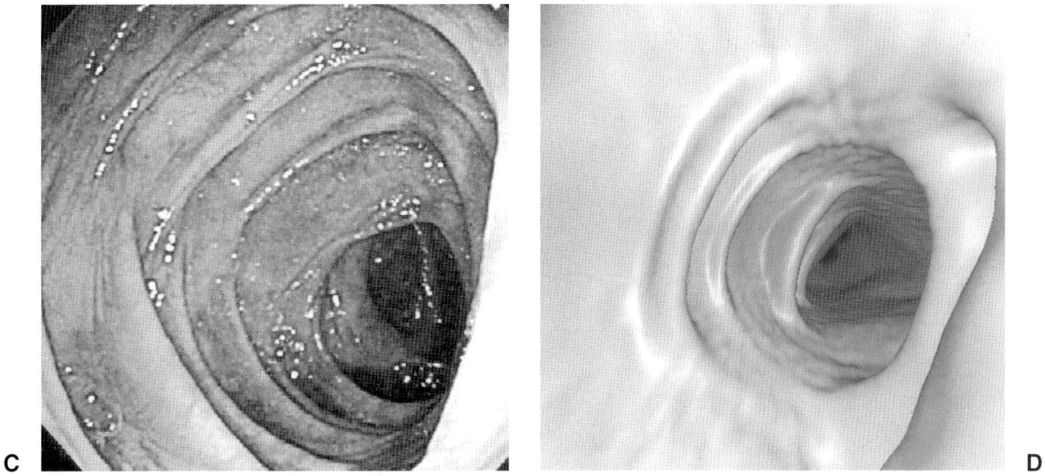

FIGURE 4.33 (*Continued*).

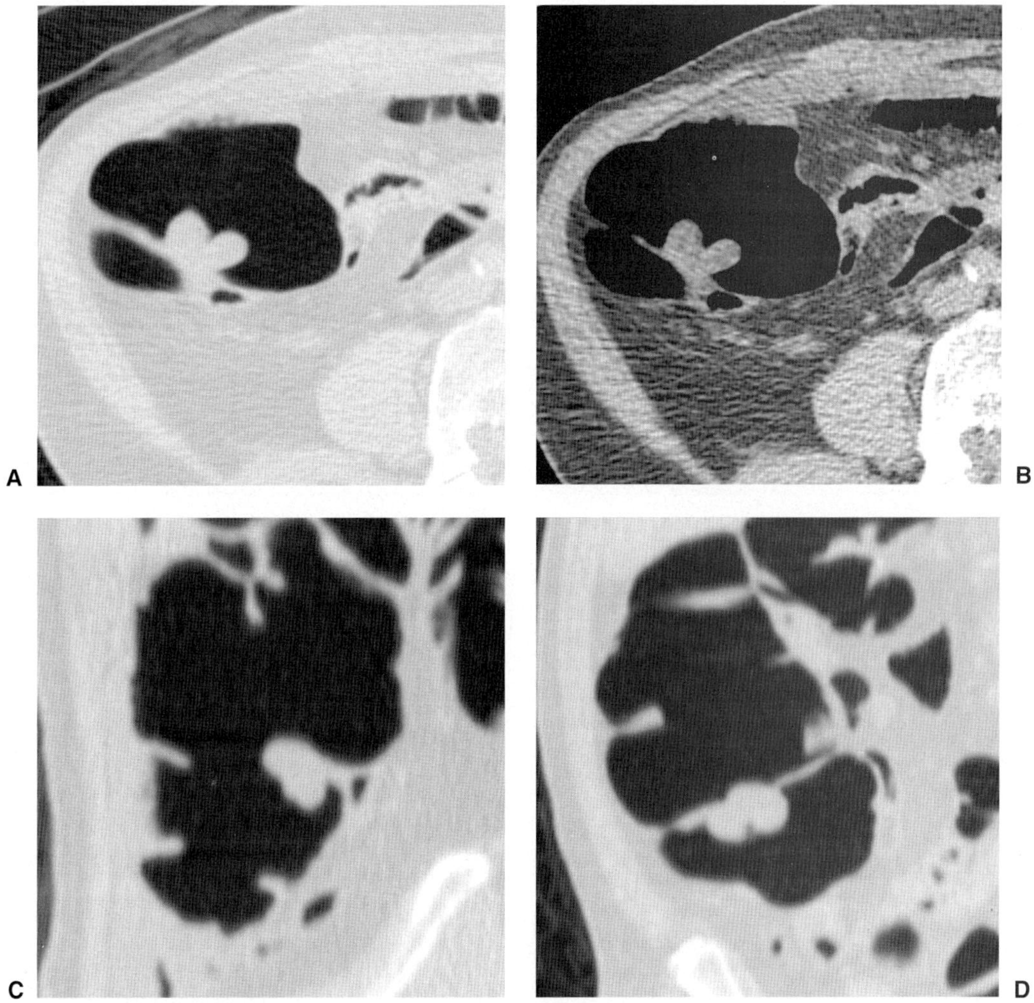

FIGURE 4.34 Papillary or polypoid ICV. The axial image in colon windows **(A)** demonstrates a prominent polypoid appearing ileocecal valve which is ovoid with a central depression. On abdominal windows **(B)**, the soft tissue attenuation of the ICV is more clearly seen. Similar bilobed morphology is seen on the sagittal **(C)** and coronal **(D)** reformats.

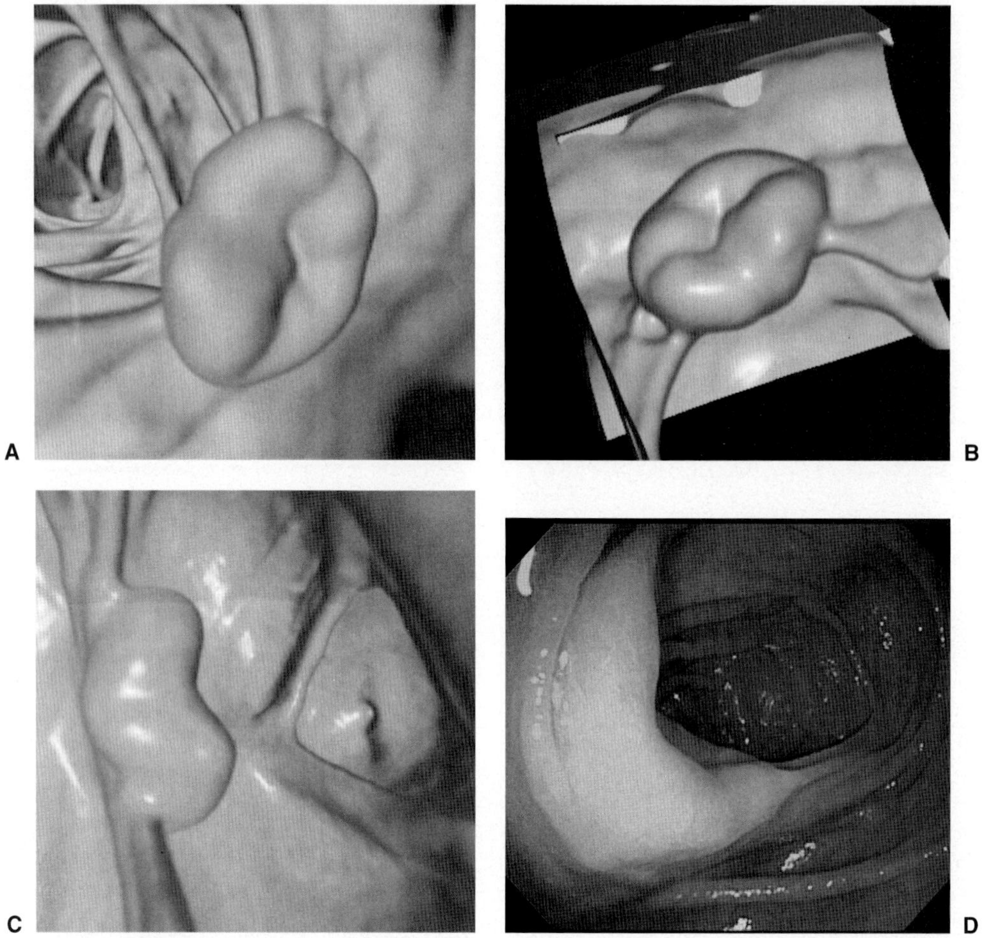

FIGURE 4.35 Papillary ICV seen *en face* on the 3D endoluminal view **(A)** and the cube view **(B)** may be mistaken for a large polyp or mass although it has a characteristic location. The valve is demonstrated in profile on the endoluminal view **(C)** and correlated with the endoscopic image **(D)**. (View D: See also color plate.)

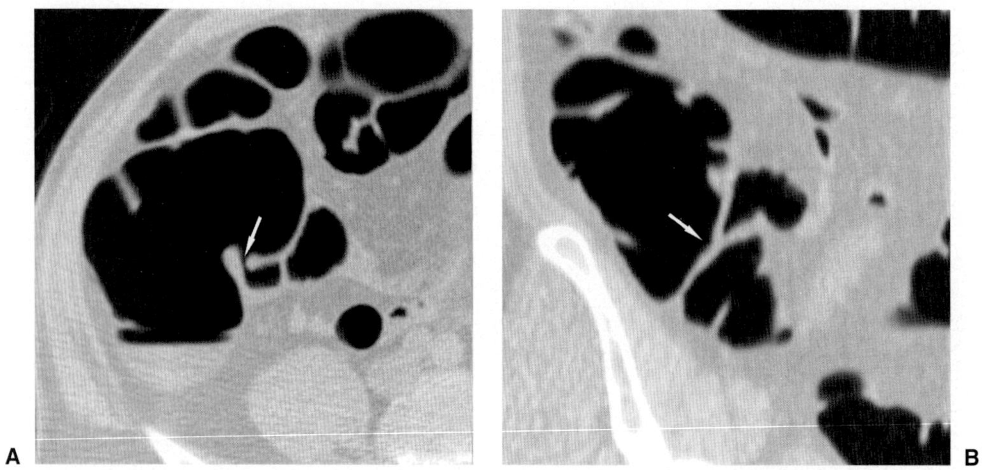

FIGURE 4.36 Labial type ICV has a slit-like appearance and may be more difficult to identify. The thin, elongated appearance of the valve is demonstrated which is seen to be partially open (arrow) on the axial image **(A)**. The valve appears closed on the sagittal **(B)** and coronal **(C)** reformats as well as on the 3D endoluminal view **(D)**.

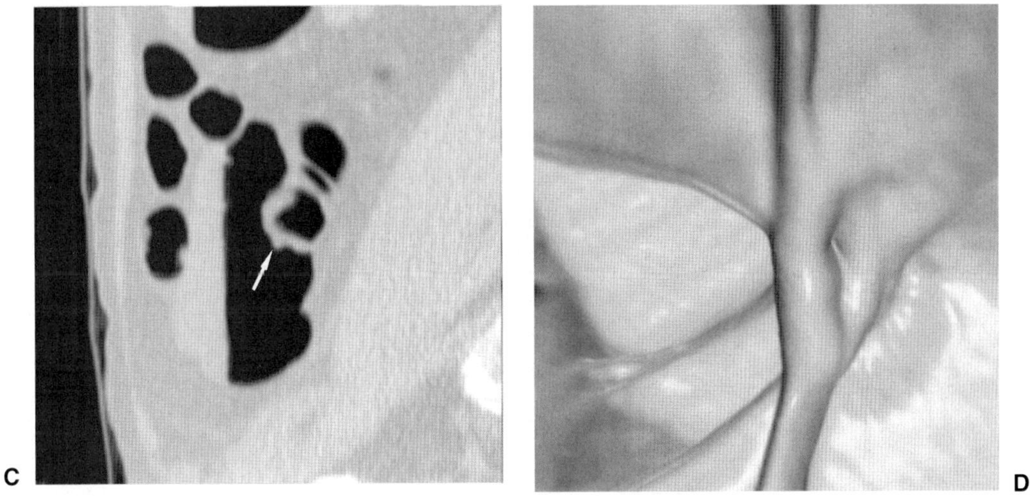

FIGURE 4.36 (*Continued*).

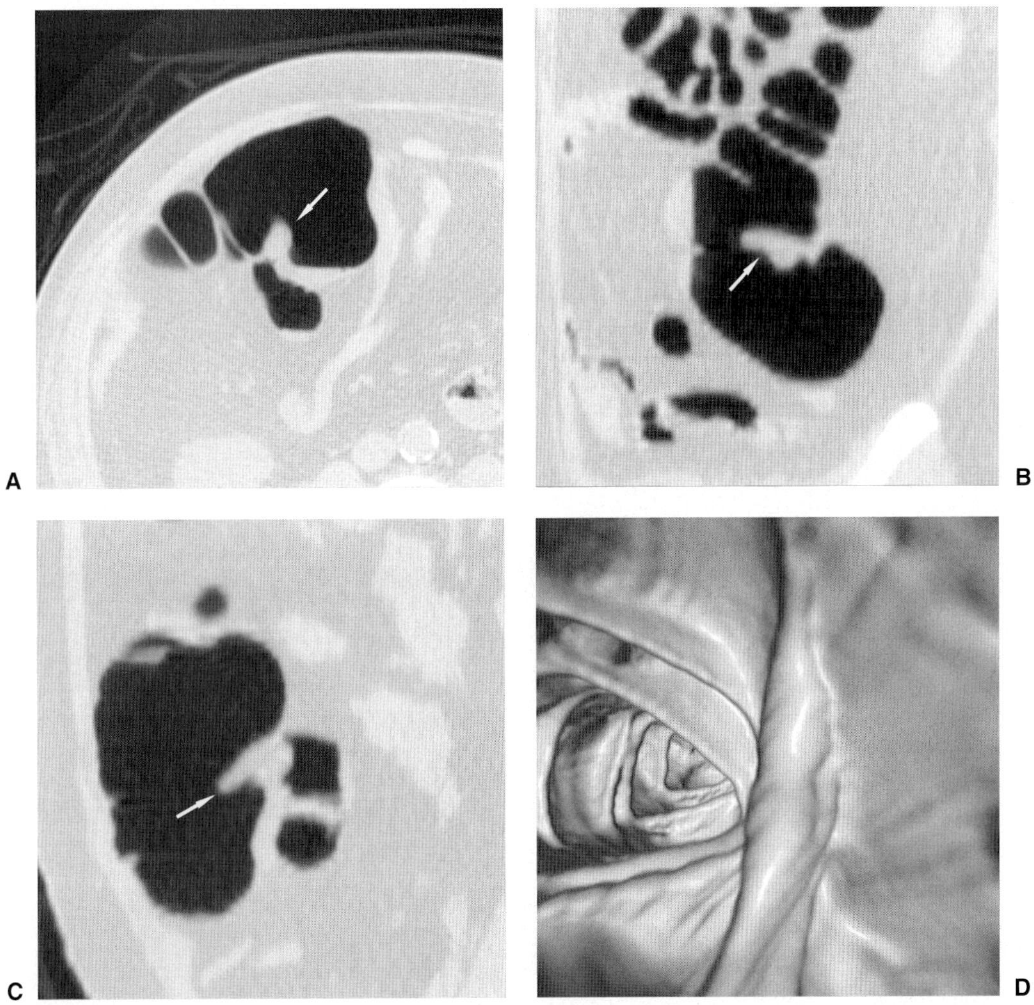

FIGURE 4.37 Intermediate type ileocecal valve with features of both the papillary and labial types is demonstrated on the axial image **(A)**, sagittal and **(B)** coronal reformat **(C)**, and on the 3D endoluminal view **(D)**.

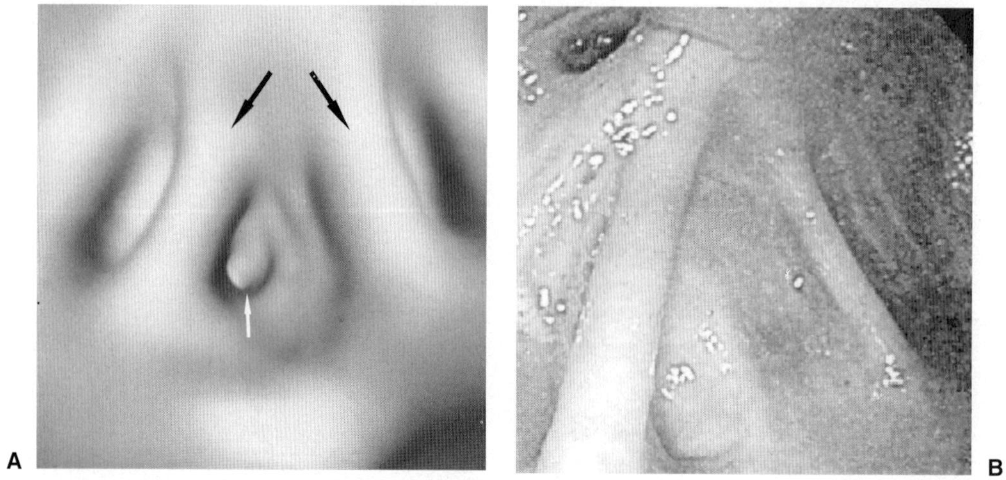

FIGURE 4.38 Convergence of the three taeniae coli in the cecum form two prominent folds called the crow's feet (black arrows) that flank the appendiceal orifice (white arrow) and is shown on the 3D endoluminal image **(A)** and correlated on endoscopy **(B)**.

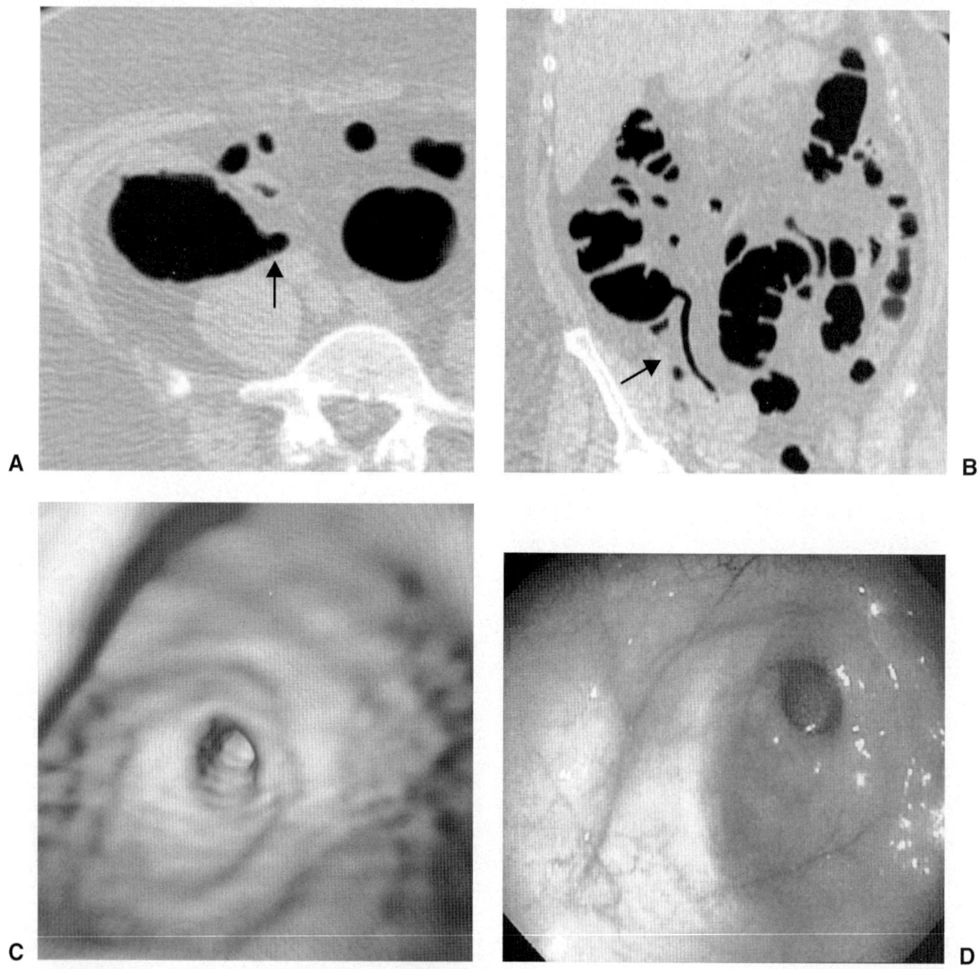

FIGURE 4.39 Appendiceal orifice is easily identified on the axial image along the medial border of the colon **(A)**. Coronal reformat **(B)** demonstrates the entire length of the normal air-filled appendix. The appearance of the appendiceal orifice on the 3D endoluminal view which simulates the appearance of a diverticulum **(C)** and on the endoscopic image **(D)**. (View D: See also color plate.)

evaluated in 212 patients who underwent CTC.[51] Mean ICV density was −26.3 +/−14 HU (range −60.1 to 18.3 HU). There was no correlation between the fat content of the ICV and patient's age or amount of body fat. Most valves (83.5%) were heterogeneous in appearance. The ICV is covered by colonic mucosa so polyps and cancer may develop on the valve. Routine identification and evaluation of the valve should be performed on both supine and prone positions to exclude pathologic lesions. Visualization of the terminal ileum entering the cecum at the site of the valve is helpful for delineating the valve from a cecal mass. This is most easily performed by scrolling through the 2D axial views or by using the coronal MPR images. If the valve has an atypical appearance on 2D images, it should be examined more closely on the 3D endoluminal view.

The cecum is proximal to the ICV and may assume a range of anatomic positions including medial, anteflexed, and retroflexed. In up to 10% of the population, peritoneal fixation of the ascending colon and cecum is absent or incomplete, allowing mobility of the cecum.[52] Cecal mobility was evaluated in 21 patients using supine and prone data sets in the axial, coronal and sagittal planes.[53] The ICV and the appendiceal origin were used to establish an ileocecal–appendiceal angle. Changes in this angle were tabulated between the prone and supine views. It was found that in 9 of 21 cases (43%), the rotational effect of the cecum could potentially affect diagnosis. A change in axis >60 degrees in a single plane corresponded to potential diagnostic dilemma.

The cecum is more capacious than the ascending colon, and thick haustral folds similar to that of the ascending colon may be present. The taeniae coli coalesce to a point in the area of the cecal tip. Two of the cecal folds flank the base of the appendix and meet a third fold located just above it. This region is called the crow's feet of the cecum because of its morphologic appearance[40,41] (see Fig. 4.38). The appendix and its orifice may have one of three appearances as seen endoscopically or on the 3D endoluminal view—closed (slit like or crescent shaped), open, or protruding into the lumen[40] (see Fig. 4.39). The appendiceal orifice may appear polypoid or mass-like if it becomes obstructed by food particles, pills, appendicolith, or tumor.[41] If the ICV is incompetent, air may reflux into the small bowel and impress upon the cecum to give the appearance of a mass on the endoluminal view.[41]

REFERENCES

1. Barish MA, Soto JA, Ferruci JT. Consensus on current clinical practice of virtual colonoscopy. *AJR Am J Roentgenol.* 2005;184:786–792.
2. Zalis M, Barish M, Choi R, et al. Working Group on Virtual Colonoscopy. CT Colonography reporting and data system (C-RADS): a consensus statement. *Radiology.* 2005;236:3–9.
3. American College of Radiology. ACR practice guideline for the performance of Computed Tomography (CT) colonography in adults. In *practice Guidelines and Technical Standards 2005.* Reston, VA: American College of Radiology; 2005; 295–299.
4. Gopalswamy N, Shenoy VN, Choudhry U, et al. Is *in vivo* measurement of size of polyps during colonoscopy accurate? *Gastrointest Endosc.* 1997;46:497–502.
5. McFarland EG. Reader strategies for CT colonography. *Abdom Imaging.* 2002;27:275–283.
6. Burling D, Halligan S, Taylor S, et al. Polyp measurement using CT colonography: agreement with colonoscopy and effect of viewing conditions on interobserver and intraobserver agreement. *AJR Am J Roentgenol.* 2006;186:1597–1604.
7. Pickhardt PJ, Lee AD, McFarland EG, et al. Linear polyp measurement at CT colonography: *in vitro* and *in vivo* comparison of two-dimensional and three-dimensional displays. *Radiology.* 2005;236:872–878.
8. Dijkers JJ, van Wijk C, Vos FM, et al. Segmentation and size measurement of polyps in CT colonography. *Med Image Comput Assist Interv.* 2005;8:712–719.
9. Pickhardt PJ, Lehman VT, Winter TC, et al. Polyp volume versus linear size measurements at CT colonography: implications for noninvasive surveillance of unresected colorectal lesions. *AJR Am J Roentgenol.* 2006;186:1605–1610.
10. Cotton PB, Durkalski VL, Pineau BC, et al. Computed tomographic colonography (virtual colonoscopy): a multicenter comparison with standard colonoscopy for detection of colorectal neoplasia. *JAMA.* 2004;291:1713–1719.
11. Rockey DC, Paulson E, Niedzwiecki D, et al. Analysis of air contrast barium enema, computed tomographic colonography, and colonoscopy: prospective comparison. *Lancet.* 2005;365:305–311.
12. Iordanescu G, Pickhardt PJ, Choi JR, et al. Automated seed placement for colon segmentation in computed tomography colonography. *Acad Radiol.* 2005;12:182–190.
13. Li H, Santago P. Automatic colon segmentation with dual CT colonography. *J Digit Imaging.* 2005;18:42–54.
14. Frimmel H, Nappi J, Yoshida H. Centerline-based colon segmentation for CT colonography. *Med Phys.* 2005;32: 2665–2672.
15. Wan M, Liang Z, Ke Q, et al. Automatic centerline extraction for virtual colonoscopy. *IEEE Trans Med Imaging.* 2002;21:1450–1460.
16. Iordanescu G, Summers RM. Automated centerline for computed tomography colonography. *Acad Radiol.* 2003;10: 1291–1301.
17. Sadleir RJ, Whelan PF. Fast colon centerline calculation using optimized 3D topological thinning. *Comput Med Imaging Graph.* 2005;29:251–258.
18. Frimmel H, Nappi J, Yoshida H. Fast and robust computation of colon centerline in CT colonography. *Med Phys.* 2004;31:3046–3056.
19. Yasumoto T, Murakami T, Yamamoto H, et al. Assessment of two 3D MDCT colonography protocols for observation of colorectal polyps. *AJR Am J Roentgenol.* 2006;186:85–89.
20. Pickhardt PJ, Taylor AJ, Gopal DV. Surface visualization at 3D endoluminal CT colonography: degree of coverage and implications for polyp detection. *Gastroenterologia.* 2006;130:1582–1587.
21. Pickhardt PJ. Translucency rendering in 3D endoluminal CT colonography: a tool for increasing polyp specificity and decreasing interpretation time. *AJR Am J Roentgenol.* 2004;183:429–436.
22. Neri E, Vannozzi F, Vagli P, et al. Time efficiency of CT colonography: 2D vs 3D visualization. *Comput Med Imaging Graph.* 2006;30:175–180.
23. Pickhardt PJ, Choi R, Hwang I, et al. Computed tomographic virtual colonoscopy to screen for colorectal neoplasia in asymptomatic adults. *N Engl J Med.* 2003;349:2191–2200.
24. Royster AP, Fenlon HM, Clarke PD, et al. CT colonoscopy of colorectal neoplasms: two-dimensional and three-dimensional virtual-reality techniques with colonoscopic correlation. *AJR Am J Roentgenol.* 1997;169:1237–1242.

25. Hara AK, Johnson CD, Reed JE, et al. Colorectal polyp detection with CT colonography: two-versus three-dimensional techniques. *Radiology*. 1996;200:49–54.
26. Yee J, Akerkar GA, Hung RK, et al. Colorectal neoplasia: performance characteristics of CT colonography for detection in 300 patients. *Radiology*. 2001;219:685–692.
27. Beaulieu C, Jeffrey RJ, Karadi C, et al. Display modes for CT colonography. Part II. Blinded comparison of axial CT and virtual endoscopic and panoramic endoscopic volume-rendered studies. *Radiology*. 1999;212:203–212.
28. Dachman AH, Kuniyoshi JK, Boyle CM, et al. CT colonography with three-dimensional problem solving for detection of colonic polyps. *AJR Am J Roentgenol*. 1998;171:989–995.
29. Macari M, Milano A, Lavelle M, et al. Comparison of time-efficient CT colonography with two-dimensional and three-dimensional colonic evaluation for detecting colorectal polyps. *AJR Am J Roentgenol*. 2000;174:1543–1549.
30. Macari M, Bini EJ, Xue X, et al. Prospective comparison of thin-section low-dose multislice CT colonography to conventional colonoscopy in detecting colorectal polyps and cancers. *Radiology*. 2002;224:383–392.
31. McFarland EG, Brink JA, Pilgram TK, et al. Spiral CT colonography: reader agreement and diagnostic performance with two- and three-dimensional image display techniques. *Radiology*. 2001;218:375–383.
32. Bruzzi JF, Moss AC, Brennan AD, et al. Colonic surveillance by CT colonography using axial images only. *Eur Radiol*. 2004;14:763–767.
33. Vos FM, Van Gelder RE, Serlie IW, et al. Three-dimensional display modes for CT colonography: conventional 3D virtual colonoscopy versus unfolded cube projection. *Radiology*. 2003;228:878–885.
34. Paik DS, Beaulieu CF, Jeffrey RB Jr, et al. Vizualization modes for CT colonography using cylindrical and planar map projections. *J Comput Assist Tomogr*. 2000;24: 179–188.
35. Fletcher JG, Johnson CD, Reed JE, et al. Feasibility of planar virtual pathology: a new paradigm in volume-rendered CT Colonography. *J Comput Assist Tomogr*. 2001;25:864–869.
36. Hoppe H, Quattropani C, Spreng A, et al. Virtual colon dissection with CT Colonography compared with axial interpretation and conventional colonoscopy: preliminary results. *AJR Am J Roentgenol*. 2004;182:1151–1158.
37. Johnson KT, Johnson CD, Fletcher JG, et al. CT Colonography using 360° virtual dissection: a feasibility study. *AJR Am J Roentgenol*. 2006;186:90–95.
38. Rottgen R, Fischbach F, Plotkin M, et al. Colon dissection: a new three-dimensional reconstruction tool for computed tomography colonography. *Acta Radiol*. 2005;46: 222–226.
39. Juchems MS, Fleiter TR, Pauls S, et al. CT colonography: comparison of a colon dissection display versus 3D endoluminal view for the detection of polyps. *Eur Radiol*. 2006;16: 68–72.
40. Schiller KFR, Cockel R, Hunt RH, et al. *Atlas of Gastrointestinal Endoscopy and Related Pathology*, 2nd ed. Tokyo: Blackwell Science; 2002:227–341.
41. Silverstein FE, Tytgat GNJ. *Atlas of Gastrointestinal Endoscopy*, 2nd ed. Philadelphia: JB Lippincott Co; 1991: 1.17–1.26.
42. Miller TA. Colon, rectum, and anus. In: Greenfield LJ, Mulholland MW, Old Hum KT, et al. eds. *Surgery: Scientific Principles and Practice*, 2nd ed. Philadelphia: Lippincott-Raven; 1997:1083–1093.
43. Chang AE. Colorectal cancer. In: Greenfield LJ, Mulholland MW, Old Hum KT, et al. eds. *Surgery: Scientific Principles and Practice*, 2nd ed. Philadelphia: Lippincott-Raven; 1997:1128–1146.
44. Hamilton SR. Structure of the colon. *Scand J Gastroenterol*. 1984;93:13–23.
45. Abramson DJ. The valves of Houston in adults. *Am J Surg*. 1978;136:334–336.
46. Fenlon HM. CT colonography: pitfalls and interpretation. *Abdom Imaging*. 2002;27:284–291.
47. Stoss F. Investigations of the muscular architecture of the rectosigmoid in humans. *Dis Colon Rectum*. 1990;33:378–383.
48. Stevenson GW. Normal anatomy and techniques of examination of the colon: barium, CT, and MRI. In: Freeny PC, Stevenson GW, eds. *Margulis and Burhenne's Alimentary Tract Radiology*, 5th ed. St. Louis: Mosby; 1994:692–694.
49. Yee J, Kumar NN, Hung RK, et al. Comparison of supine, prone and both supine and prone scans in CT colonography. *Radiology*. 2003;226:653–661.
50. Macari M, Megibow AJ. Pitfalls of using three-dimensional CT colonography with two-dimensional imaging correlation. *AJR Am J Roentgenol*. 2001;176:137–143.
51. Yitta S, Tatineny KC, Cipriani NA, et al. Characterization of normal ileocecal valve density on CT colonography. *J Comput Assist Tomogr*. 2006;30:58–61.
52. Wolfer JA, Beaton LE, Anson BJ. Volvulus of the cecum: anatomical factors in its etiology. *Surg Gynecol Obstet*. 1942; 74:882.
53. Chen JC, Dachman AH. Cecal mobility: a potential pitfall of CT colonography. *AJR Am J Roentgenol*. 2006;186: 1086–1089.

CHAPTER 5

INTERPRETATION: POLYPS AND CANCER

Gregory M. Galdino and Judy Yee

COLORECTAL POLYPS

The goal of computed tomographic colonography (CTC) is to identify the precursor lesion of colorectal carcinoma, which is the adenomatous polyp. The development of colonic malignancy through the adenoma–carcinoma sequence is commonly accepted and accounts for the vast majority of colonic adenocarcinomas.[1–4] Genetic mutations cause small adenomas to progress to large adenomas, which develop into noninvasive carcinoma and then into invasive carcinoma. Colorectal carcinoma is ideally suited for screening because there is a large window of opportunity to detect the precursor adenoma and to remove it before it becomes malignant. The relatively slow growth of adenomatous polyps is the basis for the relatively long intervals between colon screening examinations compared with other screening tests, such as mammography. It is estimated that the progression from adenoma to carcinoma takes approximately 5 to 10 years with 2 to 3 years for an adenoma <5 mm to progress to 1 cm, and another 2 to 5 years to then progress to carcinoma.[4–6] Some colon carcinomas have also been described as relatively slow-growing, requiring a 1-mm tumor approximately 6 to 8 years to reach 6 cm.[7,8] The prevalence of polyps in the adult population is high, occurring in 50% of autopsy cases and in approximately 40% of subjects on colonoscopy surveys. Of these polyps, 80% to 90% are adenomatous or hyperplastic polyps and the overwhelming majority of these (75%) are adenomas.[5] Half the number of patients with one adenoma identified are found to have a second adenoma.[7]

The incidence of degeneration of adenomatous polyps to malignancy is directly related to degree of dysplasia, villous histology, and polyp size. Polyps >1 cm demonstrate a significant increase in risk of malignancy.[5,7] Ten percent of adenomatous polyps 1 to 2 cm in size harbor malignancy, which increases to 20% to 46% for polyps >2 cm.[7] Patients with multiple adenomas and adenomas containing villous components have an even higher risk of malignancy.[5] It is therefore important to recognize the characteristics of polyps and identify polyps >1 cm on CTC.

The term polyp is derived from the Greek word (*polypous*) meaning "many-footed." However, polyp refers broadly to any lesion that extends above the colonic surface and protrudes into the colonic lumen.[5,7,9] The term polyp is typically used for those lesions measuring up to 4 cm in size, whereas lesions >4 cm are termed *masses* or *tumors*.[7] The etiology of the protrusion may result from abnormal overgrowth of the epithelial colonic mucosa or submucosal growth. Polyps may be classified according to histology, size, and morphology.

Histology

Histologically, polyps may be broadly classified into epithelial or subepithelial origins, each with neoplastic and non-neoplastic types (see Table 5.1). Neoplastic lesions may then be further subdivided into benign and malignant disease. Benign and non-neoplastic lesions of subepithelial origin can mimic true polyps or malignancies. There is currently no reliable way to differentiate between various histologic types of polyps based on their appearance on colonoscopy and CTC.

There are four main types of epithelial polyps: adenomatous, hyperplastic, inflammatory, and hamartomatous.[5] Adenomatous polyps are considered benign neoplastic lesions whereas the other types are classified as non-neoplastic polyps. Adenomatous polyps display abnormal glandular architecture (dysplasia), and therefore, have malignant potential. However, only a very small percentage (3%) of adenomas will progress to malignancy.[4,10] Dysplasia, or the degree of abnormality to the glandular architecture, is classified as mild, moderate, severe, or high grade. Severe and high-grade dysplasia are generally accepted histologically as carcinoma *in situ*.

Adenomatous polyps are divided into three histologic subtypes based on their glandular architecture: tubular, tubulovillous, and villous. Tubular adenomas contain a complex branching architecture of the glandular tissue and are the most common type. They represent approximately 85% of all adenomatous polyps and are typically smaller, measuring <10 mm.[7] Tubulovillous adenomas contain both tubular and villous glandular

TABLE 5.1 Classification of Polypoid Lesions of the Colon

Epithelial Origin

- Neoplastic
  - Benign
    - Tubular adenoma
    - Tubulovillous adenoma
    - Villous adenoma
  - Malignant
    - Adenocarcinoma
- Non-neoplastic
  - Hyperplastic polyp
  - Inflammatory polyp
  - Hamartomatous polyp

Subepithelial Origin

- Neoplastic
  - Benign lesions
    - Lipoma
    - Leiomyoma
    - Neurofibroma
    - Hemangioma
    - Lymphangioma
  - Malignant
    - Carcinoid
    - Lymphoma
    - Sarcoma
    - Metastases
- Non-neoplastic
  - Endometriosis
  - Duplication
  - Pneumotosis
  - Hematoma
  - Varix

architecture and clinically behave according to the majority component, having a higher risk of malignant degeneration when more villous components are present. Tubulovillous adenomas account for approximately 10% of all adenomatous polyps and are often larger than tubular adenomas measuring >10 mm. Villous adenomas contain short, straight glands extending to the muscularis mucosa and are associated with a 10-times greater incidence of malignancy than tubular adenomas.[7] Approximately 40% of villous adenomas will harbor infiltrating carcinoma, usually at the base of the lesion.[11] Biopsies of these lesions may not be reliable and all villous adenomas should be removed. Villous adenomas are uncommon and constitute approximately 5% of all adenomas. They occur with increasing frequency in older individuals and are often larger in size, with approximately 75% measuring >2 cm.[5,7,11] Common locations for villous adenomas are the rectum and cecum.[7] They will often display a corrugated appearance with an irregular nodular surface because of multiple villous fronds. Villous adenomas may cause a profuse watery diarrhea, resulting in severe potassium deficiency causing muscle weakness. Many polyps contain mixed histology. Tubular adenomas may contain up to 25% villous tissue, tubulovillous adenomas contain 25% to 75% villous tissue, and villous adenomas are composed of 75% to 100% villous tissue.[12] The concept of the "advanced adenoma" has developed and includes adenomatous polyps that are ≥10 mm, contains any villous component, high-grade dysplasia, or invasive carcinoma.[13] Familial adenomatous polyposis syndrome (FAPS) is a genetic disorder that includes familial polyposis coli and Gardner syndrome. Innumerable, small (≤5 mm) tubular and tubulovillous adenomas typically develop in the colon although villous adenomas can also occur. Medium-sized polyps may also be seen, but if there is a large polyp there should be high suspicion for malignancy. Colorectal adenocarcinoma will develop in almost all patients and therefore prophylactic total colectomy is usually performed.

Hyperplastic polyps are the most common non-neoplastic type of colorectal polyp and have no malignant potential. They represent a focal proliferation of the colonic mucosal epithelium, typically occurring adjacent to or on a haustral fold.[11] Hyperplastic polyps are typically small (<5 mm) and sessile and most commonly occur in the rectosigmoid colon. Most hyperplastic polyps are located in the left colon with three quarters distal to the splenic flexure and half occurring in the rectosigmoid region.[11,14] Up to 50% of polyps <5 mm are hyperplastic.[15] Colonoscopy surveillance recommendations by the US Multisociety Task Force on Colorectal Cancer and the American Cancer Society states specifically that patients with small rectal hyperplastic polyps should be considered to have normal colonoscopies and therefore the interval before the subsequent colonoscopy should be 10 years.[16]

Hyperplastic polyps often have a soft consistency and may become effaced or flattened in a well-distended colon during CTC, causing them to be missed more frequently than adenomas.[17,18] Nonadenomatous polyps accounted for 57.7% of all colorectal polyps and 39.9% of polyps ≥6 mm in a study evaluating CTC performed in a screening population.[19] Hyperplastic polyps represented the majority (75.4%) of nonadenomatous lesions ≥6 mm. The sensitivity for detection of hyperplastic polyps ranged between 72.2% to 76.2% at 6-, 8-, and 10-mm thresholds, whereas the sensitivity for adenomatous polyp detection was higher for all three thresholds at 85.7%, 92.6%, and 92.2% respectively. Hyperplastic lesions >10 mm were often found to have an elongated or flattened appearance, making them less detectable on CTC. This may have clinical significance because more recently there has been described the hyperplastic polyposis syndrome, where patients with multiple large (≥10 mm) hyperplastic polyps have been found to have increased risk for adenomas and colorectal cancer.[16,20]

Hamartomatous (juvenile) polyps occur sporadically in children younger than 10 years.[5] They affect 1% to 2% of all children and carry no significant malignant potential when solitary. These polyps are typically pedunculated and located predominantly in the rectosigmoid. In approximately one third of patients, these polyps are inherited and multiple occurring as part of the juvenile polyposis syndrome. In this situation, the hamartomatous polyps may contain foci of dysplasia and there is a 10% risk for developing colon cancer.[21] Colonic hamartomas may rarely be found in adults. A retrospective study of more than 12,000 patients found a prevalence of 0.15% in an adult population.[22] Colonic hamartomas were more common in men. Three fourths of the polyps were >10 mm and 89% were pedunculated. Two thirds were located in the rectosigmoid. Endoscopic characteristics of hamartomatous polyps are indistinguishable from adenomatous polyps. Hamartomatous polyps may also occur in adults as part of a polyposis syndrome such as Peutz-Jeghers syndrome, Cronkhite-Canada syndrome, Cowden syndrome (multiple hamartoma syndrome), and Bannayan-Riley-Ruvalcaba syndrome.

Inflammatory polyps represent focal regions of granulomatous tissue protruding into the lumen and appears as a single small lesion in adults. Rarely inflammatory polyps are large and can mimic adenomas or carcinomas. Inflammatory pseudopolyps occur in patients with acute inflammatory bowel disease (Crohn's disease and ulcerative colitis) and represent residual islands of inflamed colonic tissue in a region of denuded mucosa.[5] Inflammatory pseudopolyps are benign but may be confused with adenomatous polyps. Colonic perforation has been reported in patients with acute inflammatory bowel disease who undergo CTC.[23,24] CTC is not typically performed in the setting of acute inflammatory bowel disease. Caution is advised to avoid perforating the bowel if it is necessary to perform CTC in this setting.

One percent of polyps are serrated adenomas (mixed hyperplastic adenomatous polyps), which demonstrate hyperplastic polyp architecture with adenomatous cytology. Histologically, these lesions have a serrated, crypt architecture in association with surface epithelial dysplasia. In a study of 919 individuals there was a 1% prevalence of serrated adenomas with an average size of 5.8 mm.[25] High-grade dysplasia occurs in up to 40% of serrated adenomas and these lesions are considered to have increased malignant potential.[5,16,26,27]

Size

Polyp size is an important measurement obtained on CTC. The largest diameter of a polyp (excluding the stalk of a pedunculated polyp) is often used as a surrogate parameter for clinical importance (likelihood of harboring malignancy) upon which patient management decisions are based. The chance of malignancy in a polyp is related to polyp size and <1% of polyps <10 mm will be malignant (see Table 1.3).[15,28] Therefore, traditionally polyps measuring ≥10 mm have been considered to be clinically significant. Polyps may be classified as small (≤5 mm), medium (6 to 9 mm) or large (≥10 mm). The terms used for ranges of polyp sizes may vary with alternative classification of polyps as diminutive (≥5 mm), small (6 to 9 mm) or large (≥10 mm).[29]

Small polyps have been found to be evenly distributed throughout the colon. A higher prevalence of small adenomatous polyps has been identified proximally in the right colon with more non-neoplastic or hyperplastic polyps found in the rectum.[30] Although studies have found that the incidence of malignancy in small polyps is low, some still recommend removal of all polyps including those ≤5 mm.[30,31] Others have evaluated the multiple features of small polyps including the low risk of malignancy and suggest a focus on detection of those lesions that have more significant carcinoma risk.[32,33] The American College of Radiology Practice Guidelines for the performance of CTC in adults suggests that small polyps ≤5 mm do not need to be reported because these lesions are commonly non-neoplastic.[34] The risk of malignancy in this size range is very low at <0.01%. Additionally, many of these small polyps prove to be false positives on CTC or even if they are true lesions colonoscopy may miss 25% of them.

Small or diminutive polyps (≤5 mm) are rarely pedunculated and almost always sessile. Most of these small lesions are hyperplastic polyps. Small polyps tend to be smooth and round or ovoid in appearance rather than lobular (see Figs. 5.1 and 5.2). Medium-sized polyps (6–9 mm) are also more often sessile than pedunculated (see Figs. 5.3 and 5.4). They have an overall <1% chance of harboring malignancy. Polyps of this size category have approximately a 50% chance of being adenomatous. If adenomatous, there is a 5% to 10% incidence of malignancy within 10 years.[28] Controversy exists as to whether medium-sized polyps should be the target lesions for colorectal cancer screening rather than large polyps measuring ≥10 mm. Detection sensitivity for medium-sized polyps is higher than for small polyps and lower than for large polyps on both CTC and optical colonoscopy. Computer-aided detection of medium-sized polyps may prove to be valuable in increasing the sensitivity for these lesions.

Large polyps measuring ≥10 mm are more easily detected on CTC (see Figs. 5.5 and 5.6). Approximately 40% of large polyps have been found to have an irregular surface on CTC, which may be due to intrinsic mucosal irregularity or adherent stool (see Fig. 5.7).[35] Most large polyps will be adenomatous (>80%).[28] Although hyperplastic polyps are typically small (≤5 mm), occasionally they may be large (≥10 mm) and flat (see Fig. 5.8). Hyperplastic polyps are indistinguishable from adenomas on CTC and colonoscopy.

The prevalence of adenomatous polyps measuring 6 mm, 8 mm, and ≥10 mm was 13.6%, 6.7%, and 3.9% respectively as determined in a study evaluating CTC in a large asymptomatic screening patient population. Therefore, the likelihood of an average-risk patient having a large clinically significant polyp on screening CTC is low.[36] In this same study, it was estimated that approximately 15% of screening patients who undergo screening CTC would be referred to colonoscopy at a threshold of 8 mm, which decreases to 7.5% at a threshold of 10 mm. The higher referral rate relative to prevalence rate is likely due to the detection of false positive findings on CTC.

Morphology

Polypoid lesions in the colon should be evaluated for mobility, homogeneity (internal attenuation), and morphology to distinguish residual stool and other pitfalls

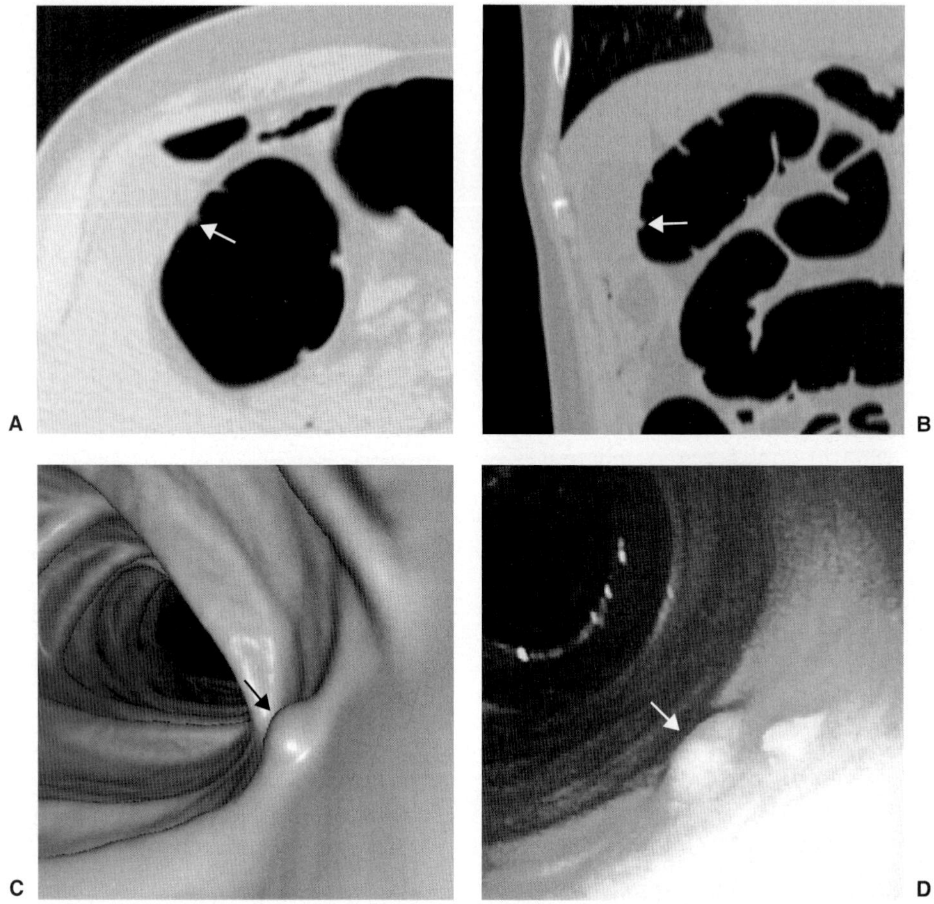

FIGURE 5.1 Small Sessile Hyperplastic Polyp. Small polyps are most commonly sessile and many are hyperplastic. Axial supine image **(A)** shows a 4-mm sessile polyp on the anterior wall of the ascending colon. Coronal reformat **(B)** shows the same polyp. 3D endoluminal view **(C)** and endoscopic view **(D)** confirm a small sessile polyp on a fold, which was found to be a 5-mm hyperplastic polyp on histology.

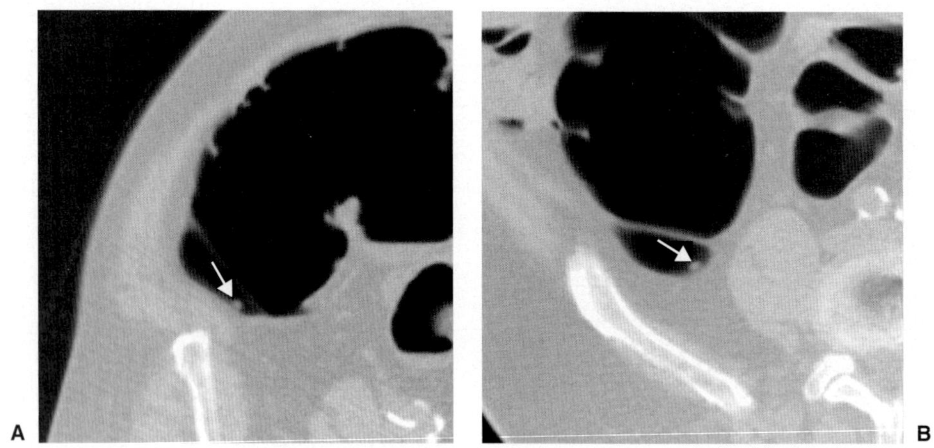

FIGURE 5.2 Small Sessile Adenomatous Polyp. Axial supine view **(A)** shows a diminutive sessile polyp in the ascending colon located along the posterior wall. The polyp is in a similar location on the prone axial view **(B)**. 3D endoluminal view **(C)** shows the polyp located between two haustral folds. 3D cube view **(D)** shows the polyp measures close to 5 mm. The polyp was found to be a 5-mm tubular adenoma on pathologic evaluation. It is impossible to differentiate adenomatous from hyperplastic polyps based on their 2D and 3D appearances.

C D

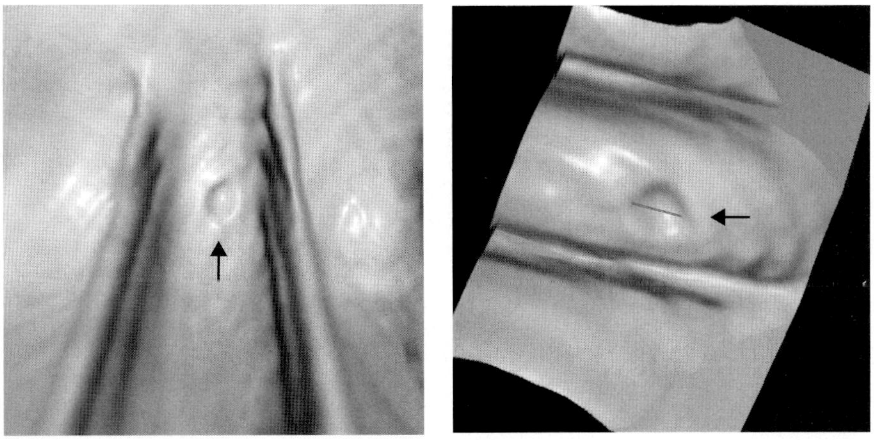

FIGURE 5.2 *(Continued)*

A B C D

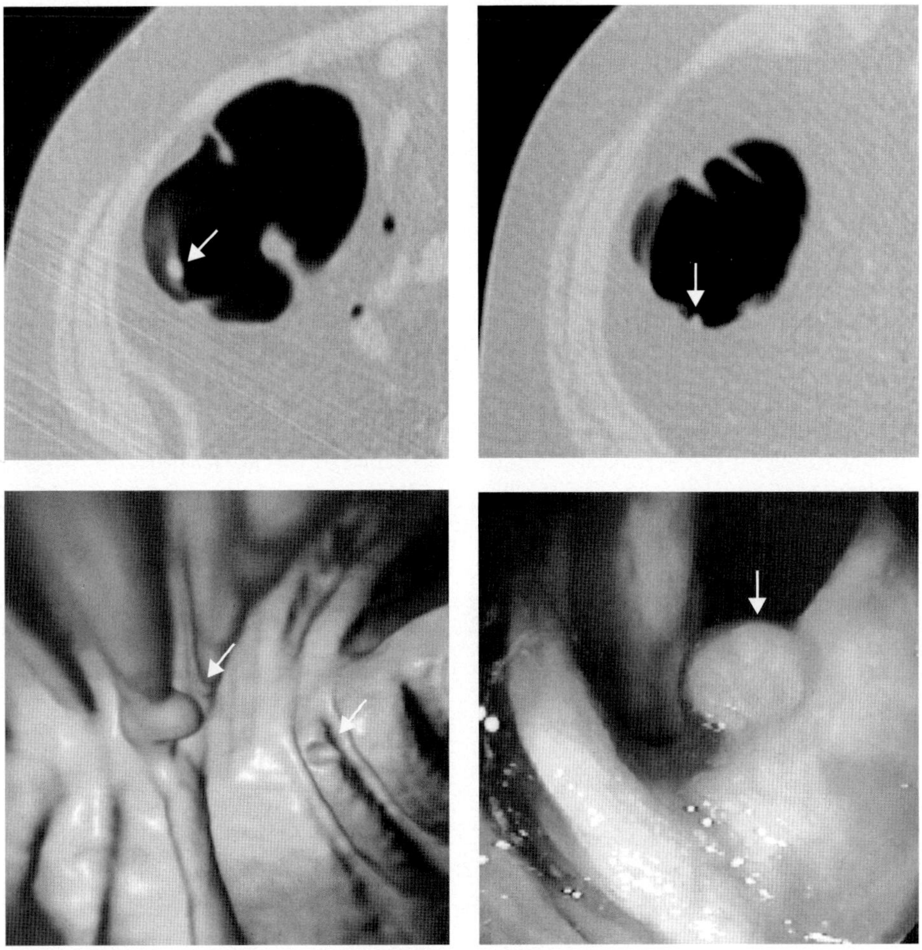

FIGURE 5.3 Small and Medium Sessile Polyps. Axial supine image **(A)** shows a medium-sized polyp located laterally on a fold in the ascending colon. Axial image **(B)** just cephalad to **(A)** shows a small sessile polyp on the posterior colon wall. 3D endoluminal view **(C)** shows the medium polyp located on a fold with a smaller polyp nearby between two folds. Endoscopic image **(D)** of the medium polyp, which was a tubular adenoma on pathology. The small polyp was also removed and was a hyperplastic polyp.

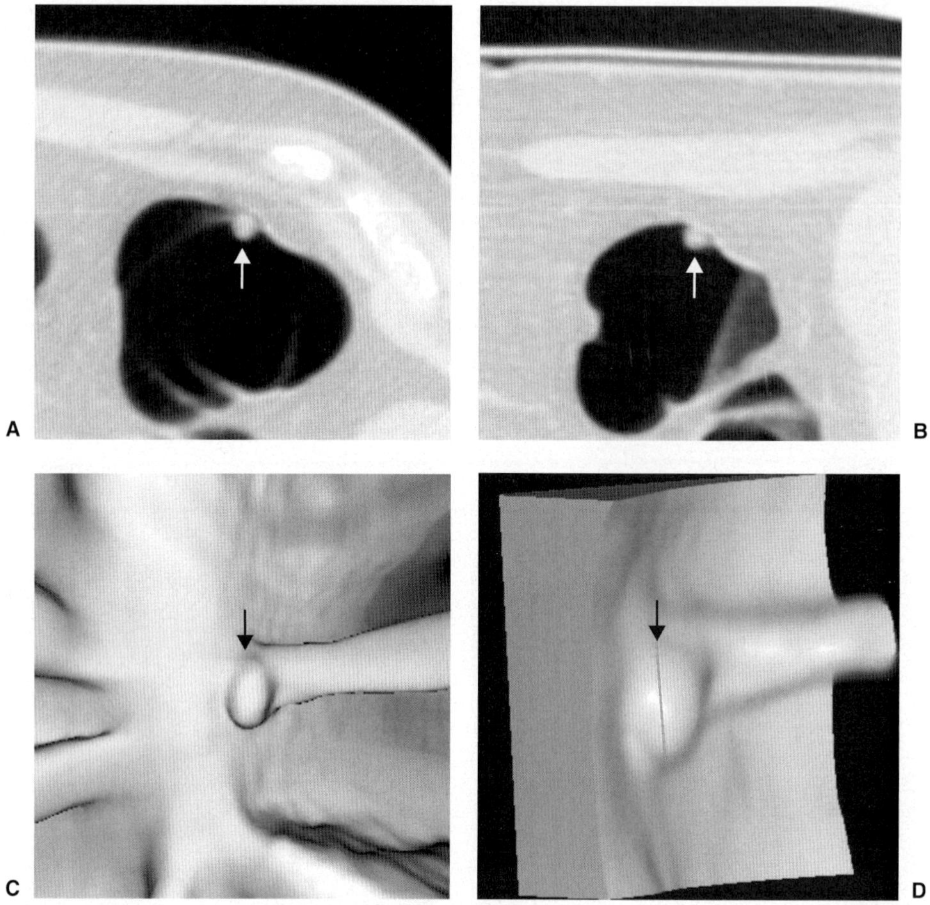

FIGURE 5.4 Medium Sessile Polyp. Axial supine image **(A)** and prone image **(B)** shows a rounded, homogeneous medium-sized sessile polyp on the anterior wall of the transverse colon. 3D endoluminal view **(C)** shows the polyp is slightly ovoid in shape at the base of a haustral fold. 3D cube view **(D)** allows easy assessment of the maximum diameter. This was a hyperplastic polyp on pathology.

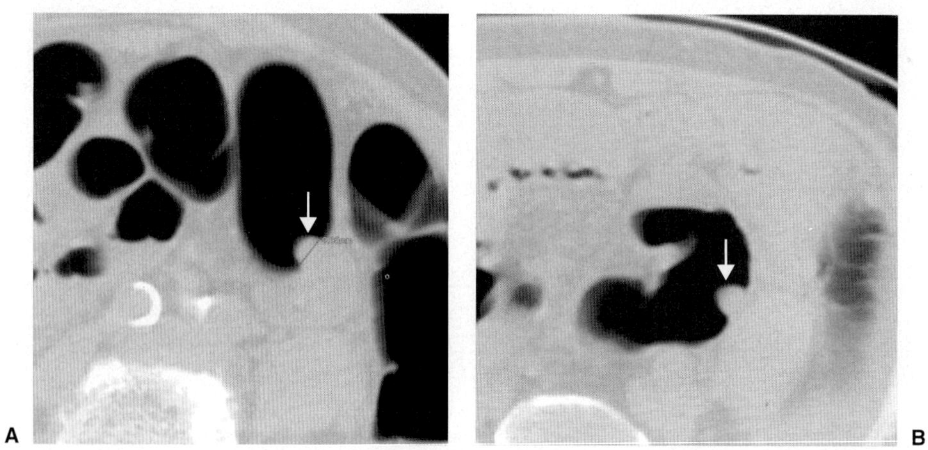

FIGURE 5.5 Large Sessile Polyp and the Importance of 3D Measurement. Axial supine **(A)** and prone **(B)** views show a large sessile polyp in the sigmoid. Polyp measurement along the base yields 10 mm. Axial prone view **(C)** in abdominal windows confirms the lesion is homogeneous soft tissue density. 3D endoluminal view **(D)** demonstrates that the lesion is ovoid and measures 18 mm in largest diameter. The polyp measured 17 mm at colonoscopy and was determined to be a tubular adenoma on histologic evaluation.

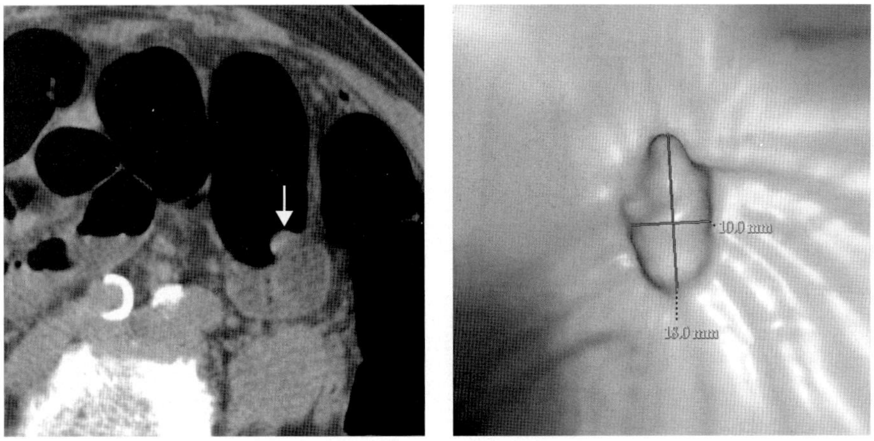

C D

FIGURE 5.5 (*Continued*)

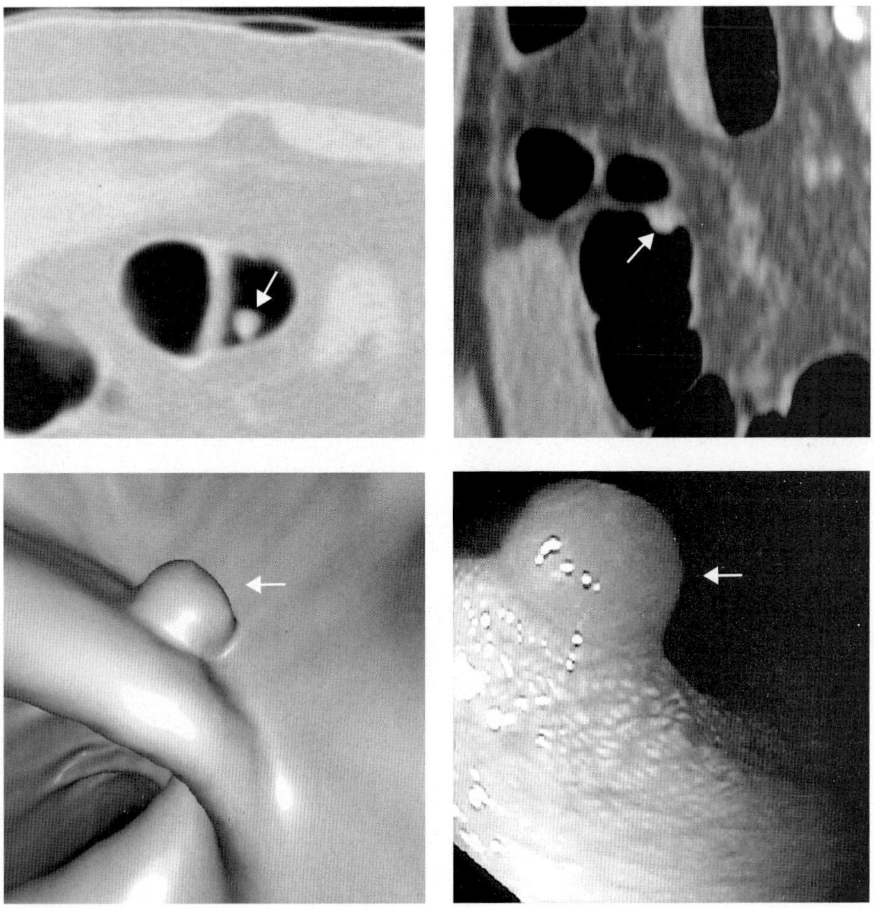

A B C D

FIGURE 5.6 Large Sessile Polyp-Tubular Adenoma. Axial prone image **(A)** shows a rounded polyp in the sigmoid. Coronal reformat in abdominal window **(B)** demonstrates the polyp is sessile. 3D endoluminal view **(C)** and colonoscopic image **(D)** show a broad-based polyp adjacent to a haustral fold. The polyp was found to be a 10-mm tubular adenoma at pathology.

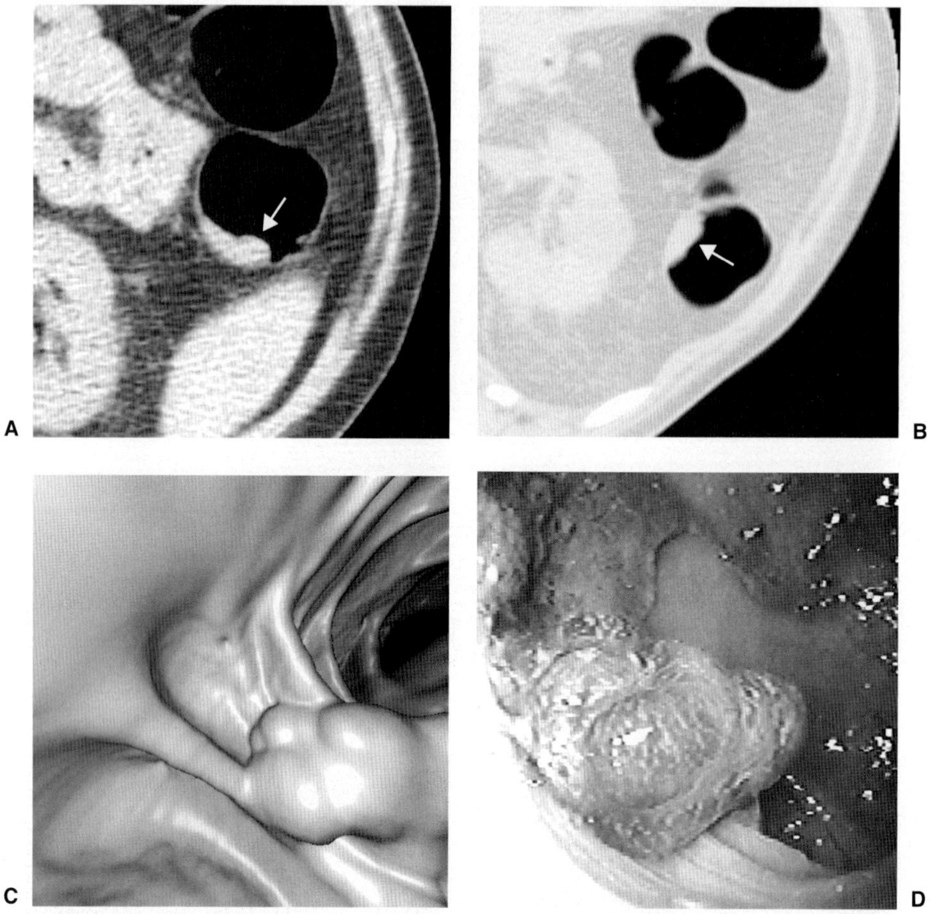

FIGURE 5.7 Large Sessile Polyp-Tubulovillous Adenoma. Axial supine view **(A)** and prone view **(B)** shows a large lobulated lesion in the descending colon, which appears to shift in location with a change in position. This is due to rotation of the segment. 3D endoluminal image **(C)** and colonoscopic view **(D)** better shows the lobulated surface. Pathologic evaluation revealed a tubulovillous adenoma.

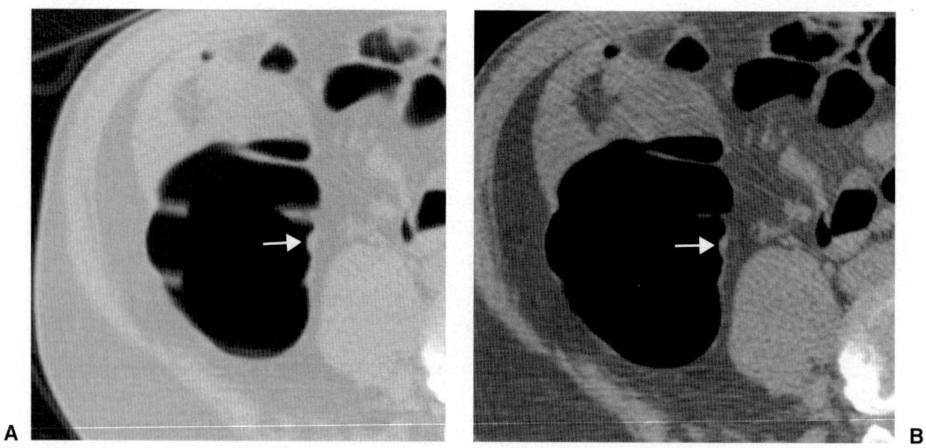

FIGURE 5.8 Large Flat Hyperplastic Polyp. Axial prone image in colon window **(A)** and abdominal window **(B)** show a large flat lesion in the well-distended ascending colon. 3D endoluminal view **(C)** and the endoscopic image **(D)** show a large flat lesion located between two haustral folds. Pathologic evaluation revealed a 12-mm hyperplastic polyp. Hyperplastic polyps may become effaced or flattened in a distended colon segment.

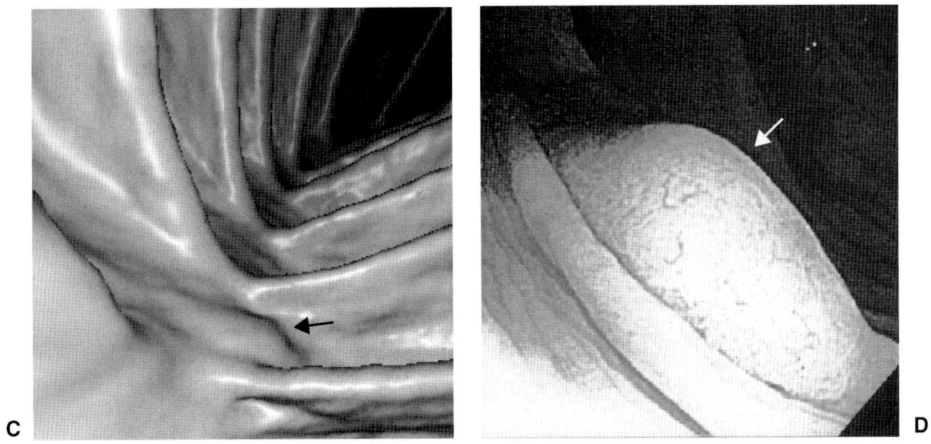

FIGURE 5.8 (*Continued*)

from polyps. Polyps typically occur in the same location within the colonic segment (nonmobile) on opposing views, demonstrate homogenous soft tissue attenuation, and are smooth, round, lobulated, or ovoid without geometric borders or sharp angles. However, polyps may be mobile, especially when pedunculated and upon a long stalk or may appear to be mobile if located within colonic segments that are mobile (sigmoid, transverse: cecum).[37] Morphologically, polyps can be classified as sessile, pedunculated, and flat lesions (see Fig. 5.9). Some lesions have also been described as "subpedunculated" when they have a mixed morphology between sessile and pedunculated.

Sessile polyps are typically hemispherically shaped lesions with a broad-based attachment to the colonic mucosa. On two-dimensional (2D) images (axials and multiplanar reformats), these lesions are homogenous in attenuation and in the same location on both supine and prone positions. The surface is typically smooth; however, with larger size or with more villous components, the lesion can exhibit a lobular or slightly irregular surface (see Figs. 5.10 and 5.11). Surface ulceration may indicate the presence of malignancy.[5,7] A distinguishing feature of sessile polyps from folds is that polyps appear and disappear during cine scrolling evaluation without the "flowing" continuity that haustral folds exhibit with the colonic wall that may be followed on multiple consecutive axial images. The surface of these polyps is smooth on 2D without angular or irregular borders characteristic of stool. Because of the broad-based mucosal attachment, there may be associated focal colonic wall thickening. Focal mucosal thickening can also help distinguish polyps from residual stool. Some sessile polyps have a narrower-based attachment to the colonic wall or an angulated attachment that may trap air or contrast in the angle between the polyp and the colonic wall and caution is advised to not confuse this appearance with air located (more centrally) within residual stool. A sessile hemispheric polyp appears as a rounded or ovoid lesion with a smooth contour protruding into the colonic lumen on the three-dimensional (3D) endoluminal view. Sessile hemispheric polyps have been described as having an incomplete dark ring surrounding the base when viewed in profile in contrast to diverticulae which have a complete ring shadow[38,39] (see Fig. 5.12). However, it should be noted that sessile polyps may demonstrate a complete ring shadow if viewed *en face*.

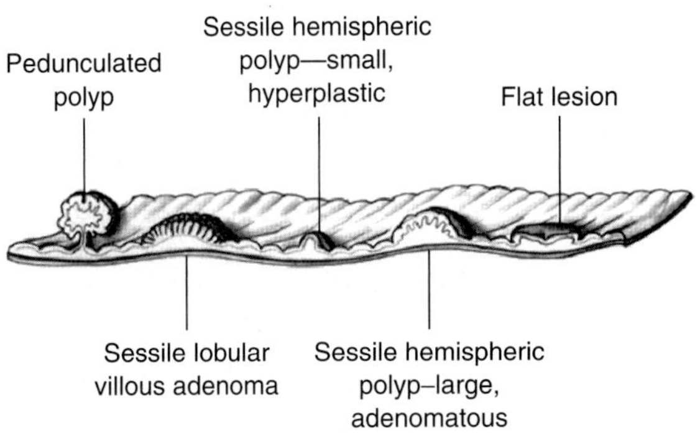

FIGURE 5.9 Polyp Morphologies.

Pedunculated polyps are composed of two parts, a spherical head and an elongated stalk (see Figs. 5.13–5.15). Traction on the colonic mucosa or a sessile polyp due to peristalsis is thought to be the mechanism for development of the stalk.[11] Pedunculated polyps have less risk of malignancy than sessile lesions because dysplastic elements are usually confined to the polyp head and distant from the colonic mucosa, unless a short thick stalk is present. A long stalk $\geq$2 cm is considered a virtually pathognomonic feature of a benign pedunculated polyp (see Fig. 5.16).[11] Invasive carcinoma has been reported to invade the polyp stalk and extend to the muscularis mucosae.[40] The appearance of the head of pedunculated polyps is similar to sessile polyps and exhibits similar characteristics. If the head of a pedunculated polyp is irregular or lobulated there is increased probability of malignancy. Pedunculated polyps are mobile with the extent of movement related to the length of the stalk. The stalk is typically visible on 2D axial and multiplanar reformation (MPR) views although often more easily

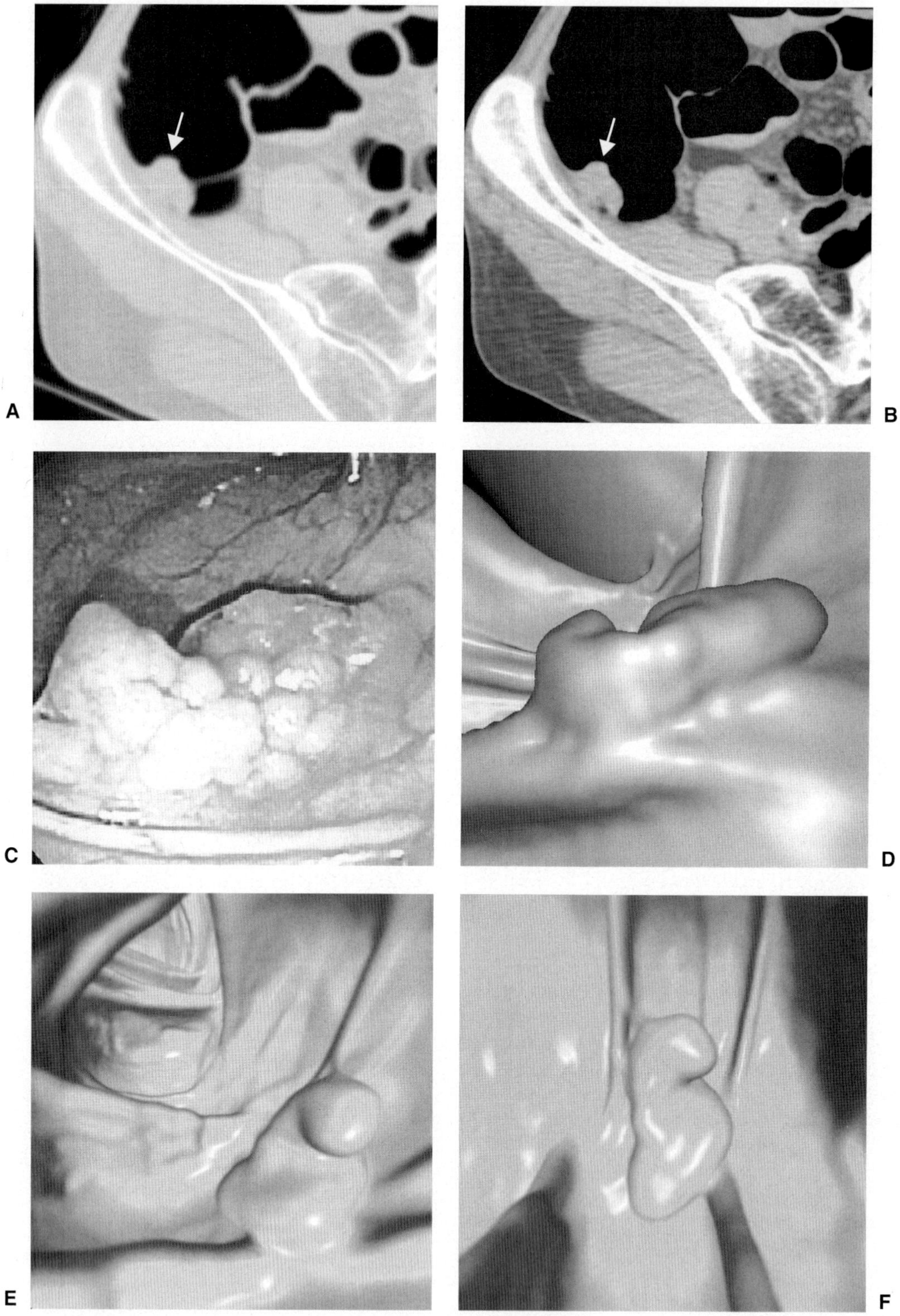

FIGURE 5.10 Large Villous Adenoma. Axial supine image **(A)** shows a large sessile polyp on the posterior wall of the ascending colon. Axial supine image in abdominal window **(B)** shows homogenous soft tissue density of the polyp with focal colonic wall thickening. Endoscopic view **(C)** shows a large sessile polyp with an irregular nodular surface. 3D endoluminal views **(D–F)** show the lobulated irregular surface of a villous adenoma.

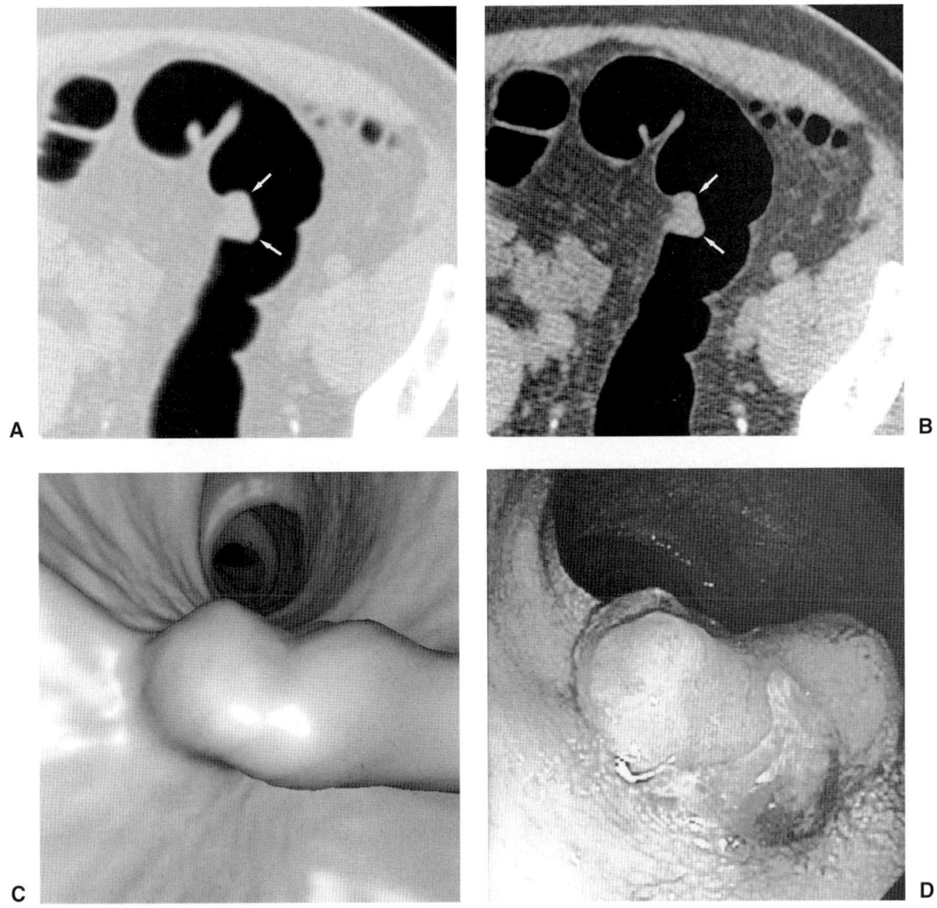

FIGURE 5.11 Malignant Polyp. Axial view in colon **(A)** and abdominal **(B)** windows show a large, homogeneous soft tissue density sessile polyp in the sigmoid. Endoluminal view **(C)** shows the lesion is lobular and broad based. Endoscopy **(D)** demonstrated a 2-cm friable lesion suspicious for carcinoma and confirmed on biopsy.

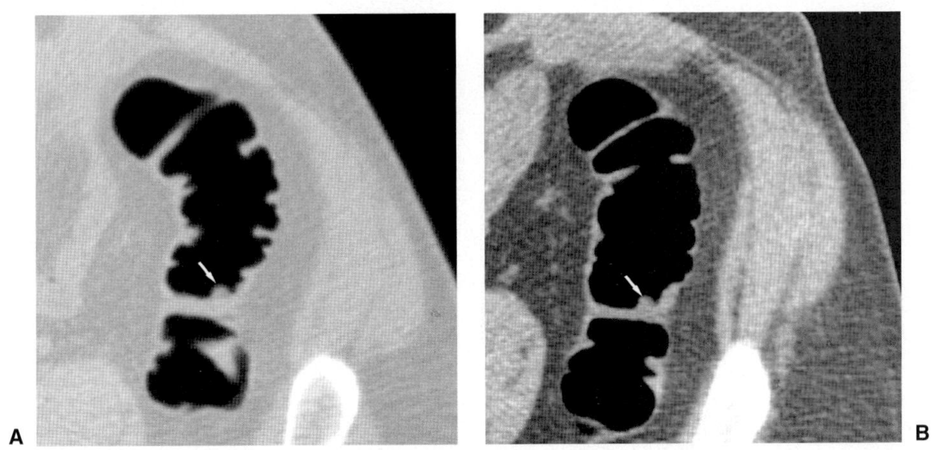

FIGURE 5.12 Polyp in Profile. Axial supine view in colon window **(A)** and abdominal window **(B)** shows a sessile hemispherical polyp. 3D endoluminal view **(C)** and colonoscopic image **(D)** shows the polyp in profile. Note that there is an incomplete ring shadow at the polyp base, which may aid in differentiating a true polyp from a diverticulum which typically have a complete dark rim. (*Views C and D are on next page.*)

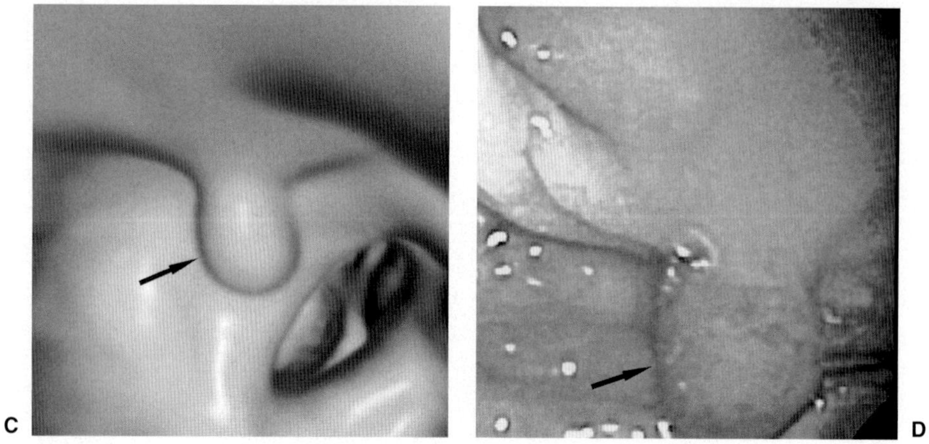

FIGURE 5.12 (*Continued*)

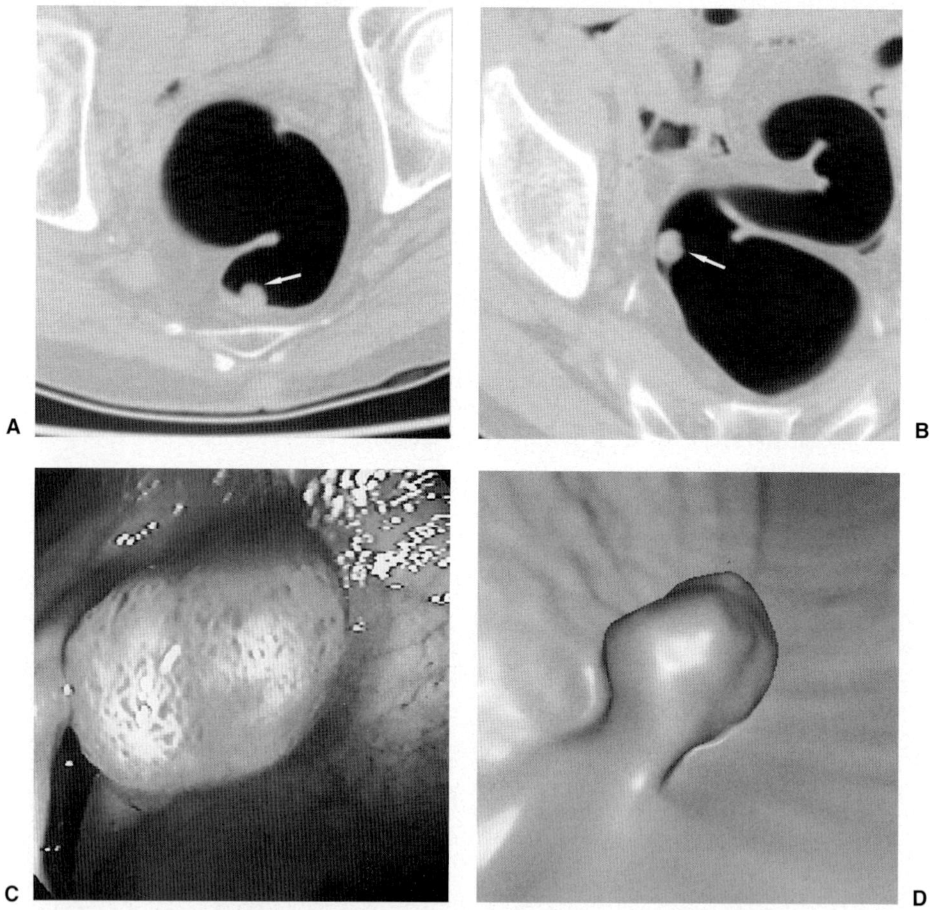

FIGURE 5.13 Large Pedunculated Tubular Adenoma. Axial supine image **(A)** shows an ovoid polyp in the rectum. Axial 2D prone image **(B)** shows the polyp has shifted in location. It has also changed appearance and now demonstrates a stalk. Endoscopic image **(C)** shows a lobular polyp with a small stalk visible inferiorly. 3D endoluminal view **(D)** more clearly demonstrates the stalk.

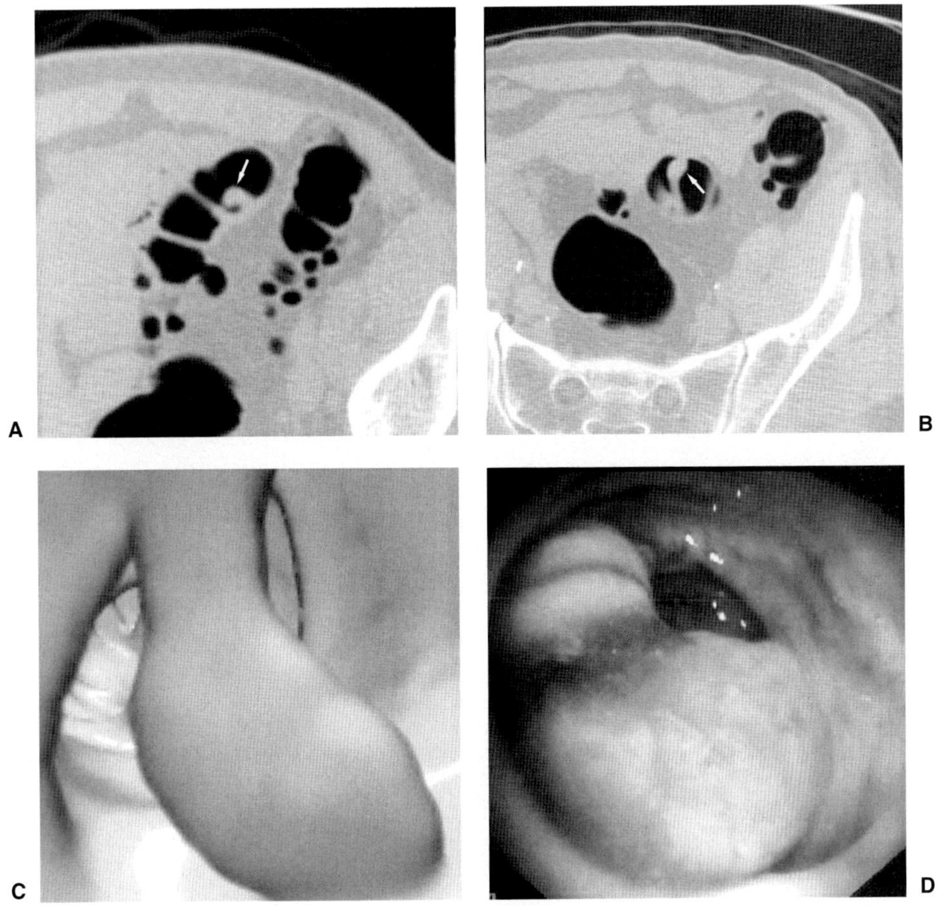

FIGURE 5.14 Large Pedunculated Tubular Adenoma. Axial supine image **(A)** demonstrates a polyp in the sigmoid. The prone image **(B)** shows the elongated stalk of a large pedunculated polyp. 3D endoluminal view **(C)** and colonoscopy image **(D)** show the stalk and large polyp head. Pathology revealed a 15-mm tubular adenoma.

demonstrated on the 3D endoluminal views (see Figs. 5.15 and 5.16). If the morphology of a polyp is in question, 3D evaluation should be utilized. Measurement of size of a pedunculated polyp is restricted to the long axis of the polyp head excluding the stalk. Mobility can lead to different morphologic appearances of the polyp because of position change. Air may be trapped between the polyp and the colon wall, which may be mistaken as heterogeneous attenuation and consequently may cause the lesion to be discounted as stool.

Flat Lesions

Flat lesions were initially thought to occur predominantly in the Japanese population and to be relatively rare in the Western population. Recent studies report that flat lesions occur in the Western population with a prevalence of 4% to 12%.[41–43] Flat colonic lesions may be adenomatous or hyperplastic polyps. In a study of 594 flat colorectal polyps, 481 (81%) were found to be adenomatous with the majority being tubular adenomas.[44] The flat adenoma has been postulated to be a more aggressive pathway than the typical adenoma–carcinoma sequence in colorectal carcinogenesis. However, the malignant potential of flat adenomatous lesions is not clearly understood. Some have reported that up to one third of flat adenomas may demonstrate foci of high-grade dysplasia.[42,45] Sessile adenomas from the National Polyp Study were evaluated histopathologically and flat adenomas represented 27% of all baseline adenomas.[46] Most importantly it was found that flat adenomas identified at baseline were not associated with a higher risk for high-grade dysplasia initially or for advanced adenomas at surveillance. Two large trials found that 38% of adenomatous lesions detected on colonoscopy were classified as flat.[41,47] Flat adenomas have been found to occur more commonly in cancer-prone families and in patients with hereditary polyposis syndromes.[5,42] Flat lesions are also being detected with increased frequency at colonoscopy because of new colonoscopic techniques such as high-magnification chromoscopy and dye spraying.[41]

Flat lesions are defined as minimally elevated polyps measuring <3 mm in height or as lesions with a height less than half of its width (see Figs. 5.17–5.21).[41] Most flat lesions are <10 mm. Some have described a distinction between lesions that appear flat and those

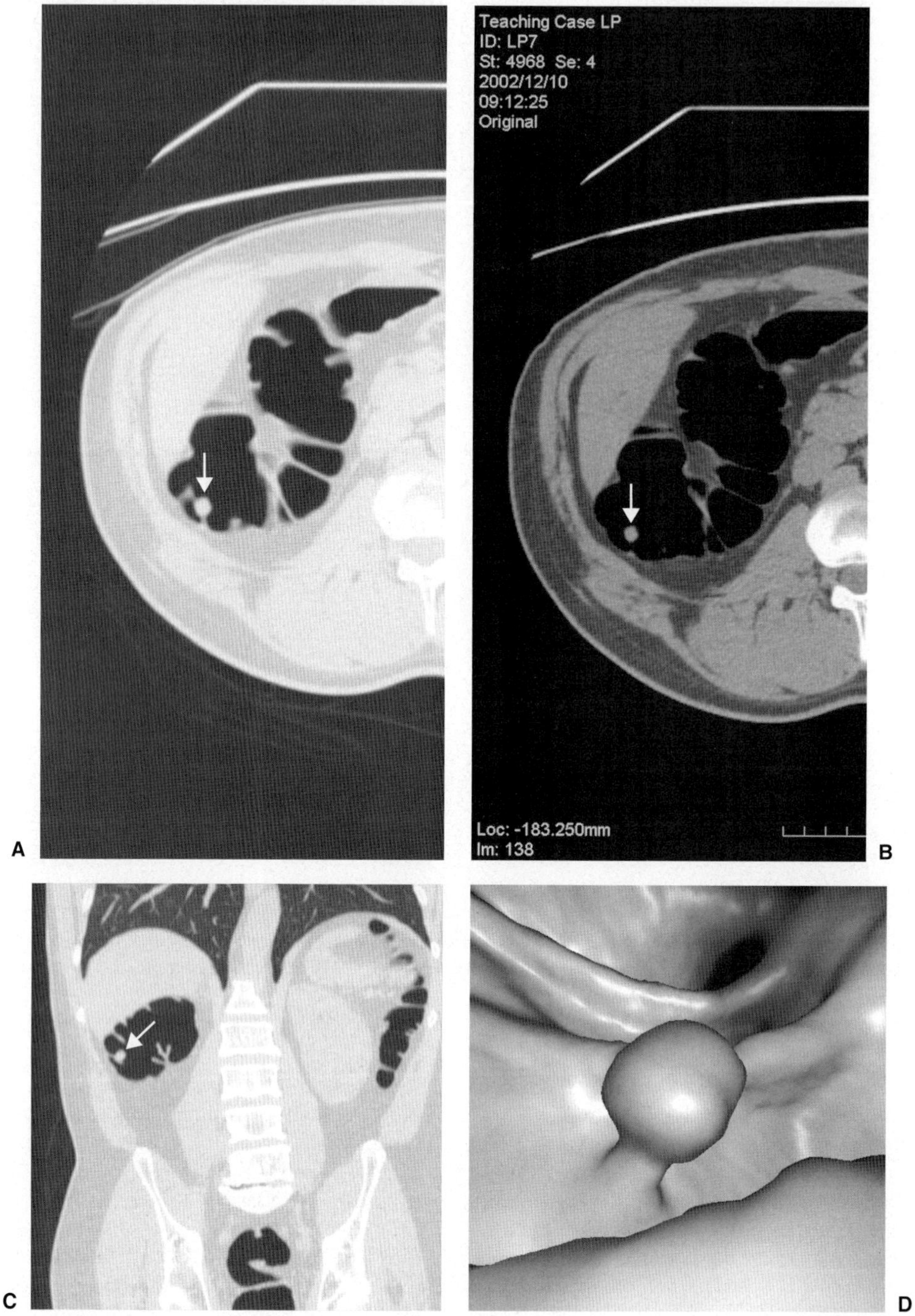

FIGURE 5.15 Large Pedunculated Tubular Adenoma. Axial supine image in colon window **(A)** and abdominal window **(B)** shows a large pedunculated polyp on a short stalk. Note that the stalk may not be visualized on the abdominal window. Coronal multiplanar reformat **(C)** shows the polyp is located in the hepatic flexure. 3D endoluminal view **(D)** shows the short stalk and large polyp head. This lesion was initially missed on first pass colonoscopy but was subsequently identified and removed.

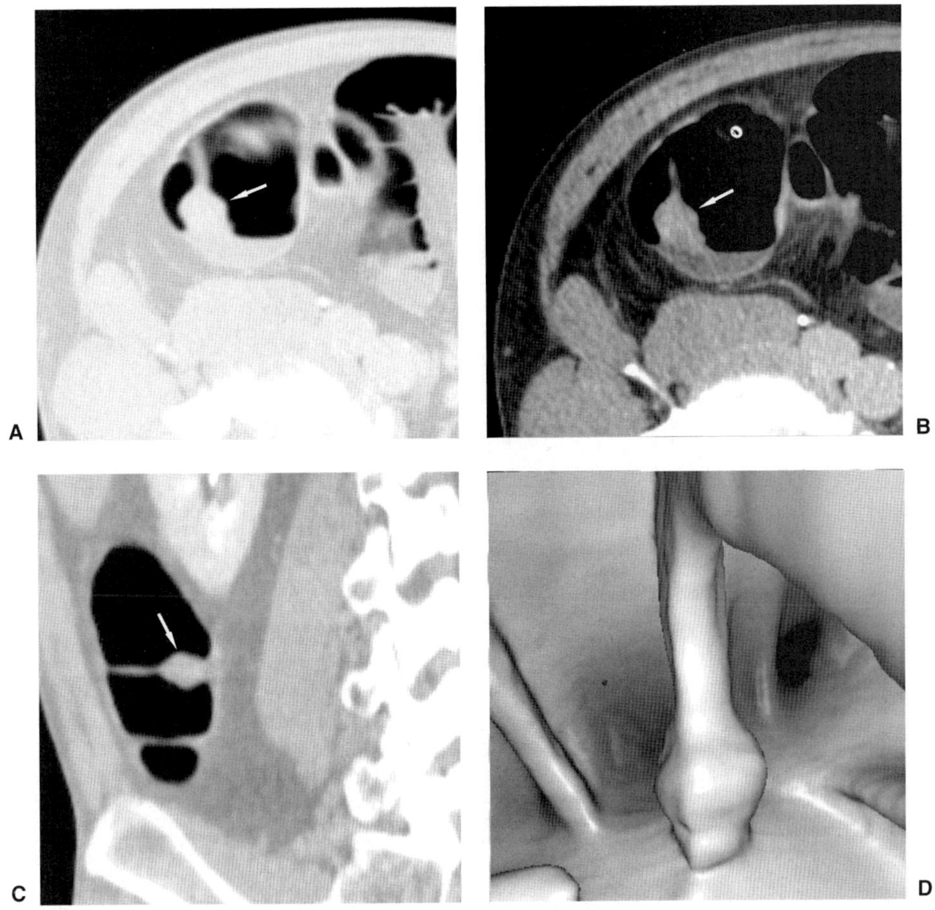

FIGURE 5.16 Large Pedunculated Tubular Adenoma. Axial supine image in colon window **(A)** and in abdominal window **(B)** shows a large pedunculated polyp on a long stalk >2 cm which is a sign of a benign lesion. The stalk is not as well visualized on the abdominal window. Coronal reformat **(C)** confirms the pedunculated polyp. The long length of the stalk is best visualized on the 3D endoluminal view **(D)**.

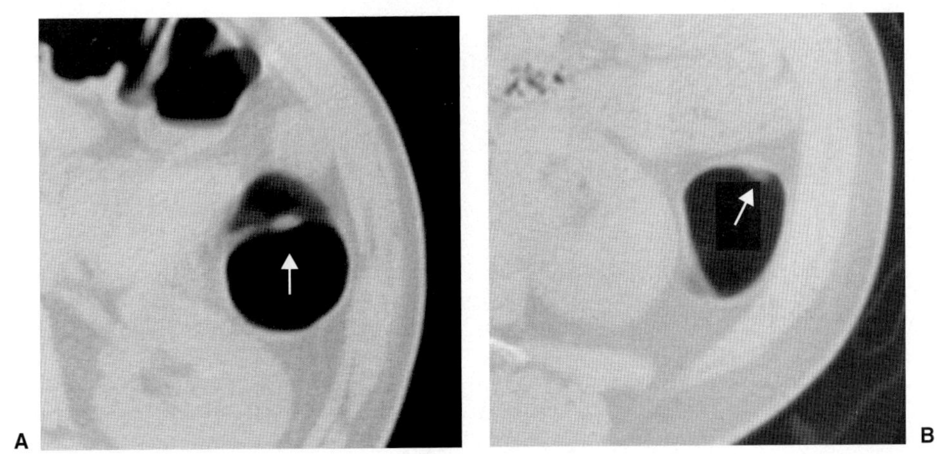

FIGURE 5.17 Flat Lesion. Axial supine image **(A)** shows a focal thickening of the haustral fold with an elliptical shape. On the axial prone image **(B)**, the lesion is barely visible along the anterior colonic wall. The 3D endoluminal view **(C)** shows a minimally elevated flat lesion. The 3D cube view **(D)** may be rotated so that the lesion is in profile and shows the height of the lesion is <50% of the width. Pathologic evaluation demonstrated a tubular adenoma. (*Views C and D are on next page.*)

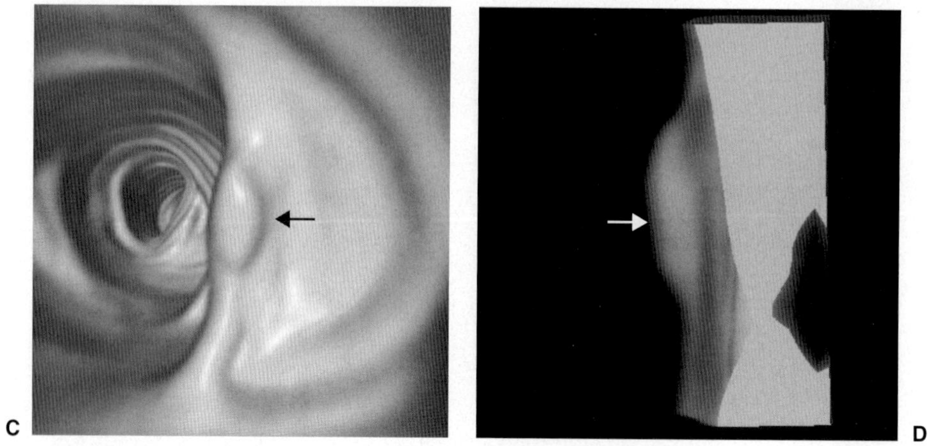

FIGURE 5.17 (*Continued*)

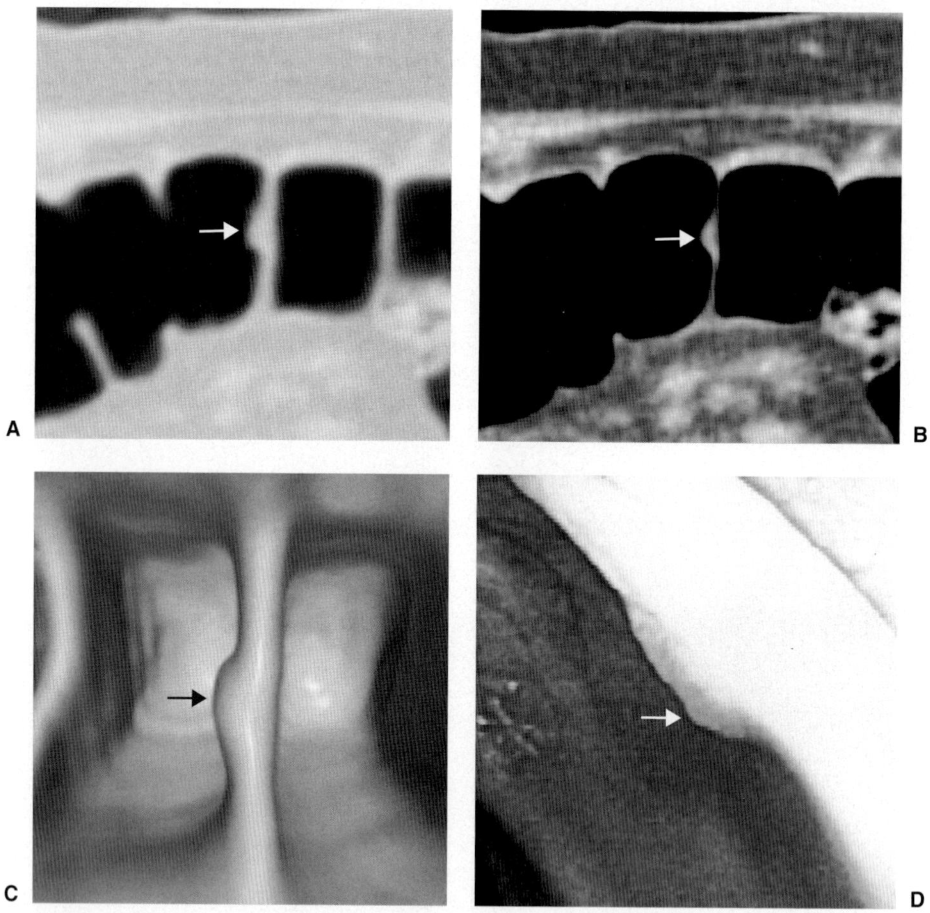

FIGURE 5.18 Flat Lesion. Axial image in colon window **(A)** demonstrates a minimally elevated lesion on a haustral fold in the transverse colon. Axial image in abdominal window **(B)** demonstrates enhanced conspicuity of the lesion. Endoluminal 3D view **(C)** and endoscopic view **(D)** show the flat lesion in profile. This was found to be a 10-mm tubular adenoma on pathologic evaluation.

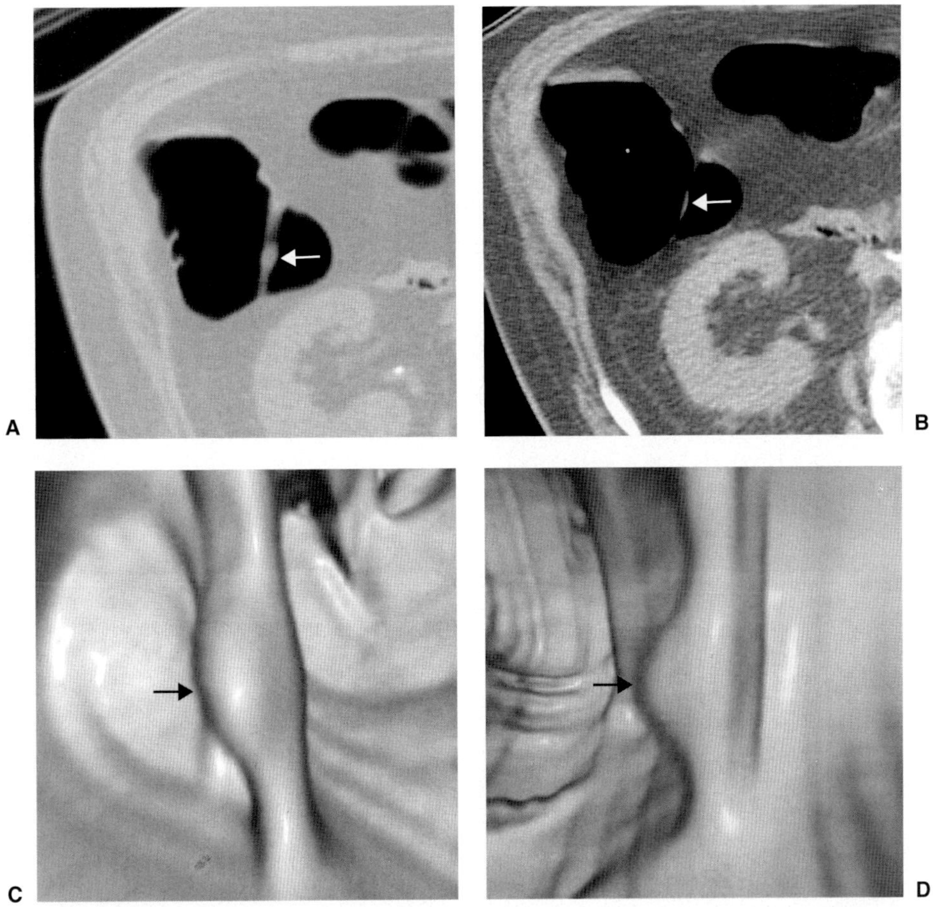

FIGURE 5.19 Flat Lesion. Axial image in colon window **(A)** demonstrates a flat adenomatous polyp in the ascending colon. The lesion appears as focal thickening of a haustral fold. On abdominal windows **(B)** the lesion is barely visible as focal wall thickening, which may in part be due to partial voluming. On 3D endoluminal views **(C, D)**, the polyp appears as a focal mild elevation on the haustral fold.

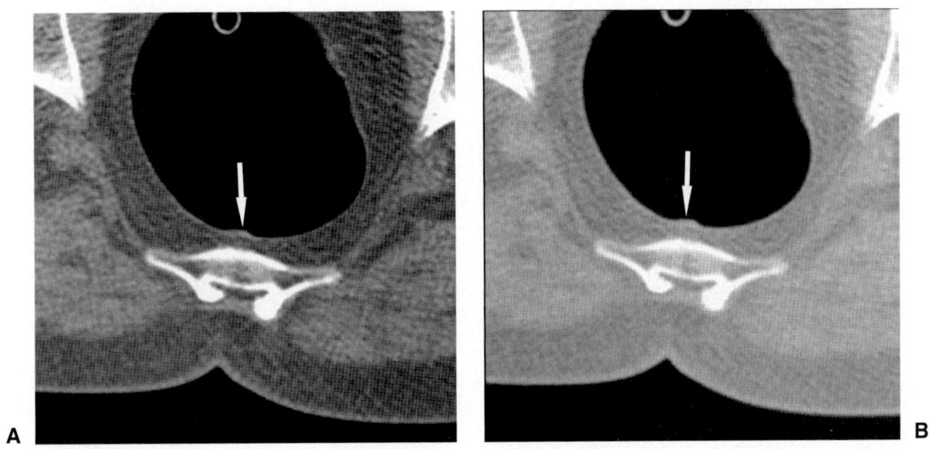

FIGURE 5.20 Flat Lesion. A subtle small flat lesion is seen on the axial image in colon window **(A)** and on abdominal window **(B)**. The sagittal reformat **(C)** shows the same lesion as a slight focal elevation of the posterior rectal wall. This lesion is best visualized on the 3D endoluminal image **(D)**. Biopsy and histologic evaluation revealed a hyperplastic polyp. (*Views C and D are on next page.*)

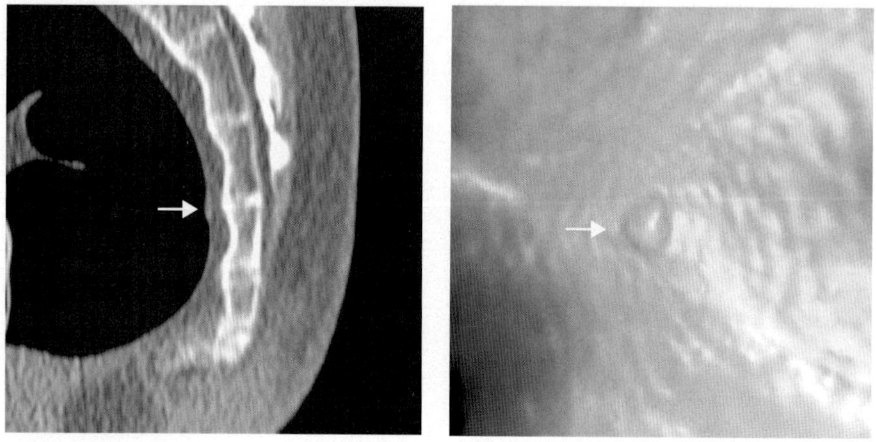

C D

FIGURE 5.20 *(Continued)*

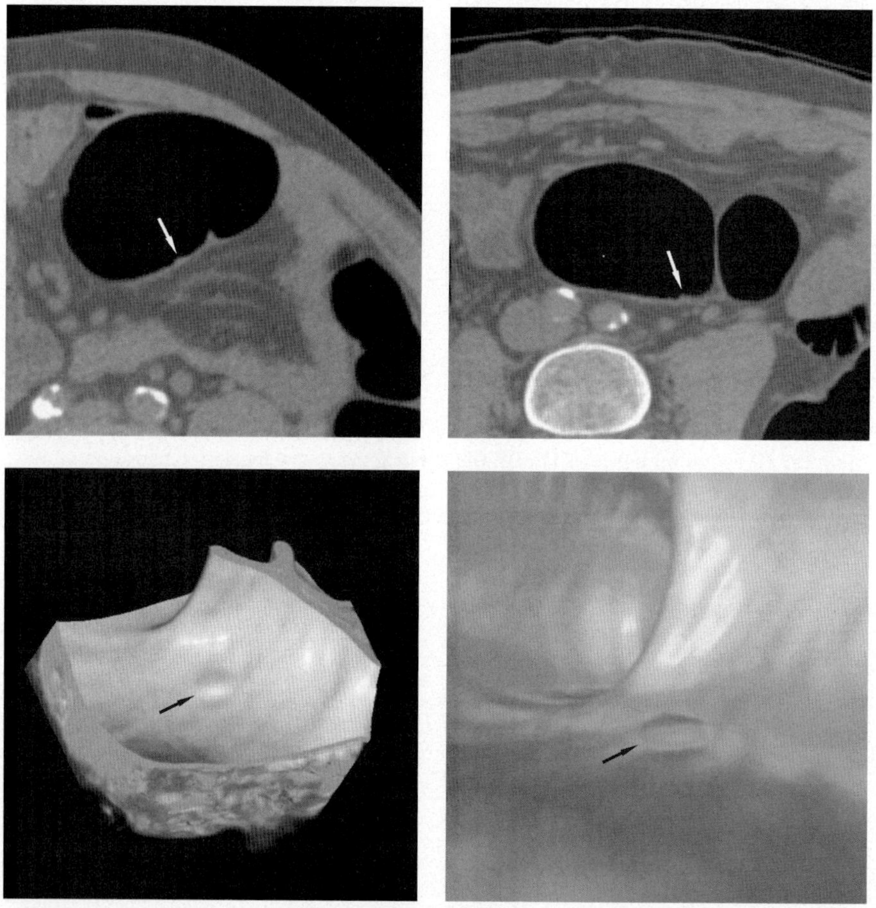

A B C D

FIGURE 5.21 Flat Lesion. A small flat lesion in the sigmoid is barely perceptible on the axial images **(A, B)** and more easily identified on the 3D cube view **(C)** and on the traditional endoluminal view **(D)**. This was a hyperplastic polyp on histologic evaluation.

that are truly flat and associated with a higher risk of dysplasia and carcinoma. These truly flat lesions are nonelevated, may be depressed or have a characteristic flat central depression, and may not be identifiable on CTC even retrospectively.[37] These lesions are thought to spread endophytically and become advanced cancers at small sizes, whereas the minimally elevated or laterally spreading adenomas are early precursors to the typical polypoid adenomas.[41]

Detection of flat lesions on CTC may be challenging. A flat lesion appears as a focal thickening of the colon wall or as a minimally elevated ovoid lesion on 2D views. They may occur on a fold or between folds and have been found easier to detect when located on a fold. Fidler et al. performed an early study using single detector CT with 5-mm slice thickness to investigate the sensitivity of CTC for the detection of flat lesions.[42] The authors found that overall, flat lesions were difficult to detect (41% sensitivity) but detection rates were higher for more experienced readers and following double reading by another reader (68% sensitivity). The authors reported that detection rates were higher for adenomatous polyps and that the use of abdominal windows in addition to colon windows was helpful in identifying those lesions that were minimally raised. Three-dimensional endoluminal views were found to be least helpful for the detection of flat lesions. Park et al. evaluated ten patients with 18 flat polyps using 16-row multidetector CT with a slice thickness of 1 mm and the administration of intravenous contrast.[48] Less than 50% of flat lesions were identified. It was found that lesions with a height of $\leq$1 mm were not detected on CTC. In order for flat lesions to be detected on CTC they had to be $\geq$2 mm in height and $\geq$7 mm in diameter. Increased lesion conspicuity was associated with contrast enhancement, location on a haustral fold, and abnormal morphology. Pickhardt et al. identified 59 flat lesions $\geq$6 mm in 52 (4.2%) of 1,233 asymptomatic patients.[43] Approximately 49% of the flat lesions $\geq$6 mm were adenomatous and they accounted for approximately 14% of all adenomas $\geq$6 mm. The sensitivity of CTC for the detection of all flat lesions and of flat adenomas was 80% and 83%, respectively compared with the detection sensitivity for all polyps and all adenomatous polyps, which was 81% and 86%, respectively. It was concluded that flat adenomas $\geq$6 mm are uncommon in a Western screening population and that the sensitivity of CTC for detecting flat lesions was similar to that of polypoid lesions.

Flat lesions may appear on 3D views as slightly elevated or irregular discoid or plaque-like lesions that may occur between haustral folds or involve a fold directly (see Figs. 5.17–5.19). Small amounts of stool or fluid can mimic these lesions and make detection nearly impossible. If a suspicious lesion is encountered using primary 3D interpretation, 2D evaluation with abdominal windows should be preformed to exclude residual stool within the segment, to evaluate for associated colonic wall thickening, and to demonstrate soft tissue attenuation.

Certain characteristics of polyps may make them less likely to be detected than others. Gluecker et al. investigated polyp characteristics (polyp size, endoscopic morphology, CT shape, surface contour) and extrinsic features (relation to folds, proximity to colonic wall, colonic flexures, colonic segments, and quality of preparation) associated with polyps that were missed on CTC using primary 2D interpretation and found that the following factors contributed to polyps being missed: identified only on one position, flat morphology, surface irregularity, occurring in a poorly prepared segment or along a thickened colonic wall.[35] Pedunculated polyps were missed more frequently than expected. Location on a fold or within a flexure had no impact on detection.

COLORECTAL CARCINOMA

The primary goal of CTC is to detect the precursor lesion of colorectal malignancy. However, CTC has also proved to be useful for the detection of colorectal carcinoma. It is important to recognize the characteristic 2D and 3D appearances of colon cancer on CTC to ensure early cancer detection when possible.

Colon cancers may be classified histologically into epithelial and nonepithelial origin. More than 90% of colon cancers are adenocarcinomas, of which nearly all are believed to develop through the adenoma–carcinoma sequence.[9,49,50] The existence of *de novo* colon cancer is an accepted but debated topic.[9] Most investigators have shown that cancers develop slowly in adenomatous precursors. In polyposis syndromes including FAPS and in hereditary nonpolyposis colorectal carcinoma (HNPCC), the morphologic sequence of dysplasia along the pathway is accelerated with minute cancers having been reported in small and flat lesions.[7,9,50] The index of suspicion for lesions of any size should be high in patients with these syndromes. Patients with inflammatory bowel disease, particularly those with ulcerative colitis, are at an increased risk of developing colorectal adenocarcinoma, and these patients often undergo rigorous screening examinations for early neoplastic lesions; however, the progression to carcinoma may not proceed along the typical adenoma–carcinoma pathway and may instead involve a dysplastic stage (flat or mass like epithelium), making screening in these patients challenging.[7] CTC should be performed with caution in patients with inflammatory bowel disease due to the risk for colonic perforation. A recent study suggests that CTC may be clinically useful when compared with other modalities such as endoscopy and barium enema for the evaluation of Crohn's colitis.[51]

Other epithelial histologic types of colon cancer include squamous cell and adenosquamous carcinomas, which may invade the distal rectum from the anal verge.[49,52] Anorectal and cloacogenic (low-lying rectal malignancies arising from cells derived from the primitive cloaca) primary carcinoma, although histologically different from colorectal adenocarcinoma, are grossly and radiolographically indistinguishable, and can appear as ulcerative, polypoid, annular, flat, or infiltrative (submucosal) lesions.[7] Squamous cell anorectal malignancy may exhibit lower attenuation than rectal adenocarcinoma.[53]

Nonepithelial carcinomas are rare and include lymphomas, carcinoid, metastases, and sarcomas.[50,52,54] Malignant lymphoma can involve the colon as a primary tumor or as part of disseminated disease. Primary lymphoma represents 0.5% to 1% of all colonic malignancies. These are typically non–Hodgkin's lymphomas of the large cell type. Colonic lymphoma often occurs in patients with acquired immunodeficiency syndrome (AIDS) or ulcerative colitis.[50] The morphologic appearance of primary lymphoma of the colon is variable and often difficult to differentiate from colonic adenocarcinoma, although lymphoma more commonly occurs in the cecum and rectum. Primary lymphoma presents as large, discrete single or multiple masses whereas systemic lymphoma usually causes longer segment involvement.[50] Lymphomatous polyposis may manifest as diffuse mucosal nodularity and can involve the entire colon, simulating familial polyposis syndromes.[7] Another appearance of lymphoma is a large bulky tumor mass with cavitation uncharacteristic for adenocarcinoma.[7]

Primary carcinoid occurs in the large bowel in 15% of cases, with the vast majority occurring within the rectum.[50] These lesions often present as small, sessile rectal polypoid lesions with sharp margins located in the lower two thirds of the rectum. Only 1% to 2% of rectal polyps >5 mm have been found to represent carcinoid. However, bulky carcinoid tumors and annular lesions have also been described.[50] Rectal carcinoid may present with rectal bleeding; however, most are asymptomatic and not associated with systemic carcinoid syndrome. Lesions >2 cm harbor a significantly increased risk of malignant potential.[49] Colonic carcinoids located proximal to the rectum are typically more aggressive and larger at the time of presentation. These are often located in the cecum and appear as bulky masses simulating adenocarcinoma.

Kaposi's sarcoma typically presents as multiple submucosal nodules, which may be identifiable on CTC using 2D or 3D techniques. However, umbilicated lesions resembling pedunculated polyps or lesions associated with thickened mucosal folds have also been described.[7] The morphologic appearance of secondary malignancy of the colon is dependent upon the route of spread and may originate from many different primary malignancies. Hematogenous spread often presents as submucosal nodules, but may ulcerate or present as fungating or polypoid lesions. Tumor spread may be directly from adjacent organs and often has the appearance of an extracolonic mass causing mass effect or an infiltrating mass that fixes the colon in place. The most common primary malignancies that directly invade the colon are from prostate, kidney, gallbladder, ovary, and uterus.[7] Gastric and pancreatic carcinomas may also spread along ligaments to invade the colon. Intraperitoneal seeding can also involve the colon typically from ovarian, gastric, and pancreatic malignancies.

Morphology

There are three main morphologic appearances of colorectal carcinoma (see Fig. 5.22). The most common appearance is an intraluminal broad-based mass which may be ulcerated and associated with a heaped-up appearance of the surrounding mucosa (see Figs. 5.23–5.26). The second type is a polypoid or fungating mass, which occurs in approximately 33% of colon cancer cases (see Figs. 5.27 and 5.28).[52] The third type is an annular (apple-core, napkin ring) mass which is associated with a higher rate of serosal invasion and lymph node metastases than polypoid types (see Fig. 5.29).[7,9,49] An atypical appearance is often seen in patients with chronic ulcerative colitis who develop an infiltrative or scirrhous carcinoma (*linitis plastica* type), which may resemble a long segment stricture due to submucosal involvement by tumor cells and fibrous reaction.[7,55] Lesions resembling large adenomas may harbor carcinoma *in situ* or invasive malignancy (termed *malignant polyps*), and the diagnosis may only be evident on histologic analysis.[9,50] Additional surgical resection, including colectomy, may be warranted in cases of invasive carcinoma in presumed adenomas.

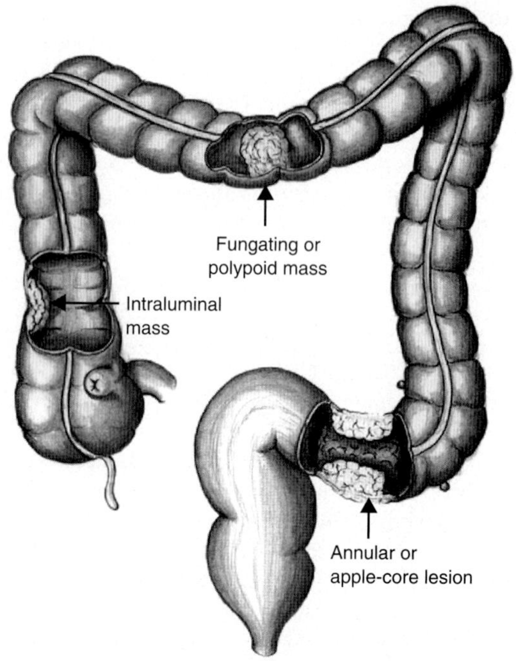

FIGURE 5.22 Carcinoma Morphologies. Intraluminal mass with a broad-based attachment to the colon wall; fungating or polypoid mass protruding into the lumen; and annular or apple-core lesion.

Controversy exists as to the characteristic distribution of various morphologic types of cancer within the colon. Fungating and polypoid masses have been described as occurring most commonly in the right colon with annular lesions typically occurring in the left colon.[56] Others have reported that the distribution is variable and specific morphologic types are unrelated to anatomic segments of the colon.[52,57,58]

Presenting symptoms of colonic carcinoma can often suggest the location of the lesion as well as indicate the degree of tumor involvement (advanced stage). Left-sided cancers tend to cause obstruction more commonly than right-sided malignancies because of the relatively smaller

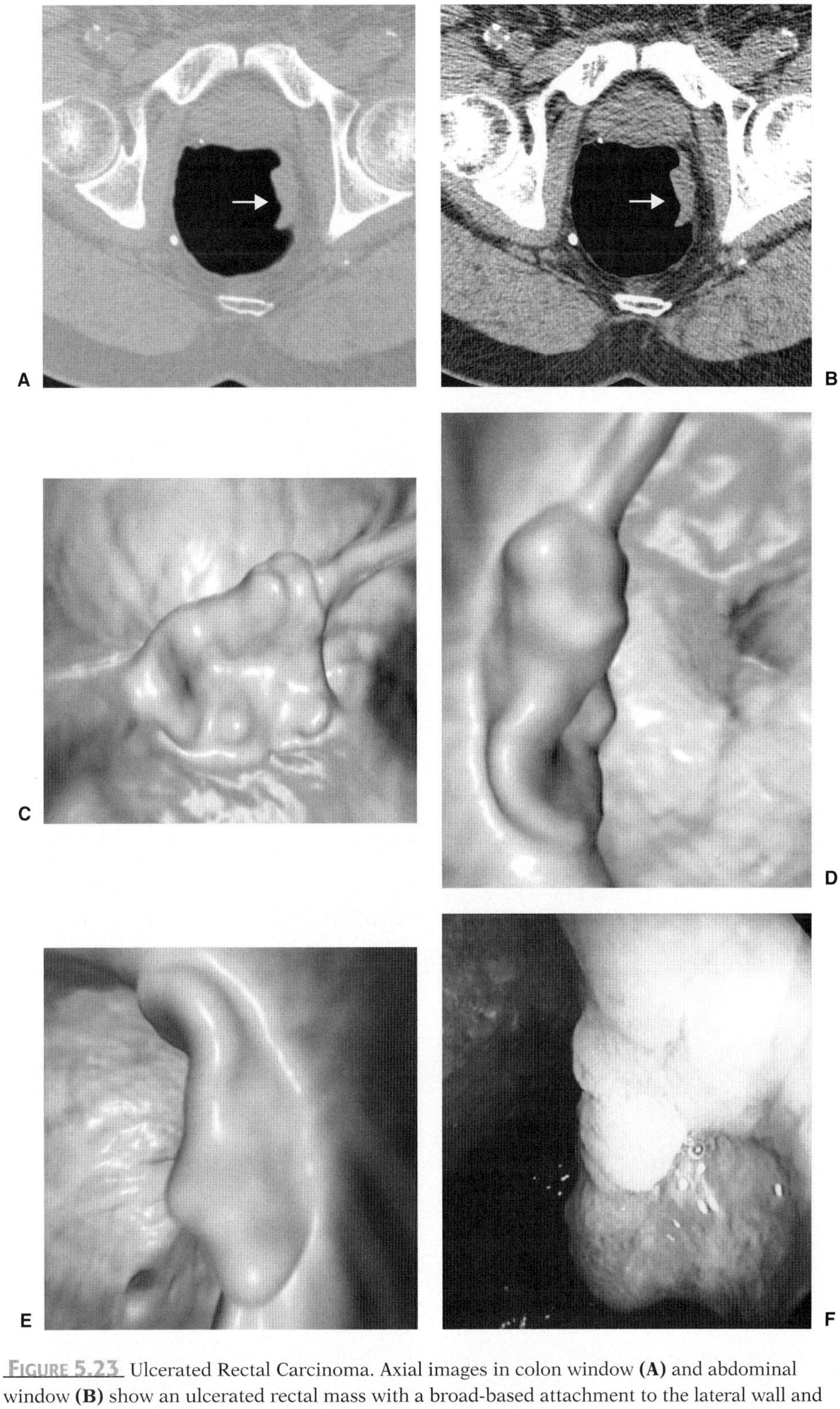

FIGURE 5.23 Ulcerated Rectal Carcinoma. Axial images in colon window **(A)** and abdominal window **(B)** show an ulcerated rectal mass with a broad-based attachment to the lateral wall and overhanging edges of tumor. Pathology revealed a 3-cm moderately differentiated adenocarcinoma. 3D endoluminal views from different viewpoints **(C–E)** show the central depression due to ulceration and the irregular border of the mass which is also well demonstrated on endoscopy **(F)**.

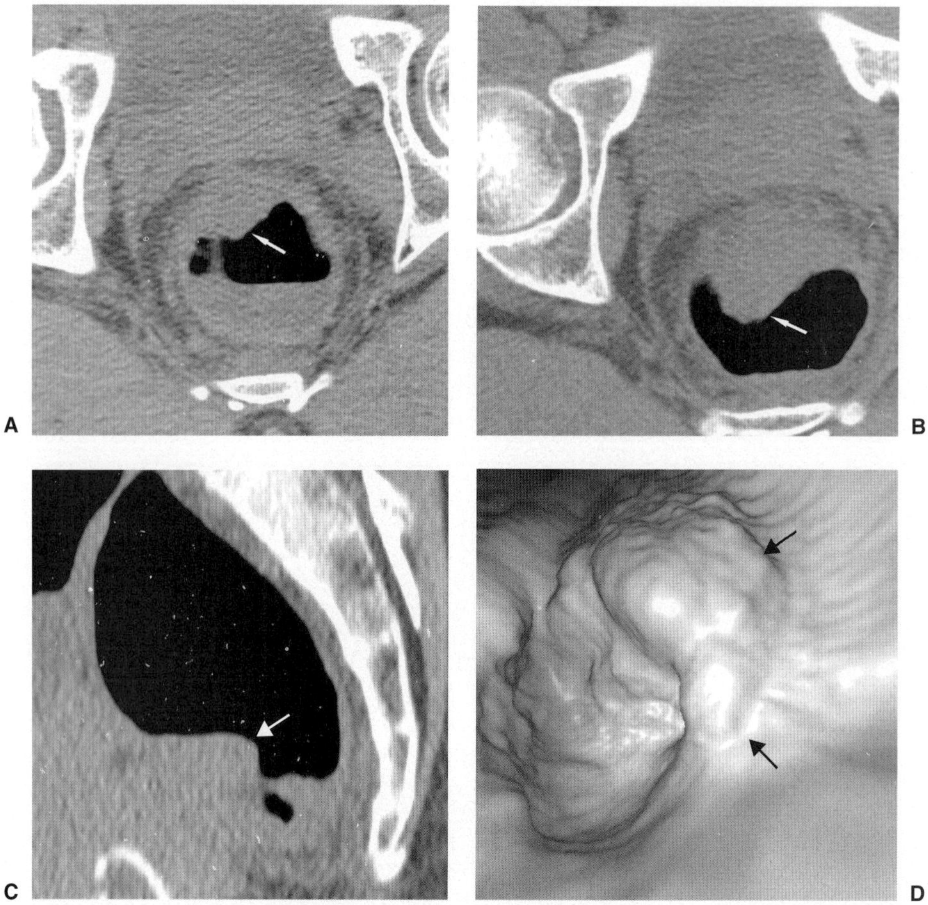

FIGURE 5.24 Large Rectal Carcinoma. Axial images in supine **(A)** and prone **(B)** positions show a large nonmobile soft tissue density mass arising from the anterior rectal wall protruding into the lumen. There is associated adjacent wall thickening. Measurement of the length of the mass is best obtained on the sagittal multiplanar reformat **(C)**. The 3D endoluminal view **(D)** shows a large mass with irregular borders.

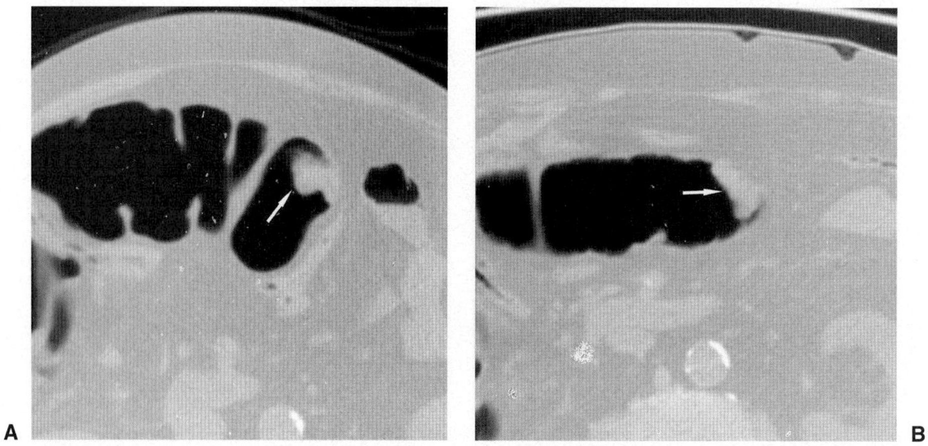

FIGURE 5.25 Transverse Colon Carcinoma. Large mass in the transverse colon which changes morphology on the supine axial **(A)** and prone axial **(B)** views. The mass has a broad-based attachment to the colonic wall and appears to protrude into the lumen more on the supine 3D endoluminal view **(C)** than on the prone 3D endoluminal view **(D)**. Prone axial view **(B)** shows a small amount of air trapped beneath the mass, which may cause it to be mistaken as stool.

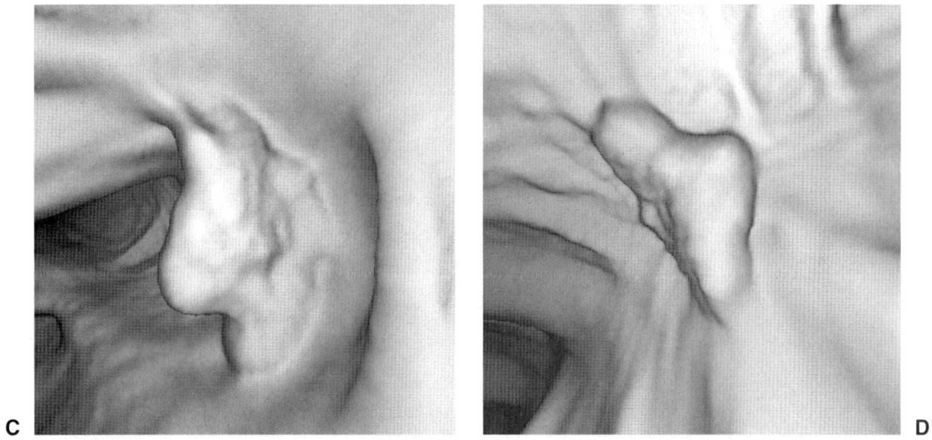

FIGURE 5.25 (*Continued*)

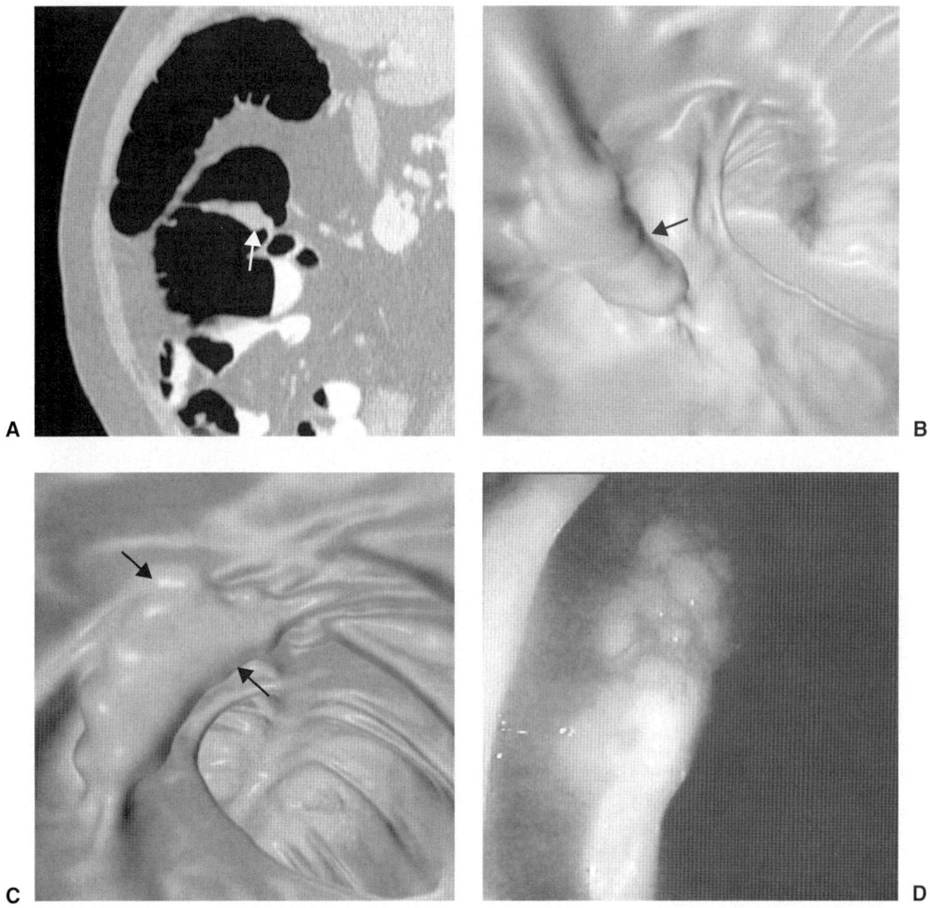

FIGURE 5.26 Ascending Colon Carcinoma Simulating Ileocecal Valve. Coronal multiplanar reformat **(A)** shows a soft tissue density mass extending along a haustral fold in the ascending colon just superior to the ileocecal valve. 3D endoluminal views from different perspectives **(B, C)** show the irregular nodular border of the mass, which is well correlated on the colonoscopic image **(D)**. The patient underwent right hemicolectomy and pathology revealed adenocarcinoma.

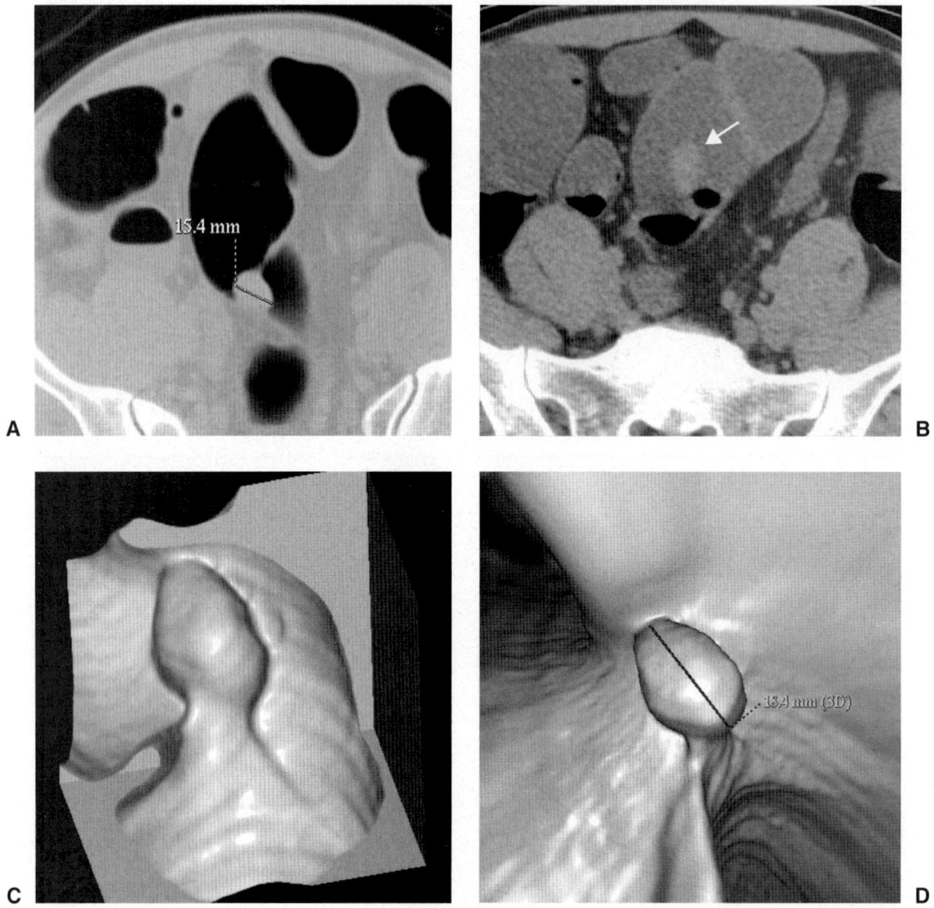

FIGURE 5.27 Polypoid Sigmoid Carcinoma. Axial supine image in colon window **(A)** shows a large pedunculated polyp in the sigmoid, which was found to contain adenocarcinoma *in situ* on pathology. Prone position **(B)** shows the denser soft tissue polypoid lesion in fluid on abdominal window. 3D cube view **(C)** and endoluminal view **(D)** demonstrate a pedunculated polyp with a short thick stalk, which may be seen with malignant polyps. Note the 3D view provided a more accurate measurement of the polyp head, which was found to be 20 mm at colonoscopy.

caliber lumen and, along with rectal cancers, tend to present with more gross bleeding. Right-sided cancers are more often clinically occult because obstruction is less common, and patients are more likely to present with anemia and advanced stage tumors.[49,50,56] Obstruction is considered to be an ominous symptom and is associated with poorer prognosis and lower long-term survival.[50] Colorectal polypoid or intraluminal masses may also serve as the lead point for intussusception.[7]

Surgical resection and paracolonic lymph node dissection may be performed for invasive colorectal carcinoma (penetration of the muscularis mucosa).[49] Large villous tumors, particularly in the rectum, may require surgical excision to assess tumor extent and presence of invasion. If pathologic evaluation of polyps from colonoscopic polypectomy demonstrates carcinoma *in situ* with negative margins and without vascular invasion, conservative treatment may be warranted. However, if the lesion is poorly differentiated, demonstrates vascular invasion, or positive margins, colectomy is recommended.[49]

Colorectal carcinomas have different characteristic appearances on 2D and 3D views. On 2D views, characteristics of masses suspicious for colorectal malignancy include fixed position on supine and prone views, morphology (including nodular, ulcerative and annular appearances), associated wall thickening, contrast enhancement, and focal narrowing or obliteration of the colonic lumen. Supportive findings on 2D axial images and multiplanar reformats include collapse distal to the cancer and the presence of lymphadenopathy or local invasion (see Figs. 5.30 and 5.31). Mucin-producing adenocarcinomas may exhibit intrinsic calcification which may be detected on 2D images.[53] All lesions should be evaluated on supine and prone axial views, MPRs and 3D endoluminal views. Abdominal windows are helpful to further evaluate for malignant characteristics. Asymmetric colonic wall thickening is abnormal if >6 mm and indeterminate if between 3 to 6 mm. Stranding of the pericolonic fat or loss of fat planes in surrounding musculature (especially in the perirectal area) may be

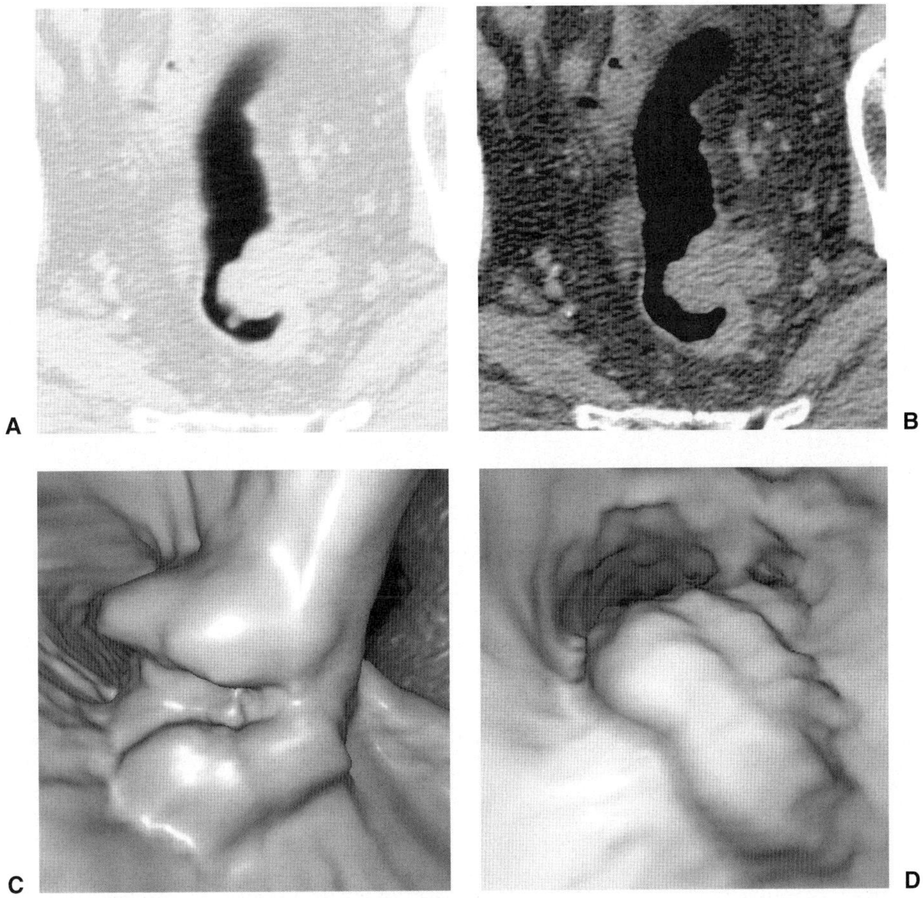

FIGURE 5.28 Polypoid Sigmoid Carcinoma with Invasion. A fungating (polypoid) sigmoid cancer is demonstrated on the supine axial image using a colon window **(A)** and abdominal window **(B)**. The mass is homogenous and has associated adjacent wall thickening. Invasion into the left pericolonic fat and adenopathy are best visualized on the abdominal windows. 3D endoluminal views show the lesion **(C)** and infiltration of the adjacent wall **(D)**. Pathology revealed a 3.2 cm moderately differentiated adenocarcinoma.

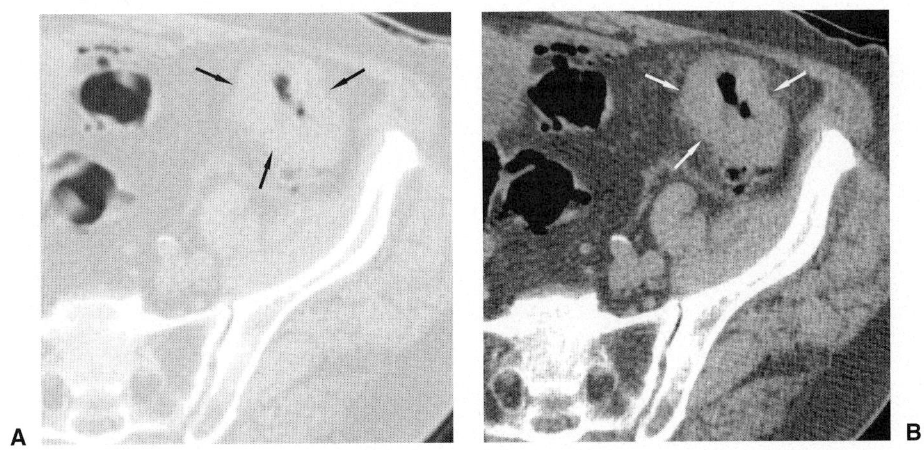

FIGURE 5.29 Annular Sigmoid Carcinoma. Axial image using a colon window **(A)** shows the focal luminal narrowing and diffuse colonic wall thickening, better seen on the abdominal window **(B)**. There is stranding of the pericolonic fat suggesting invasion through the serosa. Sagittal reformat **(C)** is the best display for measuring the length of the lesion. 3D endoluminal view **(D)** shows the characteristic luminal obliteration which limits the ability for 3D evaluation. Pathology demonstrated a moderately differentiated adenocarcinoma. (*Views C and D are on next page.*)

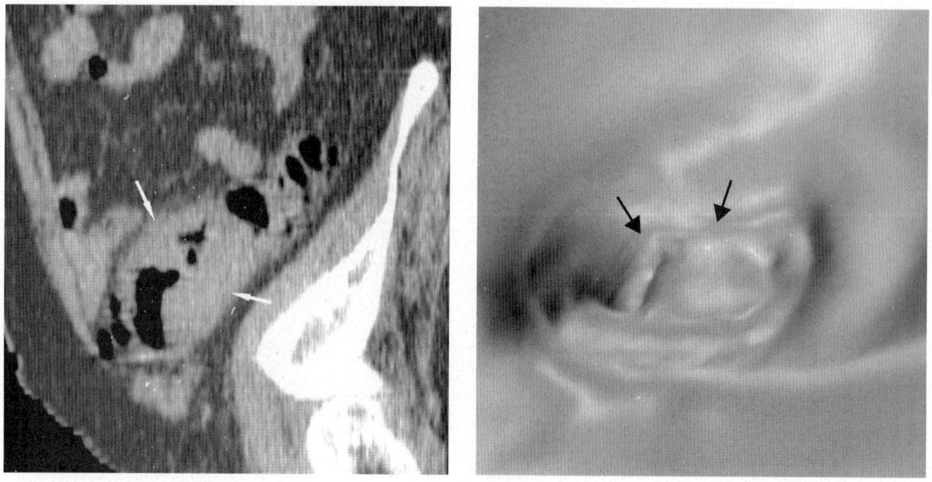

C D

FIGURE 5.29 (*Continued*)

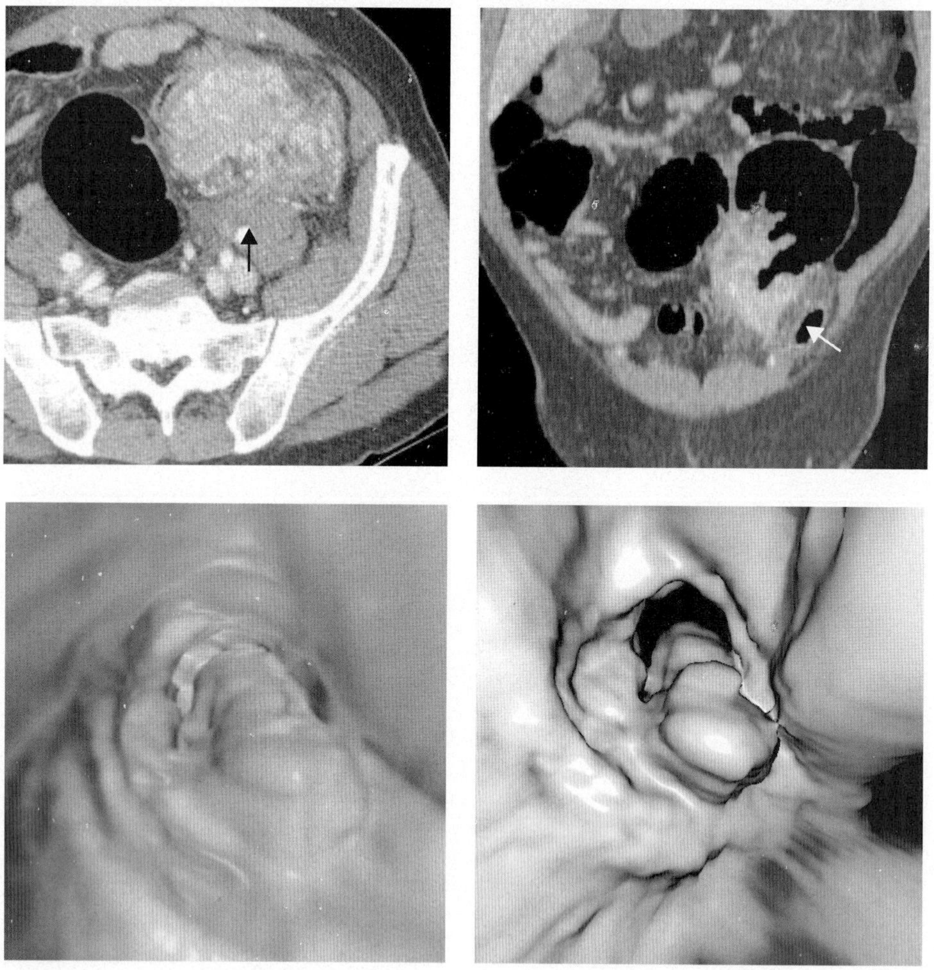

A B C D

FIGURE 5.30 Annular Sigmoid Carcinoma. Axial image **(A)** and coronal multiplanar reformat **(B)** shows a large annular mass causing obstruction. There is obliteration of the lumen noted on the 2D views and 3D endoluminal views **(C, D)**. Extensive invasion into the pericolonic fat is present. Pathology demonstrated a moderately differentiated adenocarcinoma.

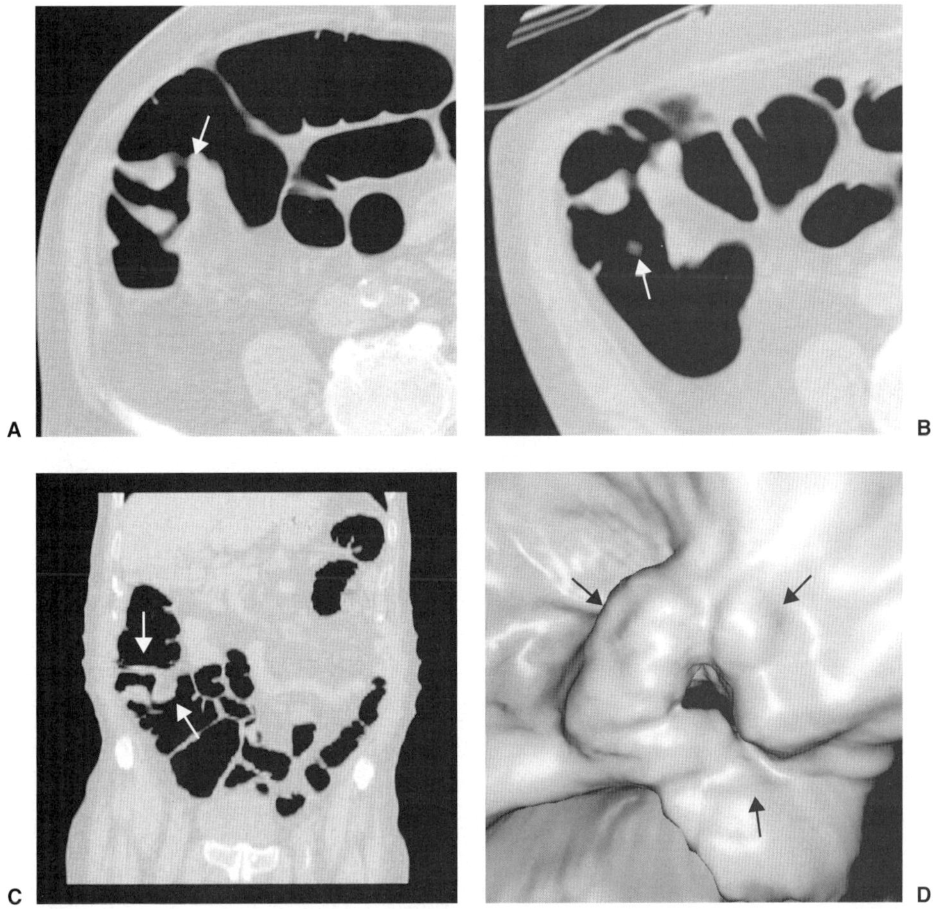

FIGURE 5.31 Near-Occlusive Ascending Colon Carcinoma. Axial image in the supine **(A)** and prone **(B)** positions shows a fixed mass causing wall and fold thickening and luminal narrowing, which is easily identified on the coronal multiplanar reformat **(C)**. The heaped up border of the tumor margin is well demonstrated on the 3D endoluminal view **(D)**.

indicative of transmural spread.[7] Lymph node size may not correlate with malignant involvement. The presence of lymph nodes in the perirectal or presacral areas are considered abnormal and are suspicious for nodal metastases in the absence of an obvious infectious etiology. Intravenous contrast may be given to more clearly delineate a potentially malignant lesion and the adjacent normal colonic wall as well as to identify and stage extraluminal extent of disease. Limited focused decubitus views may also be obtained for further evaluation if the lesion is not well characterized on one of the supine or prone positions due to retained fluid or residual stool.

The appearance of colorectal cancers on 3D views varies according to the morphologic type of the lesion (see Figs. 5.32–5.34). Ulcerative masses often demonstrate an irregular wall surface and may have sharp transition to overhanging edges. The lesions are fixed in location on both supine and prone data sets although some masses may demonstrate a different appearance with change in position due to differing degrees of luminal distention. Polypoid and lobulated masses protrude into the lumen and can cause narrowing, which is identified on the 3D endoluminal view. Annular lesions typically cause an abrupt end to the 3D endoluminal navigation with significant narrowing or obliteration of the lumen. Collapse or underdistention of a segment may mimic annular carcinoma on 3D views and 2D views are essential for differentiation. Coronal and/or sagittal multiplanar reformatted views are often the most useful images for evaluation of large malignant masses and provides the most accurate size measurements.

The differential diagnosis for masses or annular lesions on 3D endoluminal view is quite extensive. Lesions resembling masses include benign tumors, diverticulitis, inflammatory or infectious disease, colitis cystica profunda, residual stool, food, or pills, postsurgical changes, and extrinsic compression. In addition, nonepithelial malignancy may present as mass lesions.[50] Lesions resembling annular cancers include benign strictures, partial collapse, and extrinsic compression. Synchronous cancers are present in 1.5% to 6% of newly diagnosed colorectal cancer.[7,50] CTC has a definitive clinical role for incomplete fiberoptic colonoscopy, and synchronous

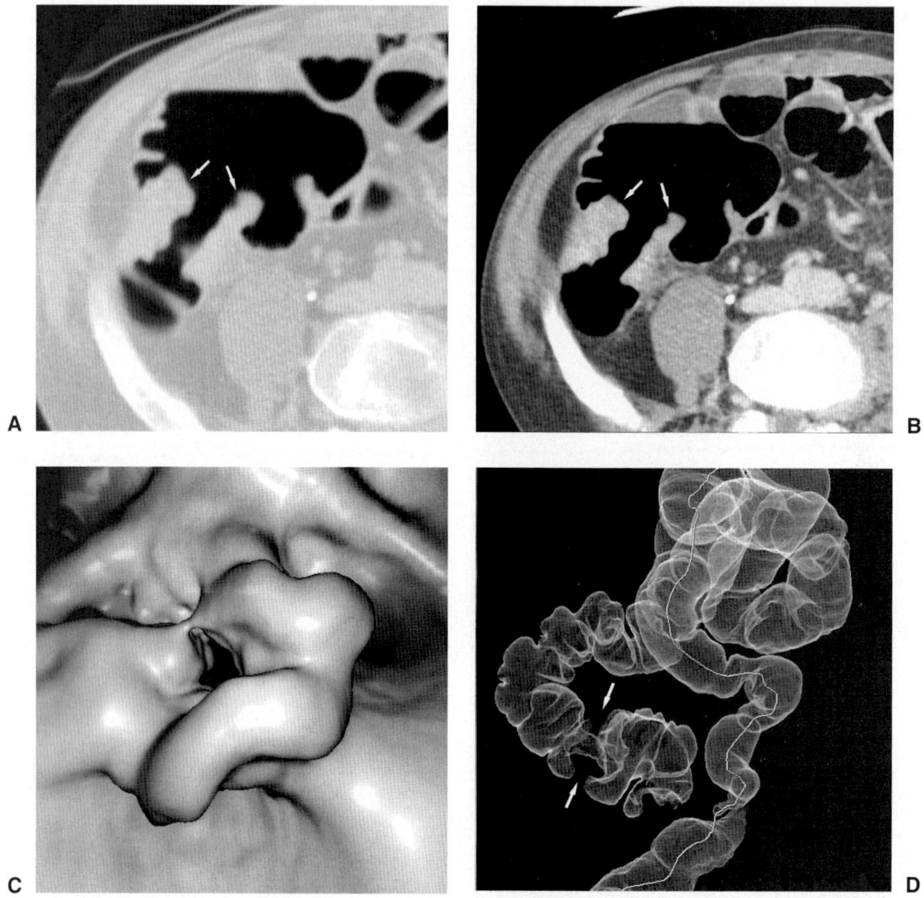

FIGURE 5.32 Annular Ascending Colon Carcinoma. Axial prone image in colon window **(A)** and abdominal window **(B)** show an apple-core lesion of the ascending colon with a narrow transition zone from tumor to normal wall (white arrows). 3D endoluminal view shows the irregular nodular border of the tumor. Volumetric reconstruction of the colon **(D)** simulating a double-contrast barium enema is useful for providing an overview and demonstrating the exact location of the tumor (white arrows). Pathology revealed invasive moderately differentiated adenocarcinoma.

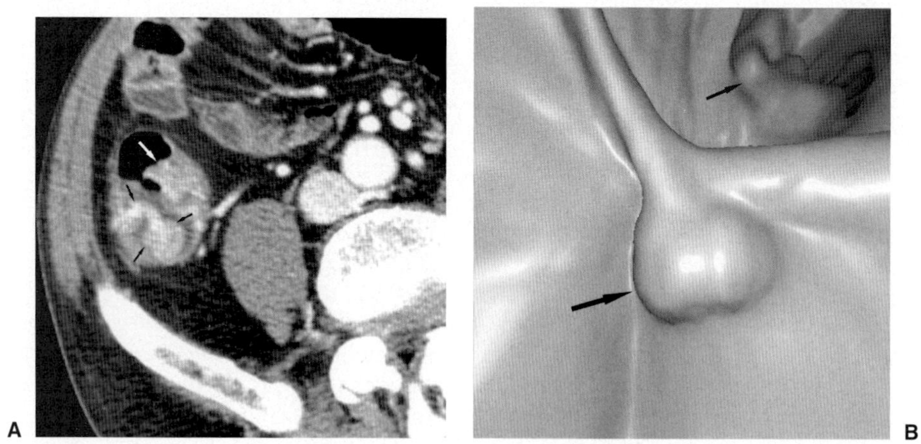

FIGURE 5.33 Ascending Colon Carcinoma and Large Pedunculated Polyp. Axial image **(A)** shows contrast enhancement of the head and stalk of a pedunculated polyp (black arrows) as well as an adjacent intraluminal mass (white arrow). 3D endoluminal view **(B)** shows the large pedunculated adenomatous polyp on a long stalk with the irregular nodular ascending colon adenocarcinoma in the background of the image. The pedunculated polyp was benign (no dysplasia), which was likely given the long length of the stalk >2 cm.

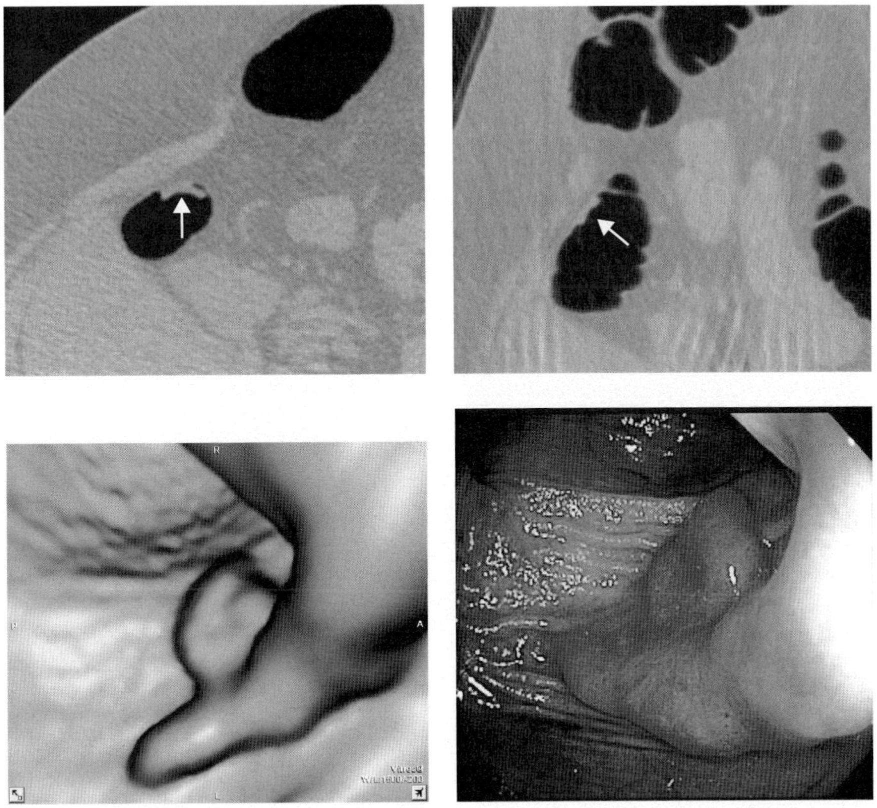

FIGURE 5.34 Atypical Adenocarcinoma. Axial images in supine **(A)** and prone **(B)** positions show a large but subtle flat lesion in the transverse colon with associated mild wall thickening. Patient also has a large ventral hernia. 3D endoluminal view **(C)** and endoscopic image **(D)** demonstrates a thickened fold with a sessile broad-based lesion. Biopsies revealed adenocarcinoma involving both the thickened fold and the polypoid component. (Views C and D: See also color plate.)

lesions may be found proximal to the primary cancer. The estimated risk of developing a metachranous cancer following the removal of a primary colonic adenocarcinoma is approximately 5% to 10%.[7,50] Particular attention should be given to surgical colonic anastamoses for signs of recurrence (irregularity, excessive mural thickening, obstruction) in patients who have undergone surgical resection of a primary colorectal malignancy. Approximately 20% of cases will demonstrate recurrence of malignancy and 20% of recurrences occur at the anastomotic site. The local lesion is the only evidence of recurrent disease in 30% of patients.[49]

The goal of CTC is to identify adenomatous polyps before degeneration into colonic malignancy. It is imperative to recognize the normal anatomy of the colon in order to communicate lesion location to clinicians and to be aware of the 2D and 3D appearances of normal anatomy to avoid potential false positives. Recognition of the common appearances of colorectal cancer is important for early identification and surgical treatment. Identification of extracolonic spread is an important finding given its impact on staging. Distinguishing between neoplastic polyps and non-neoplastic polyps and knowing the common morphologic appearances of polyps is essential to a high level of confidence in polyp detection. Particular attention should be given to identifying flat lesions as they may carry a greater malignant risk than lesions with a polypoid morphology.

REFERENCES

1. Bond JH. Clinical evidence for the adenoma-carcinoma sequence, and the management of patients with colorectal adenomas. *Semin Gastrointest Dis*. 2000;11:176–184.
2. Leslie A, Carey FA, Pratt NR, et al. The colorectal adenoma-carcinoma sequence. *Br J Surg*. 2002;89:845–860.
3. Aldridge AJ, Simson JN. Histological assessment of colorectal adenomas by size: are polyps less than 10 mm in size clinically important? *Eur J Surg*. 2001;167:777–781.
4. Muto T, Bussey HJR, Morson BC. The evolution of cancer of the colon and rectum. *Cancer*. 1975;36:2251–2270.
5. Macrae FA, Young GP. Neoplastic and nonneoplastic polyps of the colon and rectum *Textbook of Gastroenterology*, 3rd ed, Vol. 2. Philadelphia: Lippincott Williams & Wilkins; 1999:1965–1994.
6. Figel LS, Figel SJ, Wieterson FK. Roentgenologic observation of growth rates of colonic polyps and carcinoma. *Acta Radiol Diagn*. 1965;3:417.
7. Stewart ET, Dodds WJ. Neoplastic colonic lesions. Freeny PC, Stevenson GW, eds. *Margulis and Burhenne's*

Alimentary Tract Radiology, 5th ed. St. Louis: Mosby; 1994:762–800.

8. Welin S, Youker J, Spratt JS. The rates and patterns of growth of 375 tumors of the large intestine and rectum observed serially by double contrast enema study (Malmö technique). *Am J Roentgenol*. 1963;90:673.
9. Boland CR, Bresalier RS, Colonic polyps and polyposis syndromes. Greenfield LJ,Mulholland MW, Zelenock GB, Oldham KT, Lillimoe KD, eds. *Surgery: Scientific Principles and Practice*, 2nd ed. Philadelphia: Lippincott-Raven. 1997:1109–1127.
10. Eide TJ. Natural history of adenomas. *World J Surg*. 1991;15:3–6.
11. Eisenberg RL. Single filling defects in the colon.Eisenberg RL, ed.*Gastrointestinal Radiology, a Pattern Approach*, 4th ed. Philadelphia: Lippincott Williams & Wilkins; 2002:667–698.
12. Colucci PM, Yale SH, Rall CJ. Colorectal polyps. *Clin Med Res*. 2003;1:261–262.
13. Winawer SJ, Zauber AG. The advanced adenoma as the primary target of screening. *Gastrointest Endosc Clin N Am*. 2002;12:1–9.
14. Khan A, Shrier I, Gordon PH. The changed histologic paradigm of colorectal polyps. *Surg Endosc*. 2002;16:436–440.
15. Winawer SJ, Fletcher RH, Miller L, et al. Colorectal cancer screening: clinical guidelines and rationale. *Gastroenterology*. 1997;112:594–642.
16. Winawer SJ, Zauber AG, Fletcher RH, et al. Guidelines for colonoscopy surveillance after polypectomy: a consensus update by the US Multi-Society Task Force on Colorectal Cancer and the American Cancer Society. *Gastroenterology*. 2006;130:1872–1885.
17. Bertoni G, Sassatelli R, Conigliaro R, et al. Visual disappearing phenomenon can reliably predict the nonadenomatous nature of rectal and rectosigmoid diminutive polyps at endoscopy. *Gastrointest Endosc*. 1994;40:588–591.
18. Fenlon HM, Nunes DM, Schroy PC, et al. A comparison of virtual and conventional colonoscopy for the detection of colorectal polyps. *N Engl J Med*. 1999;341:1496–1503.
19. Pickhardt PJ, Choi JR, Hwang I, et al. Nonadenomatous polyps at CT colonography: prevalence, size distribution, and detection rates. *Radiology*. 2004;232:784–790.
20. Hyman NH, Anderson P, Blasyk H. Hyperplastic polyposis and the risk of colorectal cancer. *Dis Colon Rectum*. 2004;47:2102–2104.
21. Desai DC, Neale KF, Talbot IC, et al. Juvenile polyposis. *Br J Surg*. 1995;82:14–17.
22. Mesiya S, Ancha HB, Ancha H, et al. Sporadic colonic hamartomas in adults: a retrospective study. *Gastrointest Endosc*. 2005;62:886–891.
23. Coady-Fariborzian L, Angel LP, Procaccino JA. Perforated colon secondary to virtual colonoscopy: report of a case. *Dis Colon Rectum*. 2004;47:1247–1249.
24. Triester SL, Hara AK, Young-Fadok TM, et al. Colonic perforation after computed tomographic colonography in a patient with fibrostenosing Crohn's disease. *Am J Gastroenterol*. 2006;101:189–192.
25. Bariol C, Hawkins NJ, Turner JJ, et al. Histopathological and clinical evaluation of serrated adenomas of the colon and rectum. *Mod Pathol*. 2003;16:417–423.
26. Hawkins NJ, Bariol C, Ward RL. The serrated neoplasia pathway. *Pathology*. 2002;34:548–555.
27. Burgart LJ. Colorectal polyps and other precursor lesions. Need for an expanded view. *Gastroenterol Clin North Am*. 2002;31:959–970.
28. Ferrucci JT. Colon cancer screening with virtual colonoscopy: promise, polyps and politics. *Am J Roentgenol*. 2001;177:975–988.
29. Read TE, Read JD, Butterly LF. Importance of adenomas 5 mm or less in diameter that are detected by sigmoidoscopy. *N Engl J Med*. 1997;336:8–12.
30. Waye JD, Lewis BS, Frankel A, et al. Small colon polyps. *Am J Gastroenterol*. 1988;83:120–122.
31. Tsai CJ, Lu DK. Small colorectal polyps: histopathology and clinical significance. *Am J Gastroenterol*. 1995;90:988–994.
32. Nusko G, Mansmann U, Altendorf-Hofmann A, et al. Risk of invasive carcinoma in colorectal adenomas assesses by size and site. *Int J Colorectal Dis*. 1997;12:267–271.
33. Sciallero S, Bonelli L, Aste H, et al. Do patients with rectosigmoid adenomas 5 mm or less in diameter need total colonoscopy? *Gastrointest Endosc*. 1999;50:314–321.
34. American College of Radiology. ACR practice guideline for the performance of computed tomography (CT) colonography in adults. In Practice Guidelines and Technical Standards 2005. Reston, VA: American College of Radiology; 2005:295–299.
35. Gluecker TM, Fletcher JG, Welch TJ, et al. Characterization of lesions missed on interpretation of CT colonography using a 2D search method. *Am J Roentgenol*. 2004;182:881–889.
36. Pickhardt PJ, Choi JR, Hwang I, et al. Computed tomographic virtual colonoscopy to screen for colorectal neoplasia in asymptomatic adults. *N Engl J Med*. 2003;349:2191–2200.
37. Macari M, Bini E, Jacobs SL, et al. Filling defects at CT colonography: pseudo- and diminutive lesions (the good), polyps (the bad), flat lesions, masses, and carcinomas (the ugly). *Radiographics*. 2003;23:1073–1091.
38. Macari M, Megibow AJ. Pitfalls of using three-dimensional CT colonography with two-dimensional imaging correlation. *Am J Roentgenol*. 2001;176:137–143.
39. Fenlon HM, Clarke PD, Ferruci JT. Virtual colonoscopy: imaging features with colonoscopic correlation. *Am J Roentgenol*. 1998;170:1303–1309.
40. Smith TR. Pedunculated malignant colonic polyps with superficial invasion of the stalk. *Radiology*. 1975;115:593–596.
41. Rembacken BJ, Fujiti T, Cairns A, et al. Flat and depressed colonic neoplasms: a prospective study of 1000 colonoscopies in the UK. *Lancet*. 2000;355:1211–1214.
42. Fidler JL, Johnson CD, MacCarty RL, et al. Detection of flat lesions in the colon with CT colonography. *Abdom Imaging*. 2002;27:292–300.
43. Pickhardt PJ, Nugent PA, Choi JR, et al. Flat colorectal lesions in asymptomatic adults: implications for screening with CT virtual colonoscopy. *Am J Roentgenol*. 2004;183:1343–1347.
44. Rubio CA, Kato Y, Hirota Y, et al. Histological classification of endoscopically removed flat colorectal polyps: a multicentre study. *Jpn J Cancer Res*. 1996;87:849–855.
45. Togashi K, Konishi F, Koinuma K, et al. Flat and depressed lesions of the colon and rectum: pathogenesis and clinical management. *Ann Acad Med Singapore*. 2003;32:152–158.
46. O'Brien MJ, Winawer SJ, Zauber AG, et al. Flat adenomas in the National Polyp Study: is there increased risk for high-grade dysplasia initially or during surveillance? *Clin Gastroenterol Hepatol*. 2004;2:905–911.
47. Hurlstone DP, Brown S, Cross SS. The role of flat and depressed colorectal lesions in colorectal carcinogenesis: new insights from clinicopathological findings in high-magnification chromoscopic colonoscopy. *Histopathology*. 2003;43:413–426.
48. Park SH, Ha HK, Kim AY, et al. Flat polyps of the colon: detection with 16-MDCT Colonography preliminary results. *Am J Roentgenol*. 2006;186:1611–1617.

49. Chang AE. Colorectal cancer. Greenfield LJ,Mulholland MW, Zelenock GB, Oldham KT, Lillimoe KD, eds. *Surgery: Scientific Principles and Practice*, 2nd ed. Philadelphia: Lippincott-Raven; 1997:1128–1146.
50. Boland CR. Malignant tumors of the colon. *Textbook of Gastroenterology*, 3rd ed, Vol. 2. Philadelphia: Lippincott Williams & Wilkins; 1999:2023–2082.
51. Ota Y, Matsui T, Ono H, et al. Value of virtual computed tomographic colonography for Crohn's colitis: comparison with endoscopy and barium enema. *Abdom Imaging*. 2003;28:778–783.
52. Silverstein FE, Tytgat GNJ. *Atlas of Gastrointestinal Endoscopy*, 2nd ed. Philadelphia: JB Lippincott Co; 1991: 1.17–1.26.
53. Megibow AJ. Computed tomography and magnetic resonance imaging in colorectal carcinoma: staging and detection of postoperative recurrence. Freeny PC, Stevenson GW. *Margulis and Burhenne's Alimentary Tract Radiology*, 5th ed. St. Louis: Mosby; 1994:801–812.
54. Miller TA. Colon, rectum, and anus. *Surgery: Scientific Principles and Practice*, 2nd ed. Philadelphia: Lippincott-Raven; 1997:1083–1093.
55. Raskin MM, Viamonte M, Viamonte M Jr. Primary linitis plastica carcinoma of the colon. *Radiology*. 1974;113:17–22.
56. Kumar V, Cotran RS, Robbins SL. *Basic Pathology*, 5th ed. Philadelphia: WB Saunders; 1992:473–522.
57. Schiller KFR, Cockel R, Hunt RH, et al. *Atlas of Gastrointestinal Endoscopy and Related Pathology*, 2nd ed. Tokyo: Blackwell Science; 2002:227–341.
58. Geelhoed GW, Crossland SG. Carcinoma of the right colon: a change in characteristic configuration? *South Med J*. 1981;74:1436–1438.

CHAPTER 6 PITFALLS

Gregory M. Galdino and Judy Yee

The appearances of many lesions and disease processes can mimic colonic polyps and cancer on computed tomographic colonography (CTC) (see Table 6.1). Atypical appearances of polyps or cancers may resemble residual stool or other benign processes. Potential pitfalls include normal anatomic structures as well as alterations of normal anatomy, pseudopolypoid and pseudoannular lesions, diverticulae, flat lesions, external impression upon the colonic lumen, and various artifacts. Many pitfalls have typical appearances that can differentiate them from true polyps and cancer.

Certain pitfalls may be specific to two-dimensional (2D) or three-dimensional (3D) images. Pitfalls that occur on 2D images may be due to the limitations of viewing in one plane. A common pseudopolypoid pitfall encountered on 2D views that often requires 3D views for problem solving are bulbous or complex folds. Many pitfalls seen on 3D views are polypoid-appearing lesions such as residual stool or pills, which can often be distinguished from true polyps using 2D images. Some pitfalls occur on both 2D and 3D images and it may be impossible to differentiate them from true polyps or cancer. The most commonly encountered pitfall seen on all types of views is homogeneous adherent stool. Common and uncommon pitfalls encountered during CTC interpretation are reviewed in this section.

NORMAL ANATOMIC STRUCTURES

Bulbous Fold

Bulbous or complex haustral folds are a common cause of false positives on CTC, particularly on 2D images.[1–3] They may have the appearance of a polypoid or less commonly a mass-like lesion. Bulbous folds are one of the most common pitfalls seen on axial images that require multiplanar reformats or 3D views for problem solving (see Figures 6.1–6.3). These may represent haustral folds that are normally slightly thickened, complex interhaustral folds, crossing folds (see Figure 6.4), or may be due to the confluence of folds (see Figures 6.5 and 6.6). Complex folds are typically encountered at the hepatic and splenic flexures[3,4] (see Figure 6.7). Other causes of thickened folds, particularly in the sigmoid, are poor distention and muscular hypertrophy associated with diverticulosis. A suboptimally distended sigmoid may demonstrate large, thickened folds extending from both sides of the bowel wall that meet in the middle ("kissing folds")[1] (see Figure 6.8). Multiplanar reformats are very helpful for further evaluation of bulbous folds and can often quickly show the linear morphology of haustral folds. 3D endoluminal views can easily delineate the typical smooth, symmetric linear appearance of a fold as well as the convergence of folds. The subvolume cube view, which is available on many workstations, is particularly useful for rapidly focusing on an area in question and allows easy 360-degree rotation to differentiate a fold from a true polyp.

When a polypoid-appearing lesion is suspected of being a bulbous fold on 2D views, the potential lesion should be evaluated on the opposing view. The appearance of a bulbous fold may change and appear more linear with improved distention on the opposing view. Folds that have an irregular contour, appear thickened or different from adjacent folds particularly in an otherwise well-distended, well-distended colon should be approached with caution because they can represent infiltrating cancers, flat lesions, or carpet lesions.[1,5,6]

The rectum near the anal verge often has prominent longitudinally oriented folds (rectal columns of Morgagni) that may appear mass-like or polypoid on axial images, particularly with underdistention of the rectum. The 3D views are useful for problem solving these folds. Specific attention should be paid to the area surrounding the rectal tube because the catheter and/or inflated balloon may obscure findings, particularly low-lying and flat lesions at the anal verge.[7] Suspicious lesions should be confirmed in the opposing position because folds will often change appearance with a change in position. Sagittal and coronal multiplanar reformatted views are often helpful for evaluation of folds in the rectum,

TABLE 6.1 Pitfalls on Virtual Colonoscopy

Normal Anatomic Structures

- Bulbous fold
- Ileocecal valve
- Appendix–Orifice or Inverted Stump (C)

Variant Anatomy

- Congenital–malrotation
- Acquired–hernia, postsurgical
- Mobile segment (S, T, C)

Pseudopolypoid Lesions

- Stool
- Pills and seeds
- Internal hemorrhoid (R)
- Hypertrophied anal papillae (R)
- Mucous strand
- Air bubble
- Lipoma
- Gastrointestinal stromal tumor (R)

Pseudoannular Lesions

- Poor distention or collapse
- Wall thickening

Carpet Lesion (R, AC, C)

Diverticulosis (S)

- Muscular hypertrophy
- Diverticular orifice
- Impacted diverticulum
- Inverted diverticulum

Artifacts

- Respiratory
- Metallic
- Stair–step
- Digital subtraction

External Compression

- Liver
- Spleen
- Gallbladder
- Kidney
- Bowel
- Uterus
- Vasculature
- Psoas muscle
- Diaphragmatic crus

Common location(s): R, rectum; S, sigmoid; T, transverse colon; C, cecum.

which usually tapers towards the anal verge. A rectal bar representing a more prominent longitudinal fold may be visualized along the anterior rectal wall (see Figure 6.9). A subtle, small pseudopolypoid lesion may be visualized along the posterior rectal wall on the 2D views at the point of anterior angulation of the rectum (see Figure 6.10).

Ileocecal Valve

The ileocecal valve (ICV) is variable in appearance. There are three types of ICV—a polypoid (papillary) valve is a dome-like protrusion with its mouth at the apex, a labial type is the most common and appears as a thickened fold with the mouth separating the margins of the fold, and an intermediate type which has features of both[1,2] (see Chapter 4). In a study of 71 patients who underwent CTC, it was found that the ICV was at least partially visualized in 94% of cases, more frequently in the supine position.[8] Characterization of the ICV on double-contrast barium enema showed a normal mean valve height of 1.7 cm and a mean width of 2.8 cm.[9] Maximum height of the normal valve was approximately 4 cm. The valve was smooth in 85% of patients and mildly lobulated in 15% of patients.

A specific feature of the ICV is a central depression or "pit" (orifice where the terminal ileum empties into the right colon), which may be seen on 2D and 3D views. Additionally, its common location is along the medial wall of the colon where the terminal ileum enters (see Figure 6.11). If there is difficulty in identifying the ICV on axial images, it is best to locate the terminal ileum on the coronal multiplanar reformat and follow it in to the right colon. Readers should attempt to identify the ICV in each patient. The ICV may also be used as a landmark for identification of the cecum in cases where there is mobility of the segment.

Fatty infiltration (lipomatosis) of the ICV may cause it to resemble a mass on 3D endoluminal views, but 2D views will easily show its fat density (see Figure 6.12). Lipomatosis of the ICV tends to cause symmetric enlargement of the valve. Lipomas can also occur on the valve, but these are often asymmetric masses.[10] Polyps and adenocarcinoma can occur on the ICV as well because it is covered by colonic mucosa. Any disruption of the typical morphology of the ICV should be fully evaluated for possible polyp or malignancy (see Figure 6.13). Stool can also adhere to the ICV and cause angular type protrusions extending from the valve (see Figures 6.14 and 6.15). Occasionally, when the terminal ileum is distended it can prolapse into the cecum and cause an enlarged and elongated appearance of the ICV. The 2D views show protrusion of the air-filled terminal ileum into the cecum (see Figure 6.16).

Appendix: Orifice or Inverted Stump

The appendiceal orifice and cecal crow's feet have characteristic appearances that have been described in Chapter 4. The orifice of the appendix may appear closed and slit-like, open or protruding into the lumen on the 3D endoluminal views. The typical appendiceal orifice will appear as a sharply demarcated complete dark ring similar to a diverticulum (see Figure 6.17). Mass-like protrusions in the region of the appendiceal orifice should be regarded with suspicion and full evaluation should be performed for colorectal carcinoma (although rare) or carcinoid tumors. An inverted appendix or protruding appendicolith represent potential pitfalls and may resemble a polypoid or mass lesion on 2D views and on the 3D endoluminal view.[11,12]

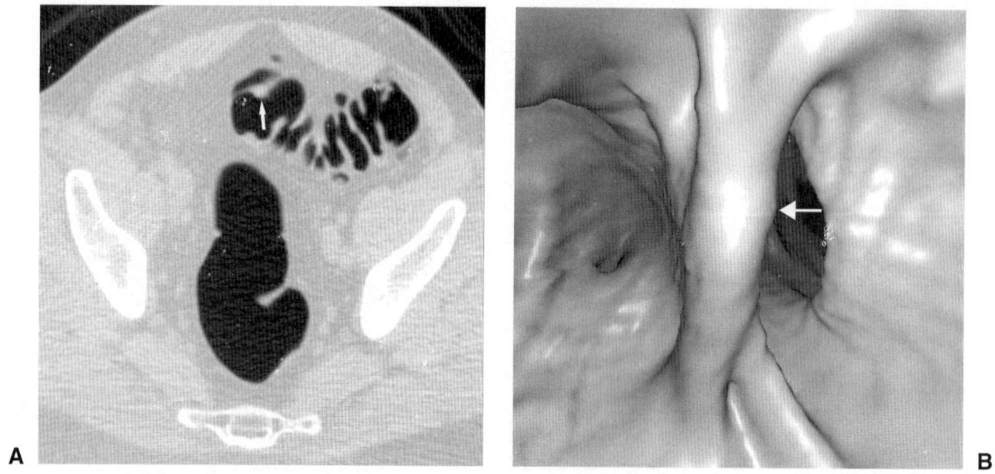

A B

FIGURE 6.1 Bulbous Fold: Axial image **(A)** reveals a polypoid lesion on a fold. The 3D endoluminal view **(B)** demonstrates a bulbous fold. No polyp was identified on colonoscopy.

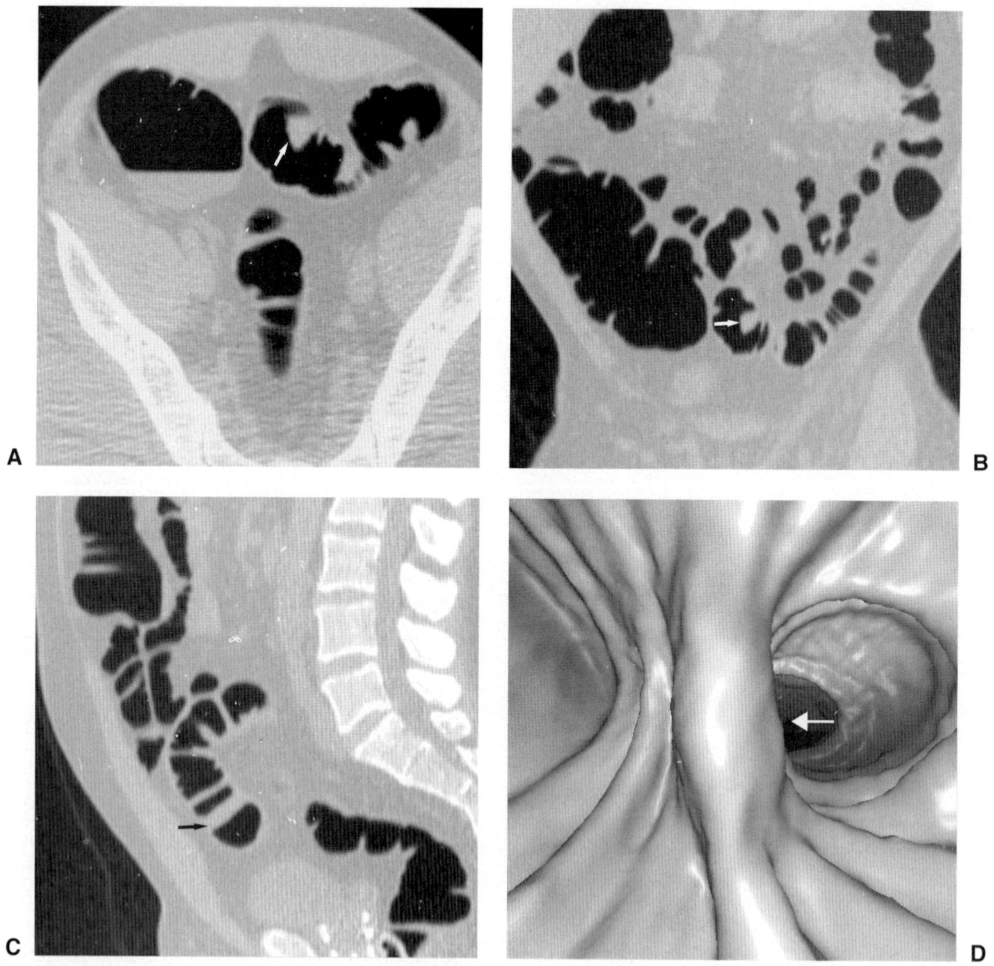

A B C D

FIGURE 6.2 Bulbous Fold: Axial supine image **(A)** and coronal reformat **(B)** reveal a homogeneous soft tissue density lesion in the sigmoid. The sagittal reformat **(C)** reveals a bulbous fold, which is also seen on the 3D image **(D)**. HINT: Note the polygonal appearance of the lesion on the first two views, which is not consistent with a true polyp.

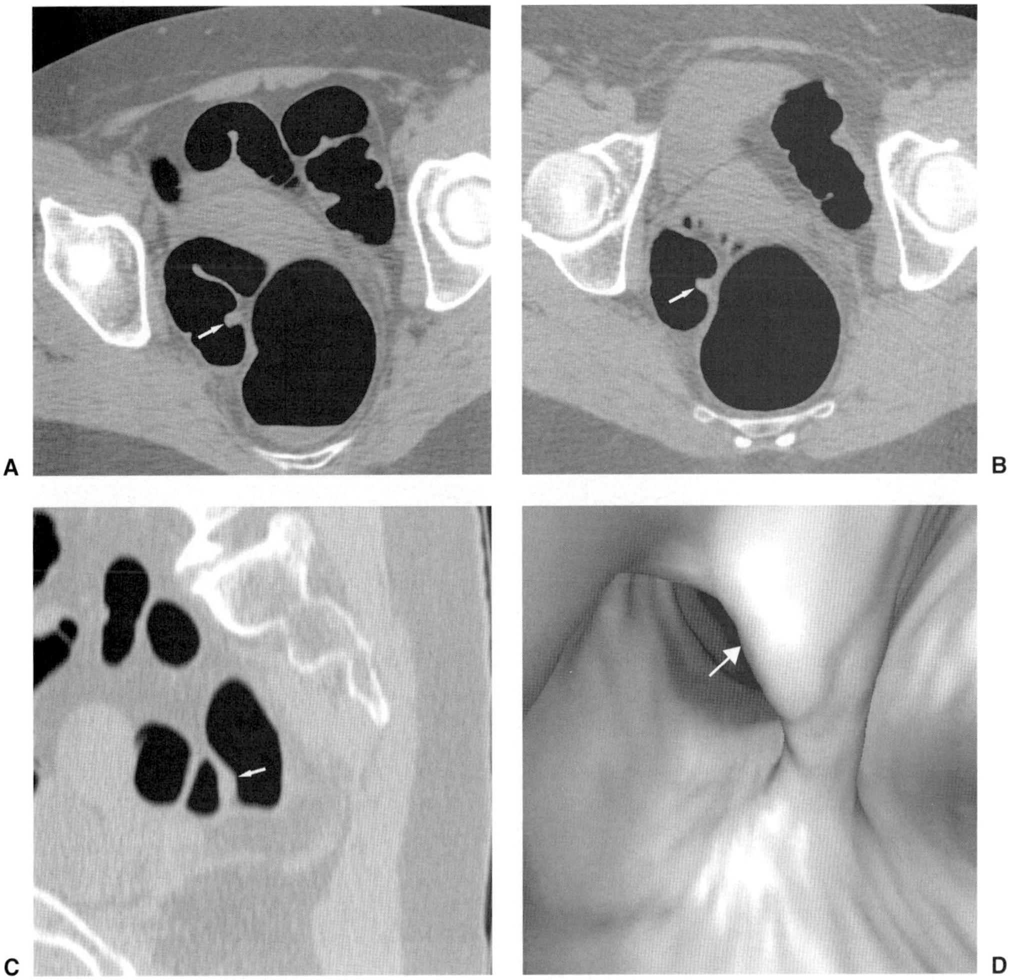

FIGURE 6.3 Bulbous Fold: Both the axial supine **(A)** and prone **(B)** images reveal a nonmobile homogeneous pseudopolypoid lesion. The sagittal view **(C)** and the 3D endoluminal view **(D)** demonstrate a bulbous fold.

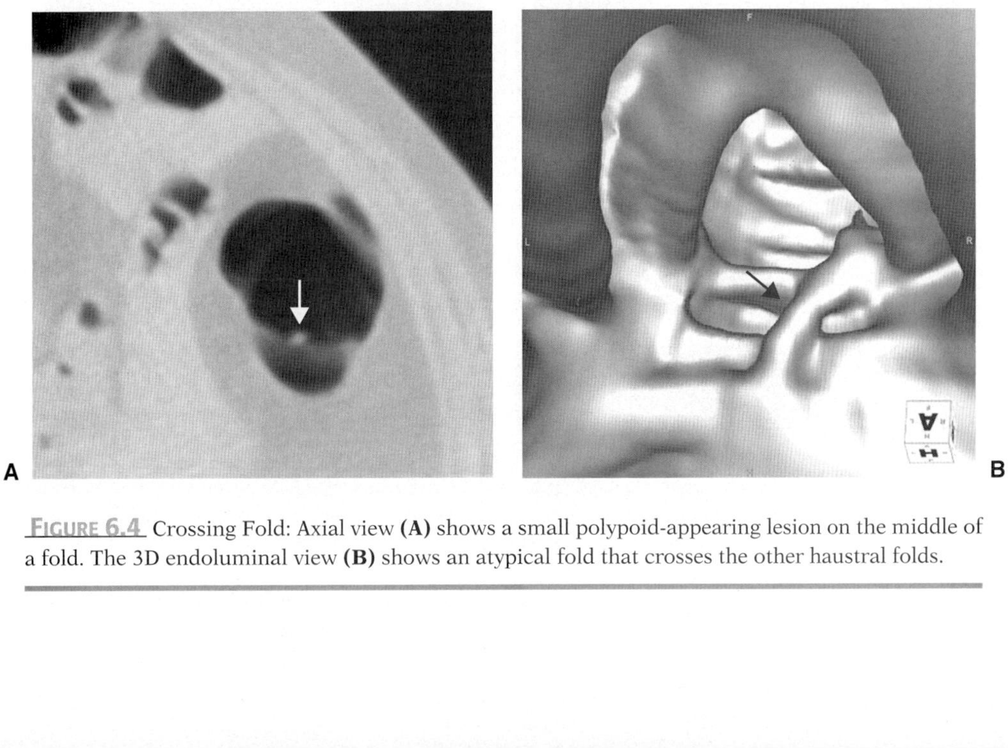

FIGURE 6.4 Crossing Fold: Axial view **(A)** shows a small polypoid-appearing lesion on the middle of a fold. The 3D endoluminal view **(B)** shows an atypical fold that crosses the other haustral folds.

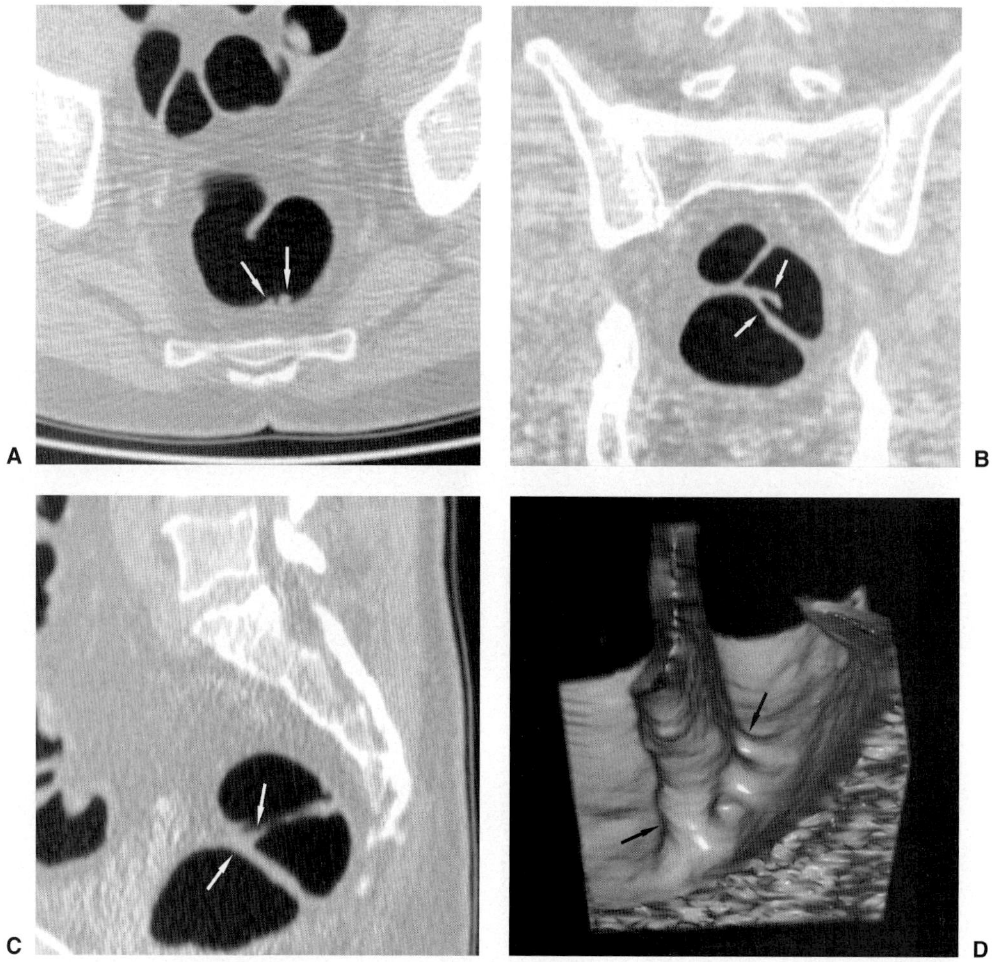

FIGURE 6.5 Confluence of Folds, Rectum: Axial image **(A)** shows two small pseudopolypoid lesions along the posterior wall. The coronal **(B)** and sagittal **(C)** reformats reveal that these represent the confluence of folds. The 3D cube view **(D)** also shows this well.

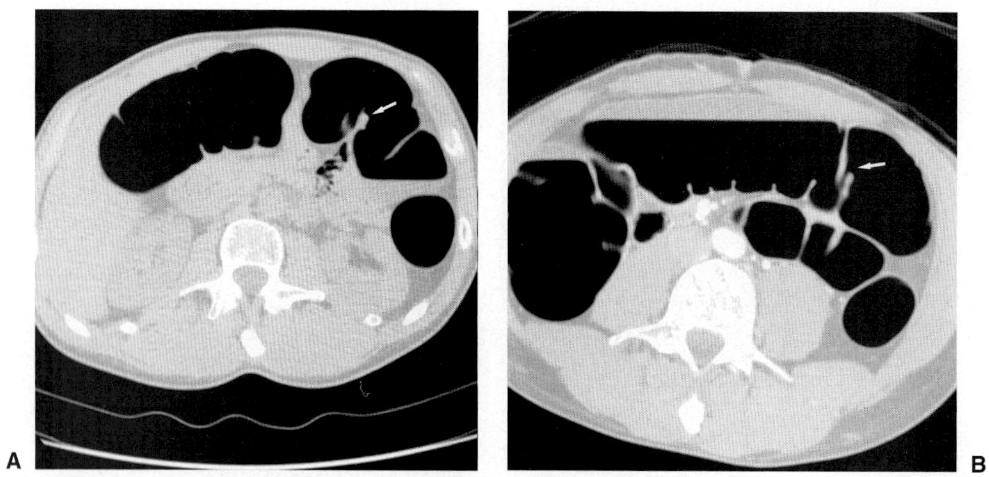

FIGURE 6.6 Confluence of Folds, Transverse Colon: Axial supine image **(A)** reveals a possible polyp. Images **(B)** and **(C)** represent consecutive slices from the axial prone series showing that this "lesion" represents a confluence of folds. The 3D endoluminal image **(D)** also shows folds converging. (*Views C and D are on next page.*)

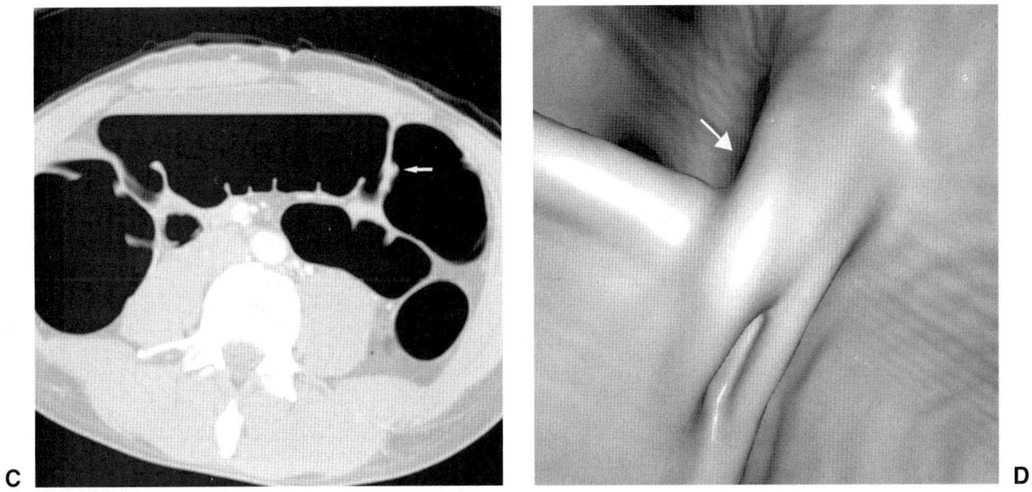

FIGURE 6.6 (*Continued*).

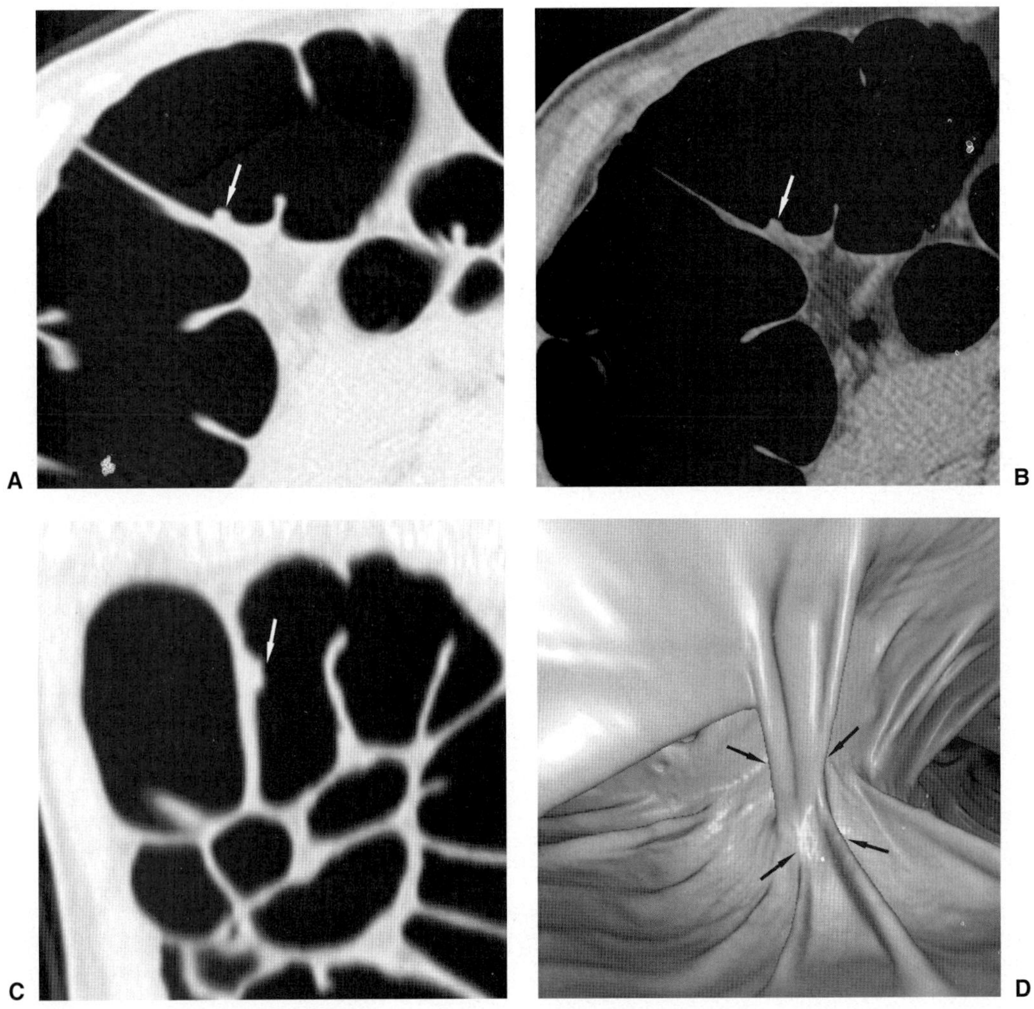

FIGURE 6.7 Complex Folds, Splenic Flexure: Axial images in colon **(A)** and abdominal **(B)** windows show a homogeneous pseudopolypoid lesion on a fold. The sagittal reformat **(C)** also shows the lesion. The 3D endoluminal view **(D)** shows a complex series of folds in an area of curvature.

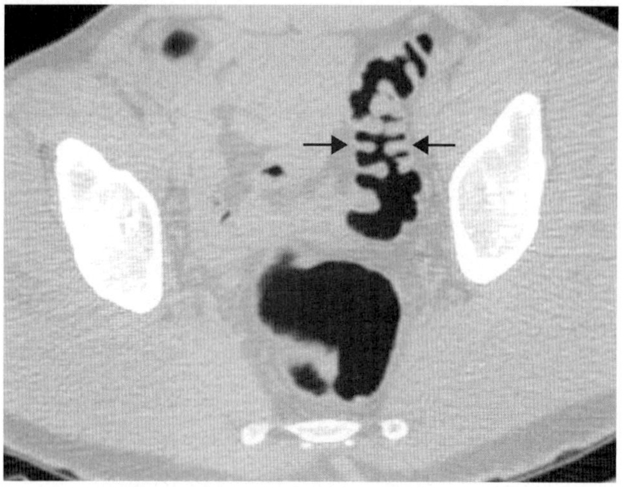

FIGURE 6.8 Kissing Folds: Axial image shows enlarged folds that may simulate polyps that extend towards the middle present in a poorly distended sigmoid.

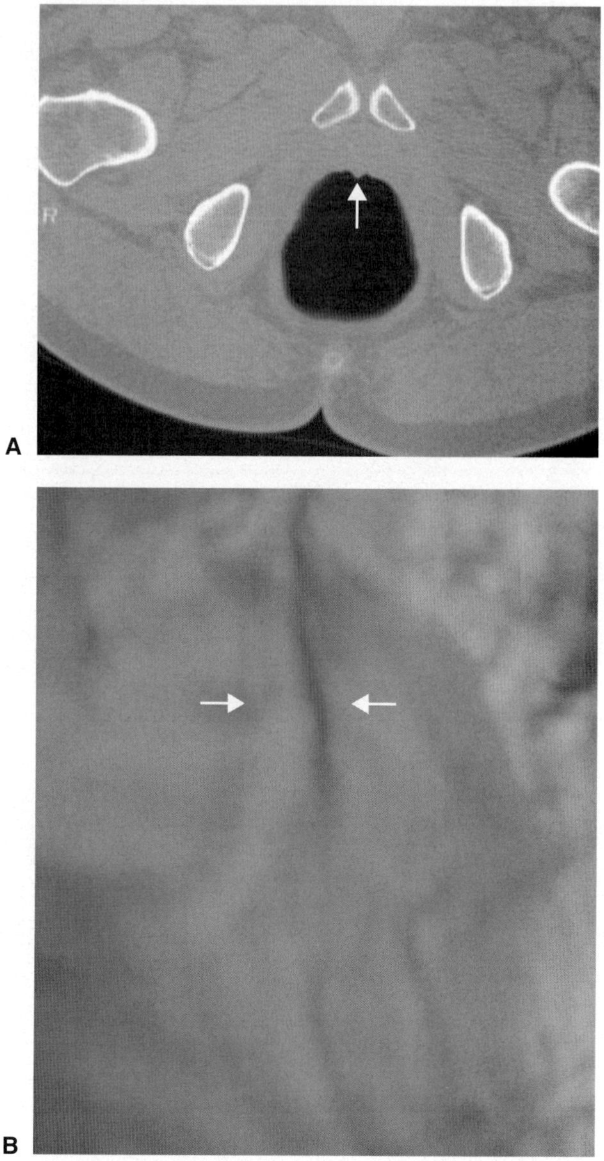

FIGURE 6.9 Anterior Rectal Bar: A small pseudopolypoid lesion is present along the anterior rectal wall on the axial image **(A)**. This correlates with a prominent fold in the same location on the 3D endoluminal view **(B)**.

The appendix may be partially or completely inverted. Use of the older inversion-ligation technique for appendectomy, which is not often used currently, will result in an appendiceal stump that may simulate a polyp.[12] If a potential polyp is identified on axial or 3D views, the reader should refer to the coronal or sagittal reformats to attempt to identify the appendix and the relation of the appendix, if present, to the lesion. History of prior appendectomy is important to obtain. An appendicolith is often also readily identifiable on 2D views. An inverted or intussuscepted cecal diverticulum has also been reported to simulate a pedunculated polyp on CT scan.[13]

VARIANT ANATOMY

Variations in colonic anatomy may be congenital (malrotation), acquired (surgical), or due to mobile segments. Alterations in the expected anatomy of the colon can make tracking the lumen difficult on axial views. The 3D transparency view (also known as *edge-enhanced view*, tissue transition projection) is helpful for demonstrating overall colonic anatomy and simulates a double-contrast barium enema in appearance. This view is not used for primary diagnosis of colonic lesions, but is helpful to the gastroenterologist and the colorectal surgeon to provide an overview of the colonic anatomy and location of lesions. When the sigmoid colon is redundant it may be difficult to track the lumen on axial images particularly if there is poor distention. Endoluminal 3D views may still be used to navigate through a redundant sigmoid unless the segment is underdistended.

Malrotation

Cecal volvulus accounts for 11% of all bowel volvulus.[14] Torsion of the cecum occurs as a result of loose fixation of the cecum and ascending colon resulting in large bowel obstruction. In general, partial malrotation is usually present in order for cecal volvulus to occur. There are two types of cecal volvulus—axial torsion and cecal bascule. Axial torsion is the most common (66%) and results in torsion (180–360 degrees) of the ascending colon and cecum around the longitudinal axis of the ascending colon resulting in obstruction and vascular compromise, usually associated with a high rate of mortality. If obstructive symptoms are present, the patient will present with obvious clinical symptoms of abdominal pain, nausea, and vomiting. The obstruction is usually a closed loop type and CTC is not indicated and should not be performed in this situation. The cecal bascule type results in the rotation of the cecum superior and anteromedial to the ascending

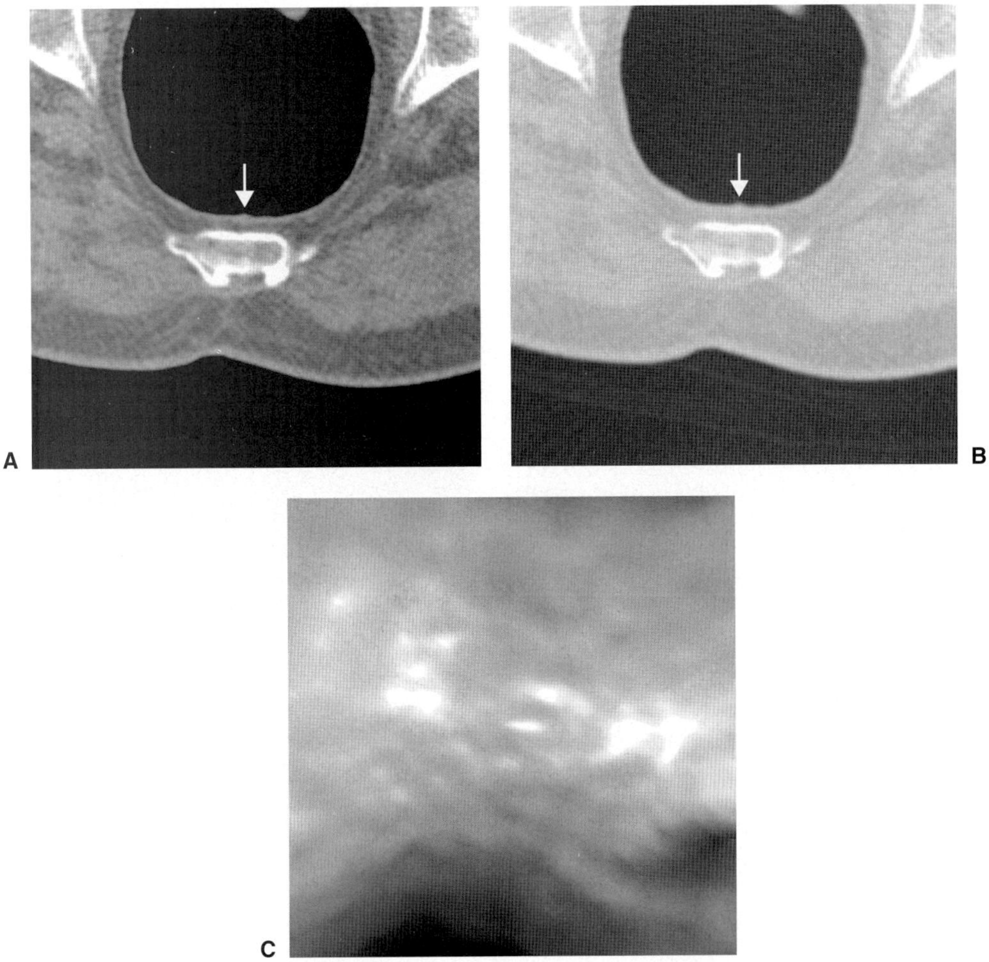

FIGURE 6.10 Posterior Rectal Wall Pseudopolyp: A minimal small protrusion can be seen on the axial images in abdominal **(A)** and colon **(B)** windows along the posterior rectal wall. No lesion is identified on the 3D view **(C)**. This finding has been described as the result of anterior angulation of the rectum.

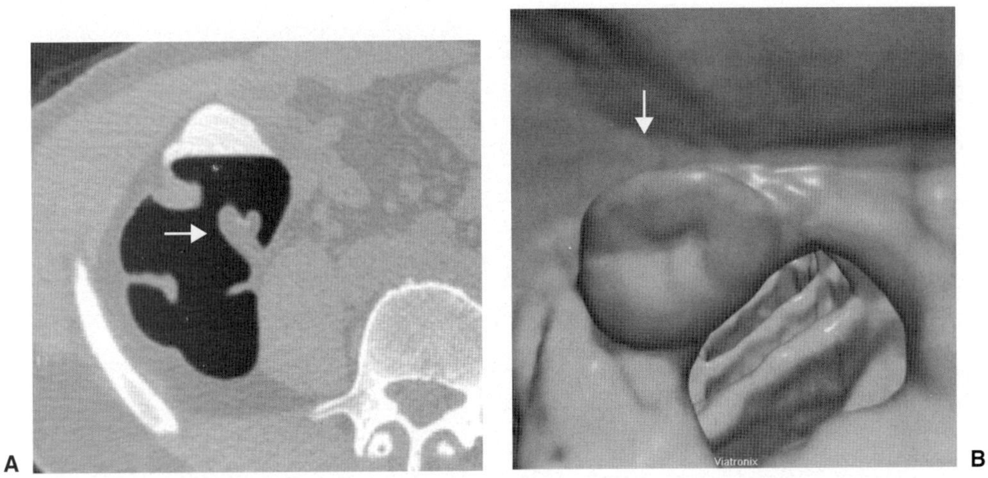

FIGURE 6.11 Normal Ileocecal Valve: Axial **(A)** and 3D endoluminal **(B)** views show the typical appearance of the ileocecal valve as rounded or ovoid with a central depression or pit.

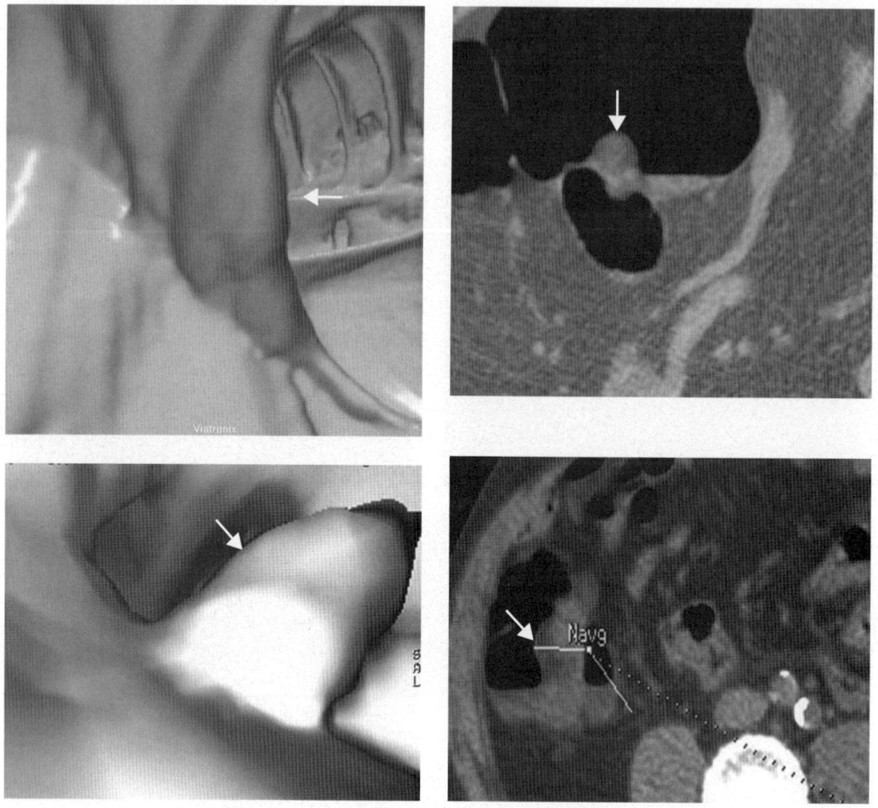

FIGURE 6.12 Lipomatosis of the Ileocecal Valve: When the ileocecal valve becomes infiltrated with fat, the central depression may not be as evident on the 3D endoluminal view **(A)**. The axial view demonstrates the fatty density of the valve **(B)**. In another patient lipomatosis causes the ileocecal valve to enlarge and appear mass-like on the 3D endoluminal view **(C)** and on the axial view **(D)**.

colon, and often occurs with a flap-valve occlusion at the site of flexion[15] (see Figure 6.18). Patients may also present with obstructive symptoms, although if the ileum undergoes passive rotation with the cecum obstruction may not occur. These patients may then present for CTC following an incomplete colonoscopy.

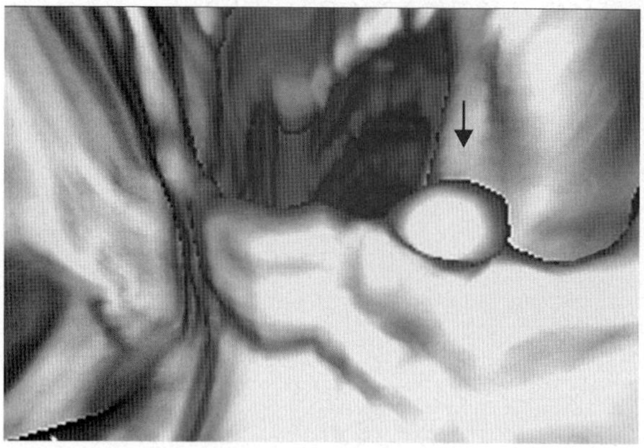

FIGURE 6.13 Polyp on Ileocecal Valve: The ileocecal valve is covered by colonic mucosa and polyps and carcinoma can develop on the valve. 3D endoluminal view shows a polyp on the ileocecal valve.

Incomplete rotation and malrotation of the bowel may contribute to difficulty tracking the colonic lumen on axial images. The 3D endoluminal view will allow easier tracking if the colon is adequately distended. The 3D transparency view is most helpful for rapidly demonstrating overall colonic anatomy. During embryogenesis, the bowel undergoes 270 degrees of counterclockwise rotation outside and inside of the peritoneal cavity. The duodenal–jejunal junction and ligament of Trietz come to lie in the left upper quadrant across the midline to the left of the second lumbar vertebral body, with the colon framing the small bowel, the jejunum residing in the left upper quadrant, and the ileum in the right lower quadrant.[16] The duodenum and colon undergo separate rotations and their position relative to the superior mesenteric artery (SMA) and superior mesenteric vein (SMV) can indicate the degree of proper rotation. Failure of proper rotation (malrotation) can occur, giving rise to a short mesenteric base and abnormal bowel anatomy which may predispose to twisting or volvulus around the superior mesenteric vessels.[16] Many cases of malrotation are associated with other congenital birth defects such as gastroschisis, omphalocele, diagphragmatic hernia, or duodenal or jejunal atresia. These entities come to clinical attention early. Malrotation is also associated with situs anomalies, which may or may not present early in life.[17]

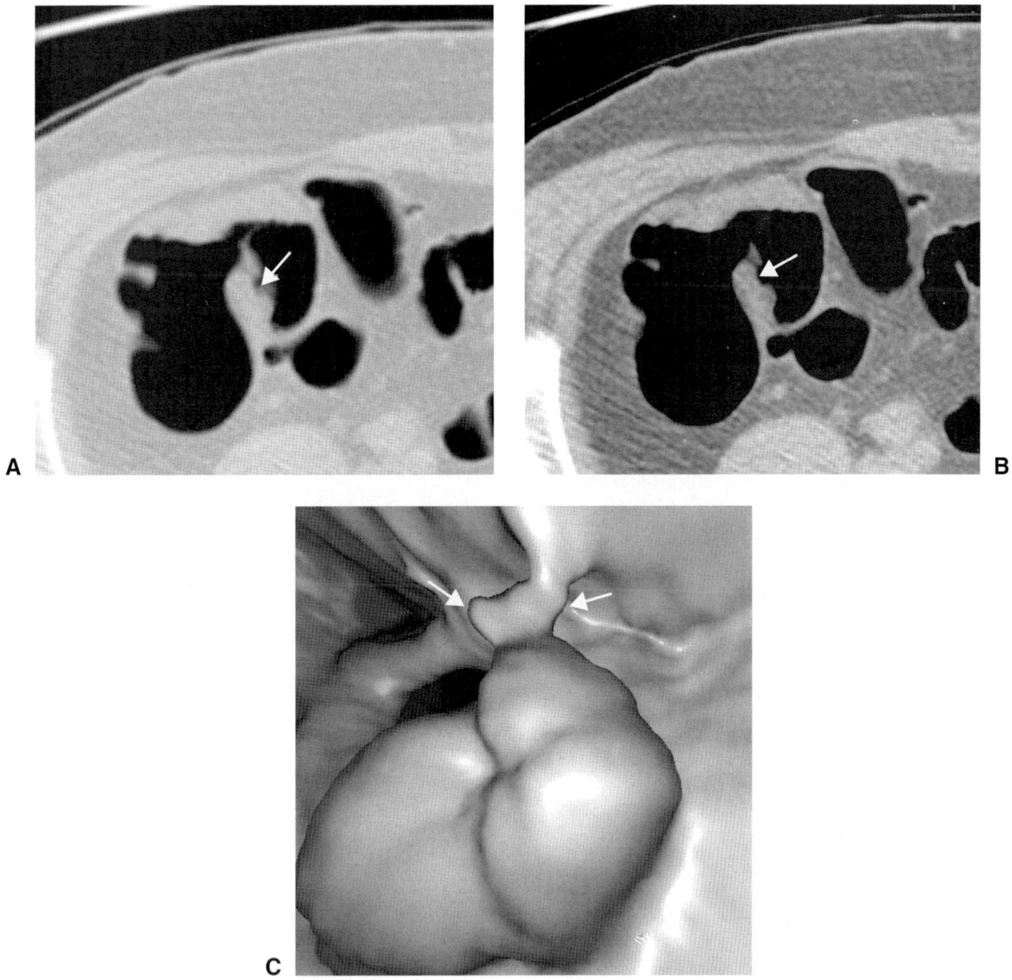

FIGURE 6.14 Stool on Ileocecal Valve: Prone axial view in colon **(A)** and abdominal **(B)** windows shows an angulated contour of the ileocecal valve. 3D endoluminal view confirms irregular surface of the valve due to adherent stool **(C)**.

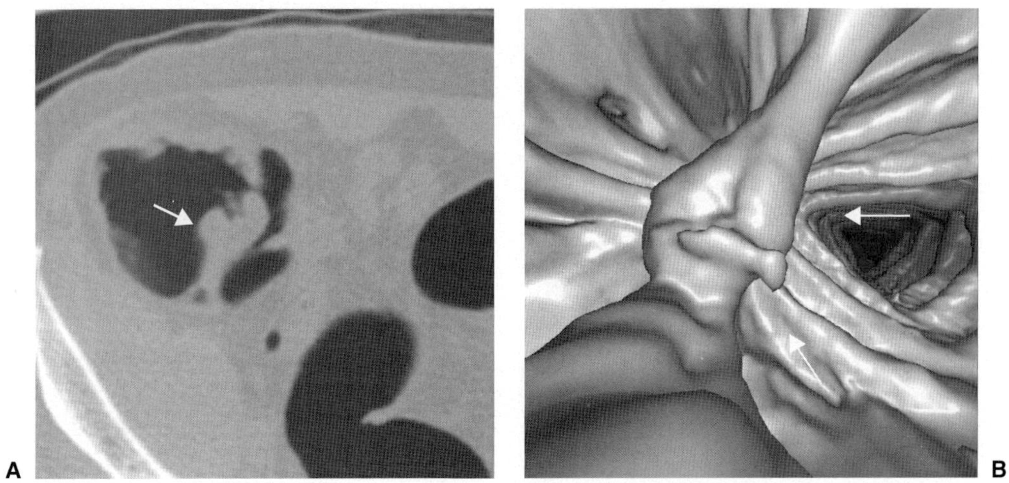

FIGURE 6.15 Stool on Ileocecal Valve: Axial view **(A)** shows an extra "lip" on the ileocecal valve. 3D endoluminal view **(B)** shows an irregular contour of the ileocecal valve with a linear and lobulated appearance due to adherent stool.

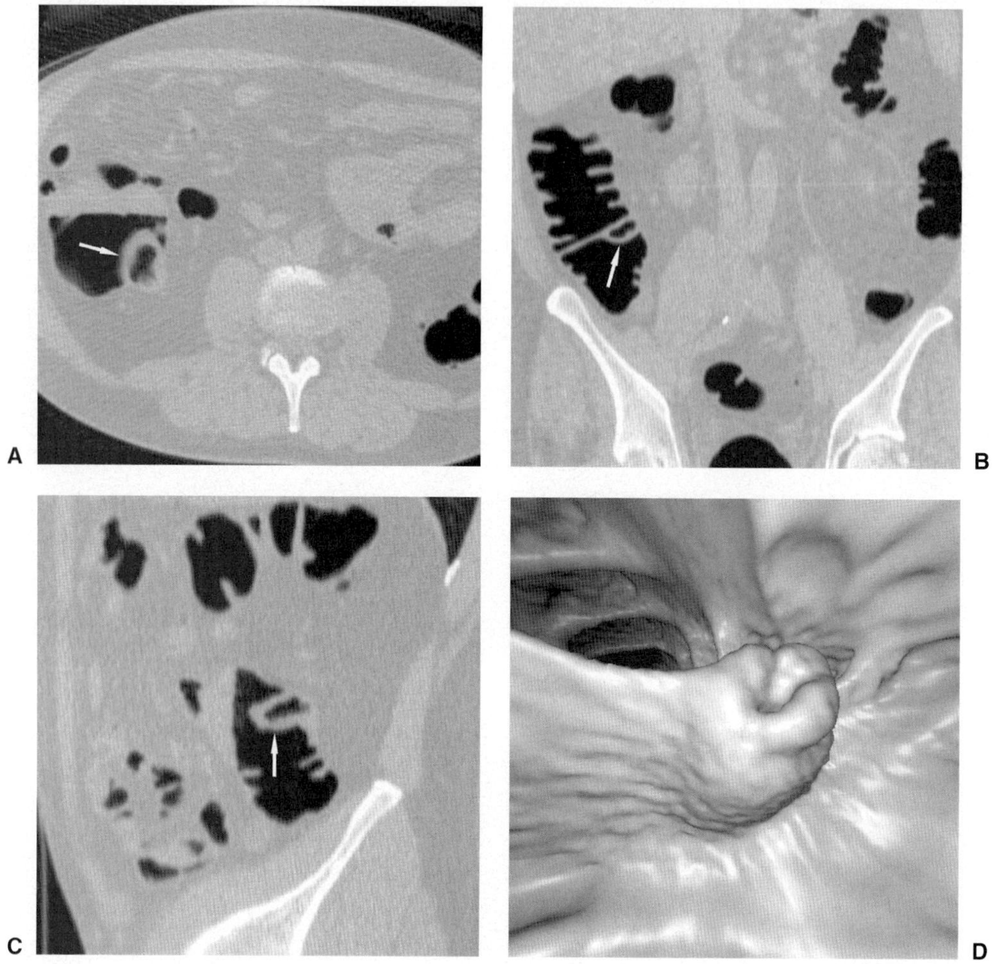

FIGURE 6.16 Prolapsed Terminal Ileum: Axial view **(A)**, coronal reformat **(B)** and sagittal reformat **(C)** demonstrate an air-distended terminal ileum (white arrow) bulging into the right colon, causing an elongated appearance of the ileocecal valve on the 3D endoluminal view **(D)**.

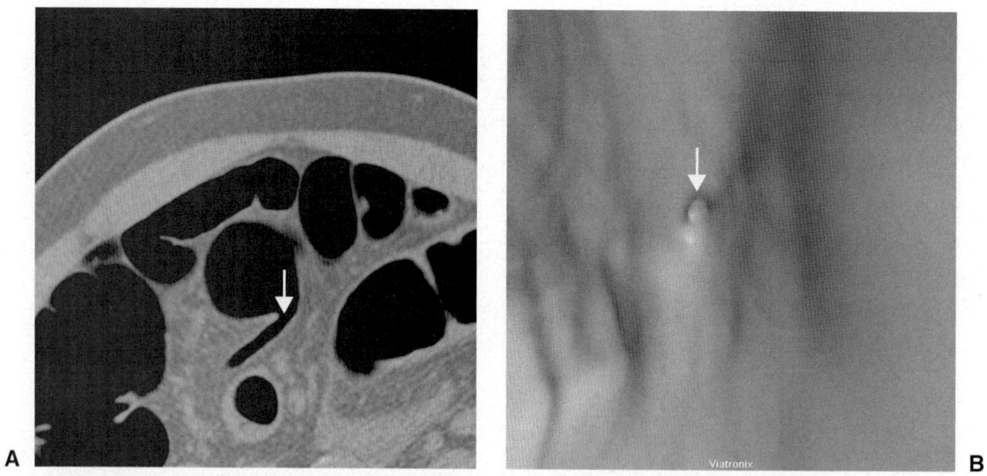

FIGURE 6.17 Appendiceal Orifice: Axial view **(A)** shows an air-filled appendix extending from the cecal tip. The open appendiceal orifice appears as a dark ring on the 3D endoluminal view **(B)** similar to a diverticulum.

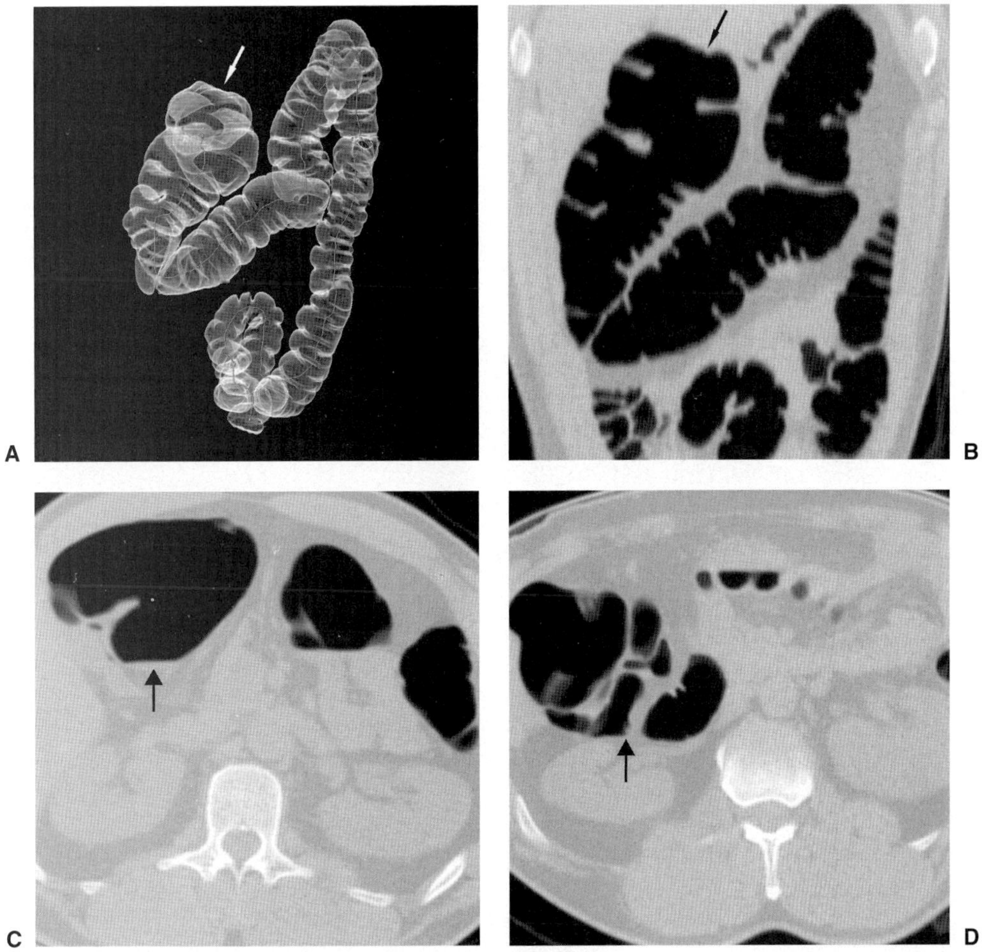

FIGURE 6.18 Cecal Bascule: The cecum rotates superior and anteromedial to the ascending colon. These patients can present for CTC after incomplete colonoscopy. The 3D transparency view **(A)** and the coronal multiplanar reformat **(B)** are best for showing the course of the right colon and the location of the cecum relative to the ascending colon. The axial supine **(C)** and prone **(D)** views demonstrate the high location of the cecum.

However, if malrotation occurs without clinical consequence, patients may present for CTC because of failed colonoscopy (see Figure 6.19). Findings that suggest malrotation are failure of the duodenum to cross midline to the left, vertical, or reversed orientation of the superior mesenteric vessels, and unusual position of the cecum and large bowel, or small bowel.[16,18]

Hernia

Acquired or congenital hernias involving the colon may cause incomplete colonoscopy and can often be easily evaluated with CTC. Patients who have had prior abdominal surgery with a ventral incision are prone to developing ventral hernias through a defect of the peritoneum and fascia at the incision site (see Figure 6.20). Umbilical hernias may also contain portions of the colon. These hernias may not be detectable by physical examination in large or obese patients and the diagnosis may not be known before CTC. Patients with hernias containing colon may develop strangulation with subsequent bowel ischemia, which is a contraindication to CTC due to the risk of perforation.

The 3D transparency view is helpful for demonstrating colon-containing hernias. Hernias containing colon may make it difficult to achieve sufficient colonic distention proximally. Hernias may also make tracking the colonic lumen difficult on axial views. Multiplanar reformats should be employed to track colon located in the hernia or the 3D endoluminal view may be used unless there is inadequate distention in the herniated segment or proximal to it. In patients with known ventral hernias, a decubitus position may be helpful for improved distention and better patient comfort compared with the prone position. The major advantage of CTC in these cases is the ability to evaluate the colon proximal to the hernia.

Inguinal hernias occur much more commonly in men and more typically involve small bowel loops. Indirect inguinal hernias are the most common type of groin hernia and occur through the inguinal ring lateral to the inferior

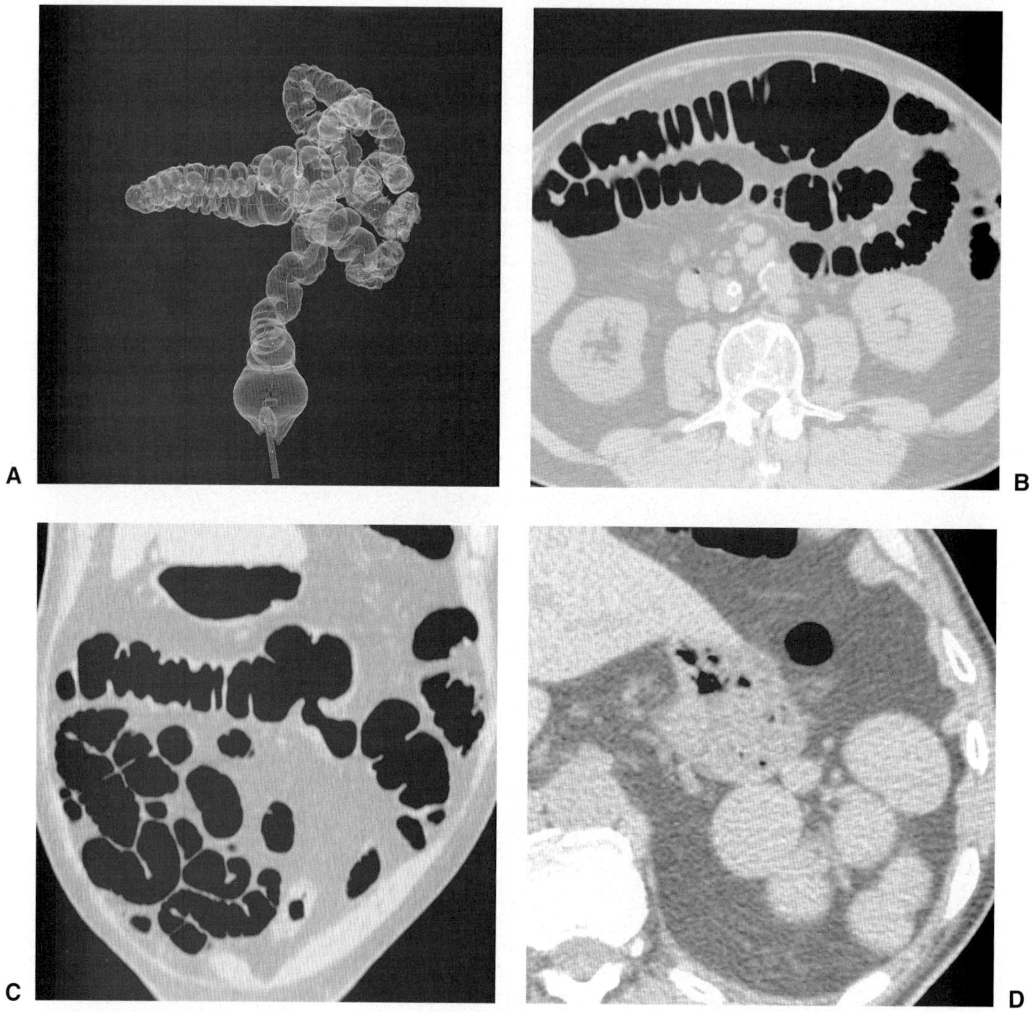

FIGURE 6.19 Polysplenia: 3D transparency view **(A)** shows malrotation of the colon with the right colon located anterior to the transverse colon. Axial supine image **(B)** demonstrates the cecum in the left upper quadrant and the acute bend of the colon in the right upper quadrant causing for failed colonoscopy. Coronal multiplanar reformat **(C)** demonstrates small bowel loops in the right lower quadrant. The axial supine image in abdominal window **(D)** demonstrates multiple small spleens in this patient with previously undiagnosed polysplenia.

epigastric vessels (see Figure 6.21). Direct inguinal hernias occur through a weakened area of the transversalis fascia within an area referred to as *Hesselbach's triangle*. The sac of a direct hernia is typically located medial to the inferior epigastric vessels. In a study by Sosna et al. four of seven patients who developed colonic perforation at CTC had left inguinal hernias that contained sigmoid colon.[19] It was postulated that incarceration of the sigmoid occurred at the hernia site which was likely caused by the insufflation of air. Practice patterns were changed so that in patients with known inguinal hernia special attention was given to the inguinal region during the insufflation process and if there was increase in size of the hernia sac, air insufflation was halted. Patients with less common hernias that may involve the colon, such as Spigelian hernias (anterior abdominal wall along lateral margin of the rectus abdominus muscle), internal hernias, or hernias occurring as a result of trauma or other surgery, may present for CTC due to incomplete colonoscopy or may be detected incidentally on CTC (see Figure 6.22).

Postsurgical Appearance

The postsurgical appearance of the colon can cause pitfalls on both 2D and 3D CTC views. Surgical resection (partial or subtotal colectomy) results in alterations of conventional anatomy. Typical segmental resections include a right colectomy (cecum to hepatic flexure, absent ICV), transverse colectomy (hepatic flexure to splenic flexure), left colectomy (splenic flexure to sigmoid), low anterior resection (LAR: descending colon to rectosigmoid), and abdominal–peroneal resection (APR: resection of the left colon, usually portion of sigmoid including the rectum, anal sphincter, and anus with resultant colostomy).[20]

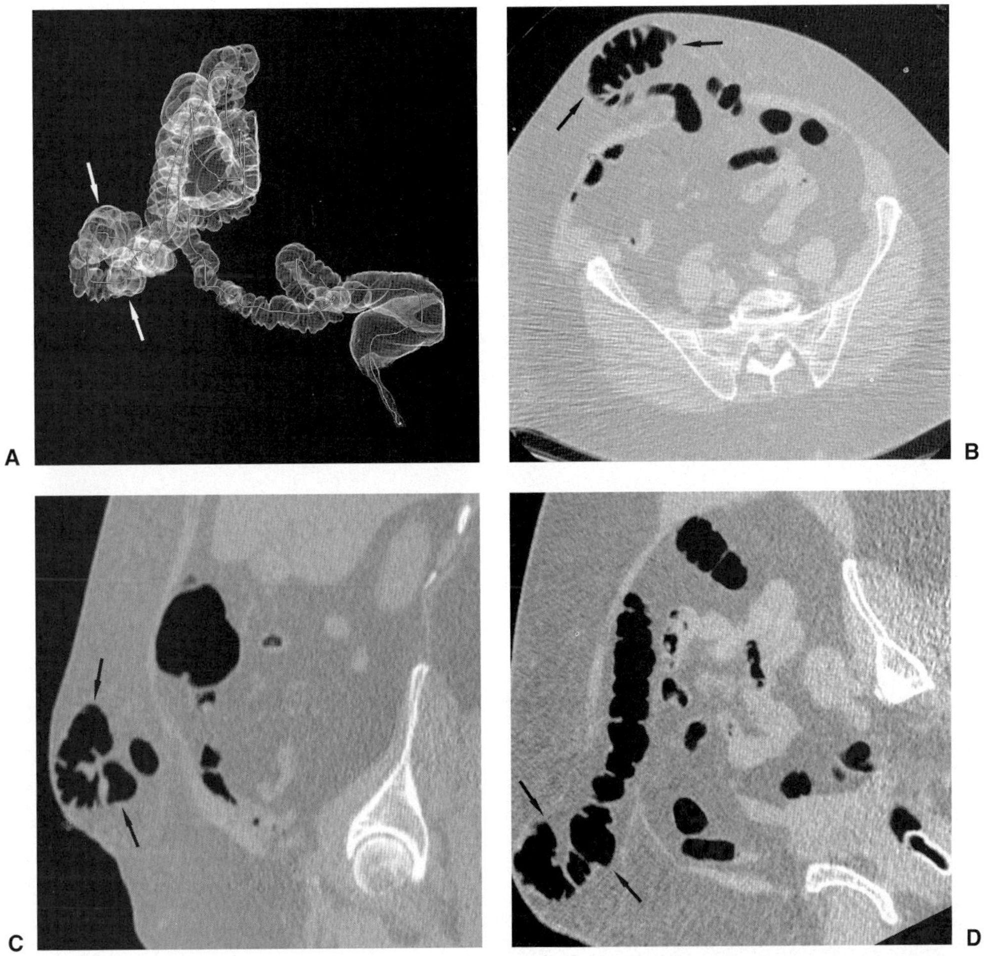

FIGURE 6.20 Ventral Hernia: 3D transparency view **(A)** from a patient referred for an incomplete colonoscopy shows an abnormal position of the transverse colon. Axial image in colon window **(B)** shows herniation of the transverse colon into the fat of the anterior abdominal wall. Sagittal **(C)** and parasagittal reformats **(D)** shows exact location of the herniated transverse colon and easy evaluation.

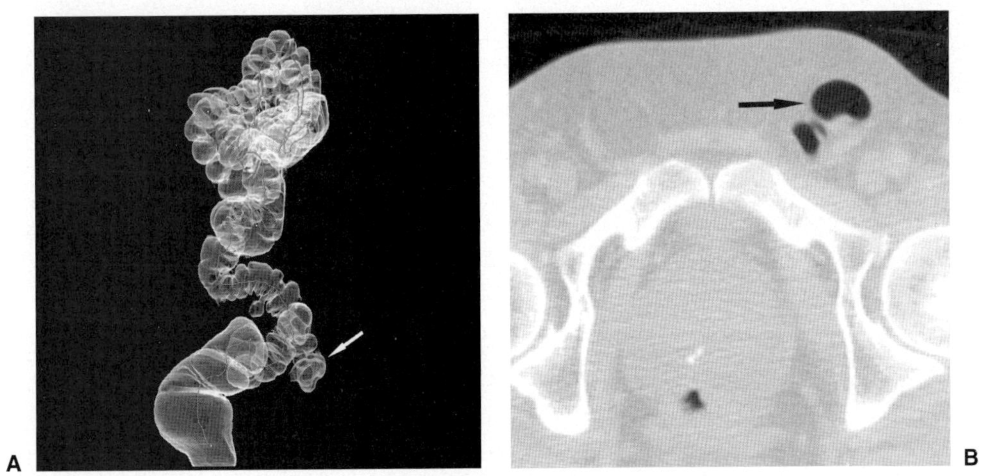

FIGURE 6.21 Inguinal Hernia: 3D transparency view **(A)** shows a left inguinal hernia containing sigmoid colon. Axial **(B)**, sagittal **(C)**, and coronal **(D)** reformats delineate the portion of the sigmoid located in the hernia sac and allows for evaluation for lesions. (*Views C and D are on next page.*)

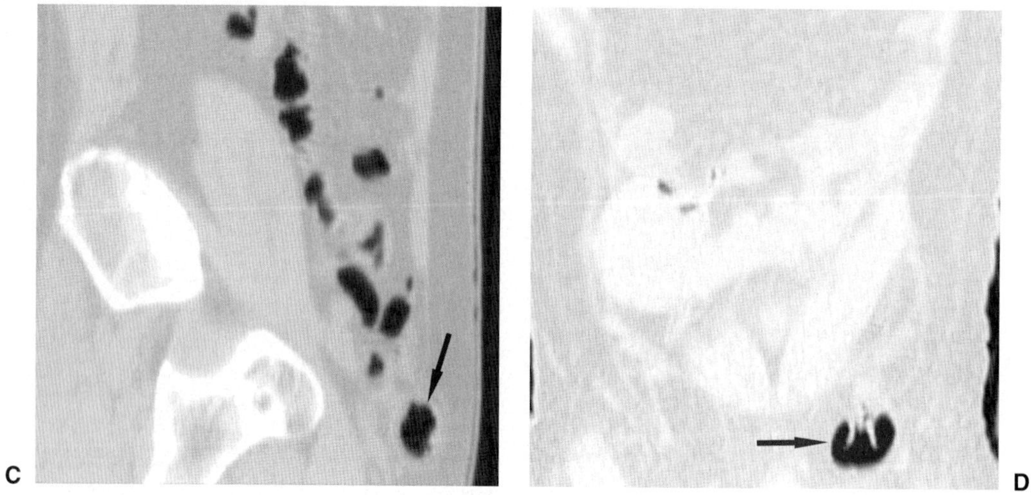

FIGURE 6.21 (*Continued*).

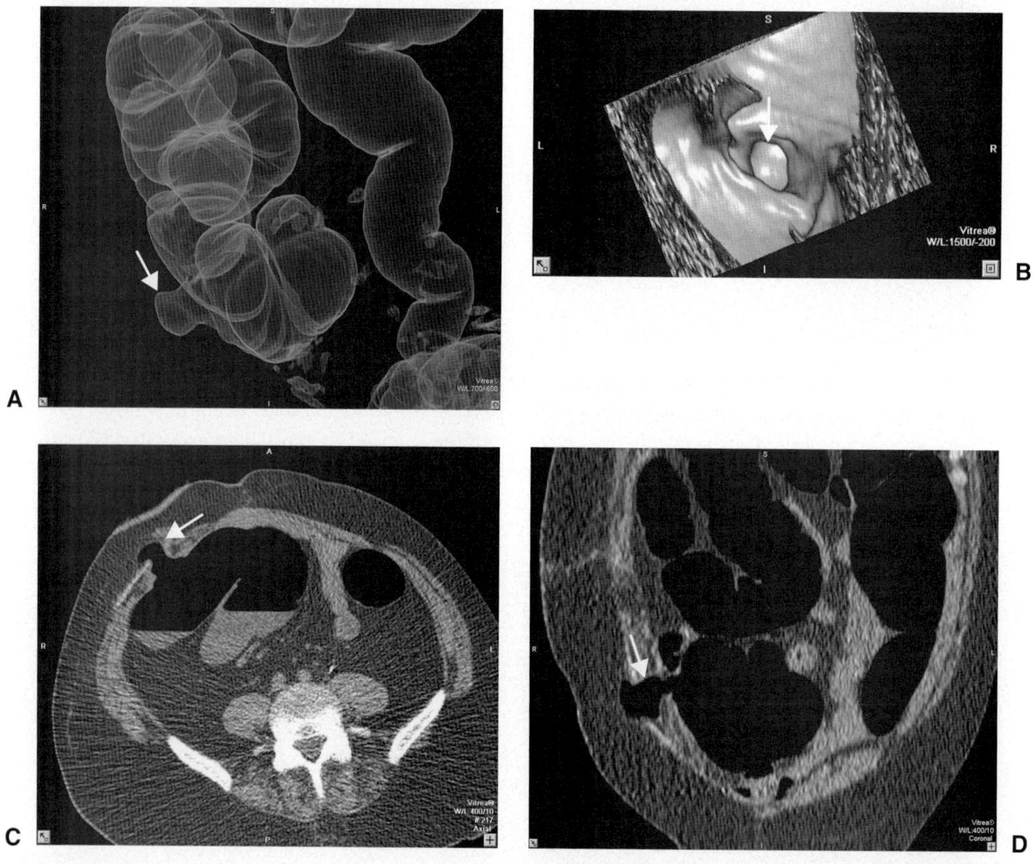

FIGURE 6.22 Stomal Hernia: 3D transparency view **(A)** shows focal herniation of ascending colon through an old ostomy site which appears as a large black ring simulating a diverticulum on the 3D endoluminal view **(B)**. The axial **(C)** and coronal reformat **(D)** shows clearly the protrusion of a knuckle of ascending colon through the abdominal wall defect.

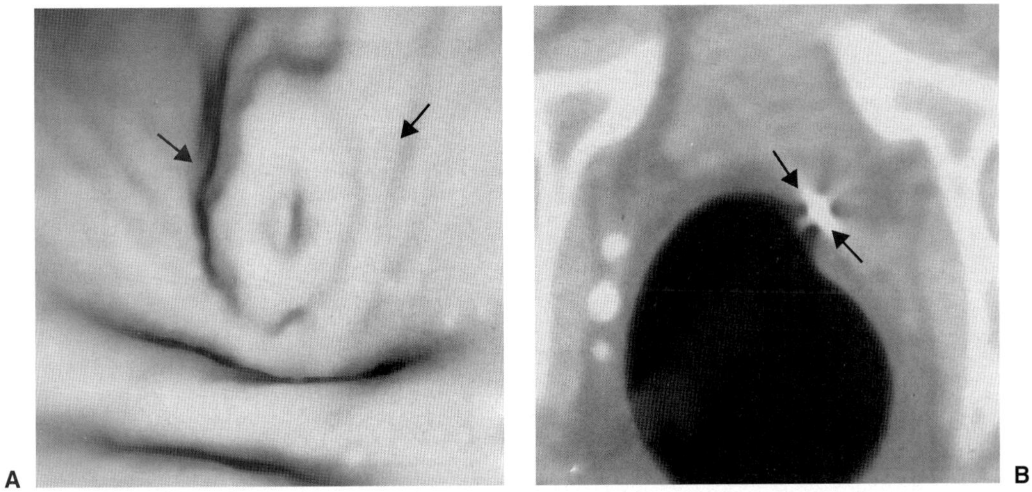

FIGURE 6.23 Postsurgical Deformity: 3D endoluminal view **(A)** reveals an ovoid lesion with a central defect which is seen to represent deformity with puckering of the colon wall due to a surgical clip on the axial view **(B)**.

CTC has not been advocated for patients with a colostomy following APR. In a study by Burling et al. perforation of a rectal stump occurred in a patient who underwent CTC inadvertently because adequate surgical history was not communicated or elicited.[21] Perforation occurred at the suture line at the apex of the rectal stump (patient presumably had prior LAR). This emphasizes the importance of obtaining a complete surgical history before performing CTC.

Following colonic surgery, scarring with fibrous and granulation tissue can develop at the site of resection or anastomosis which may resemble polypoid lesions, annular carcinomas, or focal recurrences on both 2D views and 3D endoluminal views. The 2D views typically provide evidence of prior surgery, such as metallic surgical clips, staples, or a caliber change of the bowel. Although most gastrointestinal anastomoses are currently performed with stapling devices, suture anastomoses performed in the past may not be conspicuous to suggest prior resection. Patients who have had prior resections dues to colon cancer are at increased risk of developing recurrence at the anastomotic site and special attention should be paid to these areas on any follow up imaging. Surgical clips can also cause pseudopolypoid lesions and colon wall deformities, which may be a pitfall on 3D views (see Figure 6.23). The 2D views are helpful for demonstrating the proximity of the metallic clip to the colon wall.

Mobile Segment

The mobility of colonic segments may cause false-negative examinations. In particular, the sigmoid, transverse colon, and right colon have loosely attached mesentery and can demonstrate mobility with a change in position from supine to prone (see Figures 6.24–6.27). The mobility may be complex in orientation about the x-, y-, or z-axis. Rotation about the z-axis can occur with little change in position in the other planes. The 3D transparency view is helpful for demonstrating mobility of a colonic segment. Residual stool is usually differentiated from polyps by internal heterogeneity and demonstration of mobility with a change in patient position. However, homogeneous stool can be differentiated from a sessile polyp because it is often mobile. Rotated or mobile colonic segments may cause the reader to misinterpret a true polyp as mobile homogeneous stool (see Figure 6.28).

Laks et al. performed a study evaluating positional change in colon polyps on CTC.[22] Eleven of 41 polyps (27%) measuring 5 mm or larger demonstrated movement with a change in patient position. Five of the 11 polyps were pedunculated and movement was due to the stalk. The remaining six polyps were sessile and located in mobile segments (sigmoid, transverse colon, ascending colon, and cecum) so that polyp movement was related to positional changes of the colon in the mesentery and was not true mobility of the polyp. It was concluded that a mobile lesion should not be assumed to be stool at CTC.

The cecum usually lies in the right iliac fossa, inferior and anterior to the ascending colon.[23] Approximately 10% of the population have an incompletely fixed cecum and ascending colon permitting a wide range of mobility including a number of variant anatomic positions, such as medial, anteflexed, or retroflexed in location[24] (see Figure 6.29). Patients with a mobile cecum may present with chronic right lower quadrant pain with associated abdominal distention. Cecopexy, using a lateral peritoneal flap for fixation, can relieve symptoms and prevent subsequent cecal volvulus.[25] Chen and Dachman studied the mobility of the cecum on supine and prone data sets in 21 patients.[26] The authors analyzed the position of the cecum based on the ICV and the appendiceal orifice. The measurement of a line along an axis connecting the ICV and appendiceal orifice relative to a vertical was used to determine cecal motion between the two data sets. Axial rotation was also assessed by comparing a line drawn through the center of the cecum and another from the

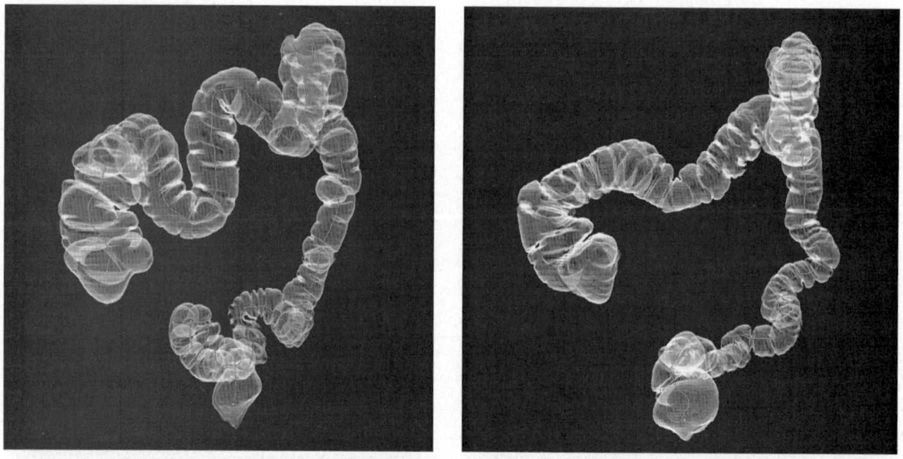

A B

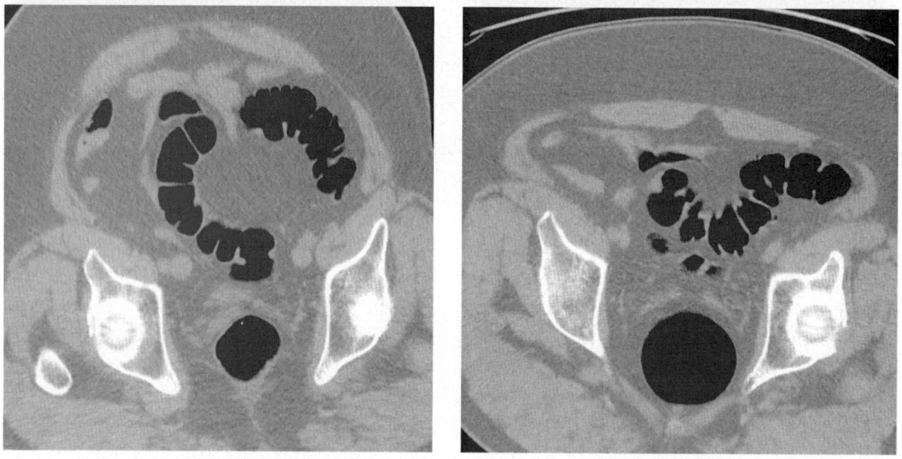

C D

FIGURE 6.24 Sigmoid and Transverse Colon Mobility: 3D transparency views in the supine **(A)** and prone **(B)** positions show straightening of both the sigmoid and transverse colon. Axial views in the supine **(C)** and prone **(D)** positions shows relative movement of a portion of the sigmoid colon more posterior.

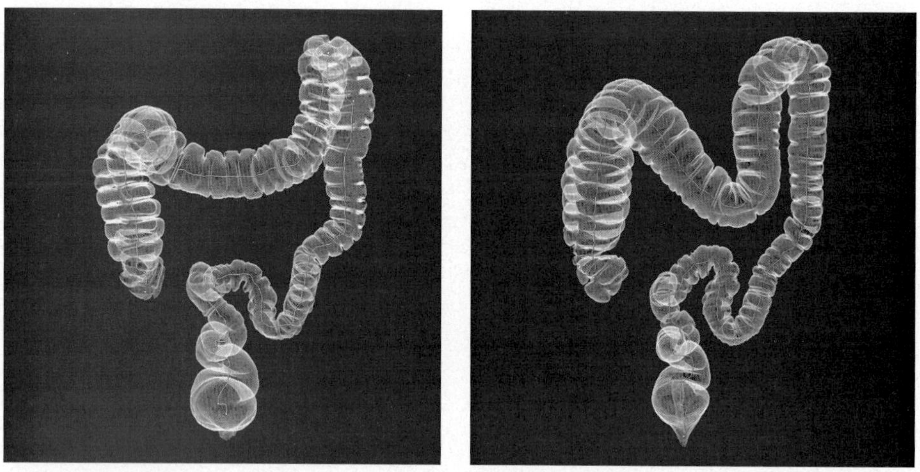

A B

FIGURE 6.25 Sigmoid and Transverse Colon Mobility: 3D transparency views in the supine **(A)** and prone **(B)** positions show straightening of the sigmoid colon in the prone position but the transverse colon moves inferiorly. This is also depicted on the coronal reformats in the supine **(C)** and prone **(D)** positions.

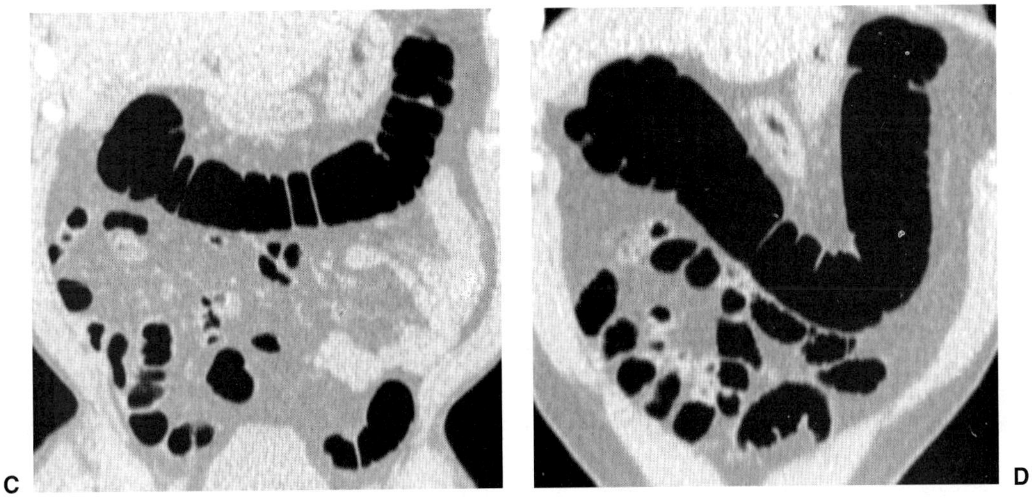

FIGURE 6.25 (*Continued*).

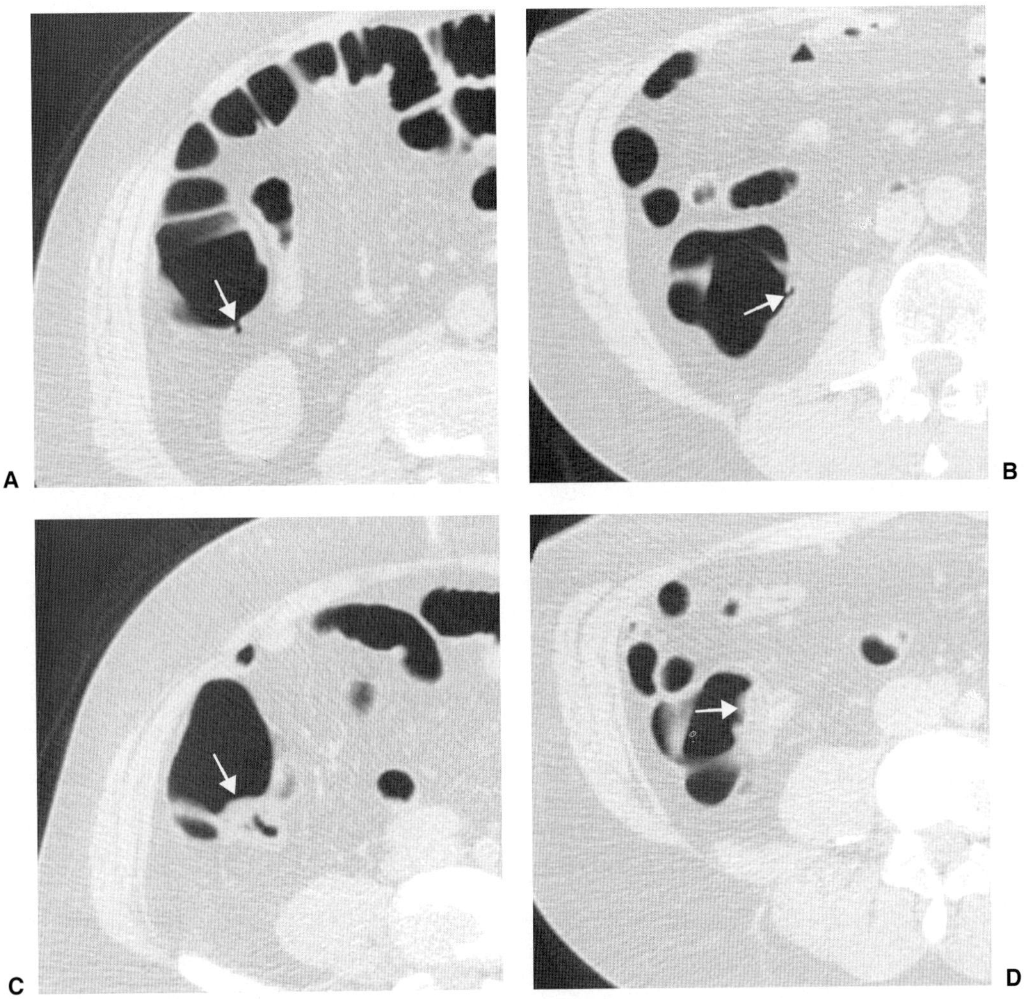

FIGURE 6.26 Right Colon Mobility: Note the position of the same diverticulum located posterior on the supine view **(A)** and medially on the prone view **(B)**. The position of the ileocecal valve posterior on the supine view **(C)** and located medially on the prone **(D)** view confirms rotation of the ascending colon and cecum.

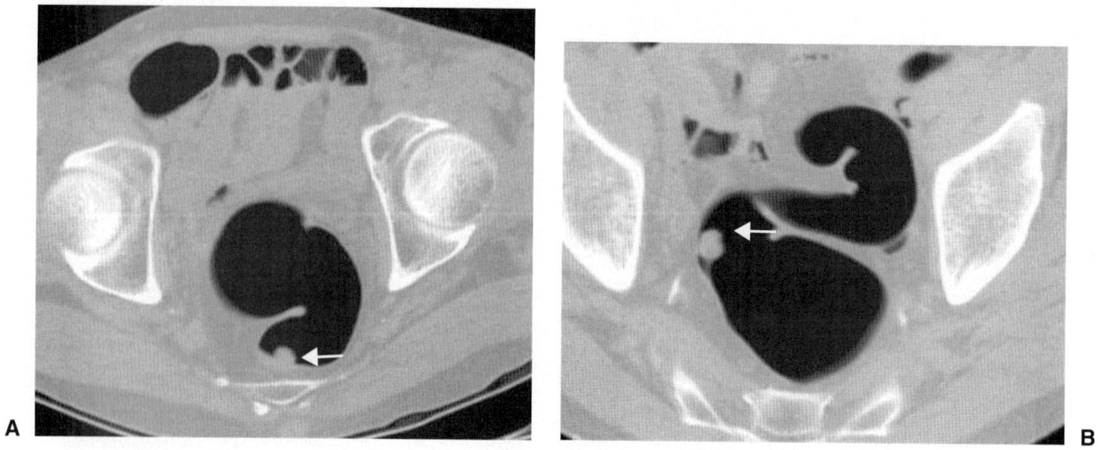

FIGURE 6.27 Mobile Sigmoid with Polyp: Supine axial view **(A)** shows a polyp along the posterior wall of the distal sigmoid colon. The stalk of this pedunculated polyp is seen on the prone view **(B)** and there is an apparent shift in location of the polyp due to mobility of the sigmoid with a change in position.

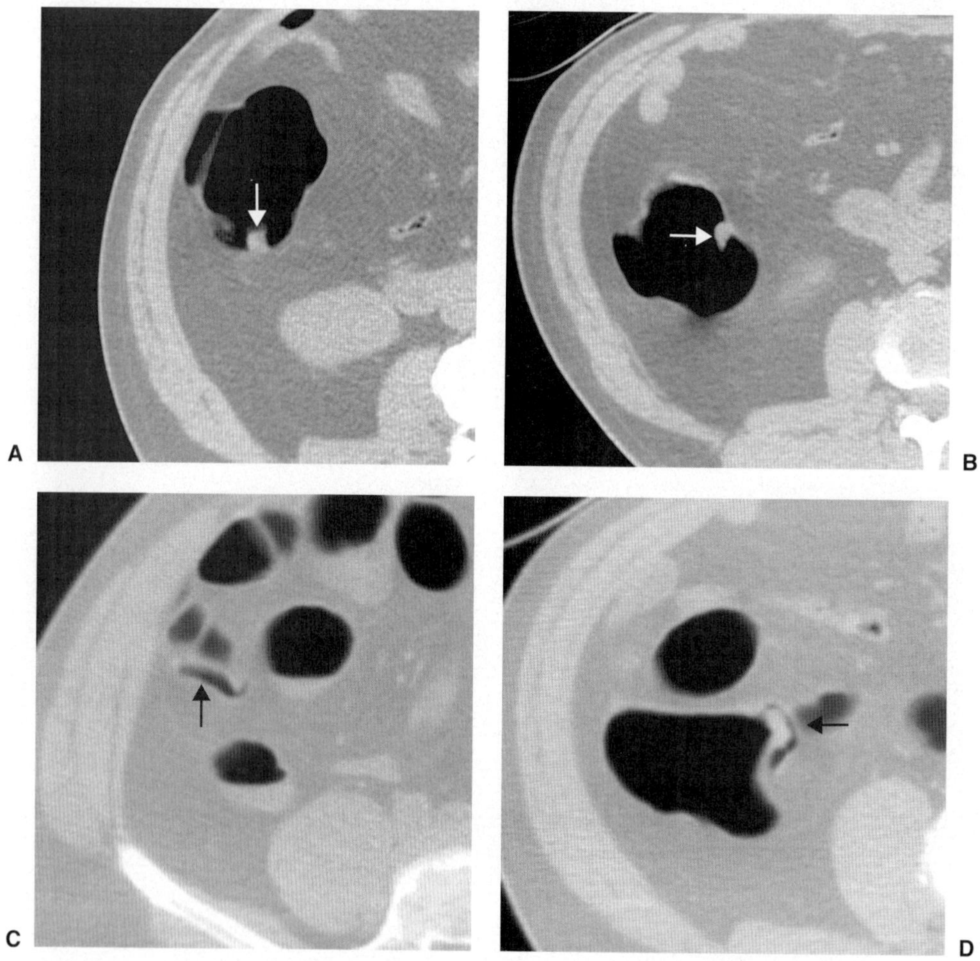

FIGURE 6.28 Mobile Ascending Colon with Polyp: The same polyp appears to be located on the posterior wall on the supine view **(A)** and then along the medial wall on the prone view **(B)**. Location of the appendix is also posterior on the supine view **(C)** and medial on the prone view **(D)**, which confirms mobility of the right colon.

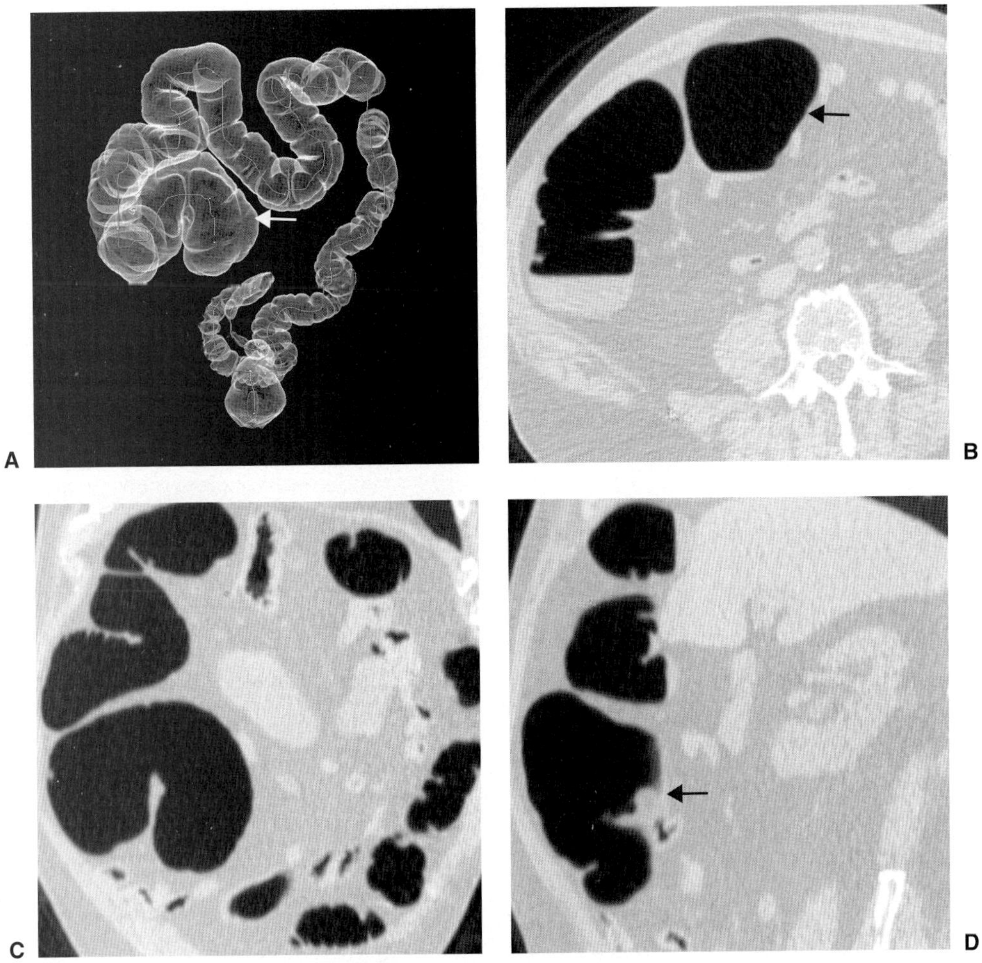

FIGURE 6.29 Mobile Cecum: 3D transparency view **(A)** and axial image **(B)** shows variant location of the cecum which is located medially. Coronal **(C)** and sagittal **(D)** reformats demonstrate the inferior and posterior location of the ileocecal valve and terminal ileum.

center of the cecum to the ICV. Any degree of rotation of this line was interpreted as axial mobility. Rotation that could impact the diagnosis was found to occur in 9/21 (43%) cases with an average rotation of 78.9 +/−27.4 degrees. In the 12 cases that did not pose a diagnostic dilemma, the average rotation was still 22.5+/−12 degrees. In addition, the main axis of rotation was varied, occurring predominantly in coronal (6 cases), sagittal (4 cases), or axial (11 cases) planes. It was concluded that rotation of the colon occurs frequently, is geometrically complex, and occurs in several planes. Multiplanar reformatted views are helpful when solid stool is suspected in the cecum to assess for rotation.

PSEUDOPOLYPOID LESIONS

Stool

Residual stool is one of the most common causes for both false-positive and false-negative findings on CTC.[1–3,27] Residual stool may be misdiagnosed as a polyp, particularly if homogeneous and adherent to the colon wall. Stool can also obscure polyps and cancer. Residual stool may be classified into four categories based on mobility and internal density: (a) heterogeneous mobile, (see Figures 6.30–6.33) (b) heterogeneous adherent, (see Figure 6.34) (c) homogenous mobile, (see Figures 6.35 and 6.36) (d) and homogeneous adherent (see Figure 6.37). Residual stool is often mobile with a change in patient position. However, mobility is also a feature of pedunculated polyps and apparent mobility of a lesion may be seen with rotation of a colonic segment. Residual stool typically has heterogeneous density and shows internal air attenuation. Other characteristics of stool include irregular, odd, or uneven geometric shapes or borders, and internal residual contrast material that help distinguish it from true polyps or malignancy (see Figures 6.38–6.41). However, it should be noted that if stool and fluid tagging is performed there may be contrast coating a polyp which may cause an irregular contour of the polyp.

Stool may resemble polyps morphologically; however, focal lesions in segments without other residual stool

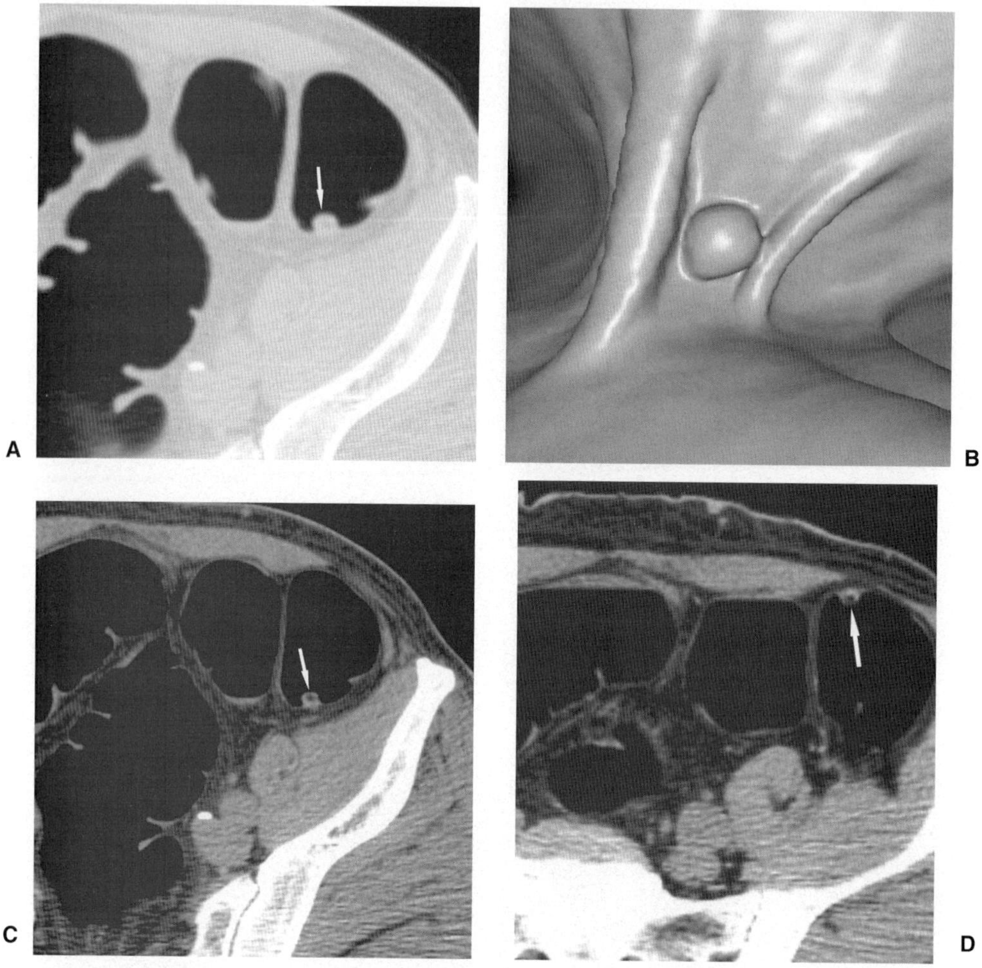

FIGURE 6.30 Heterogeneous Mobile Stool: Supine axial image in colon window **(A)** shows an ovoid lesion with central low density. This lesion simulates a polyp between folds on the 3D endoluminal view **(B)**. Axial images in supine **(C)** and prone **(D)** abdominal window show the central low density more clearly, indicating this is stool. Note movement of the stool to the dependent wall on the prone image.

should be regarded as suspicious and fully evaluated using 2D views.[10] Lesions demonstrating internal heterogeneity on 2D views that lack mobility (adherent) are typically residual stool. However, one common pitfall is trapping of air underneath a polyp or mass (between the lesion and colon wall), which may give the false appearance of heterogeneity and residual stool. Careful evaluation should be made for the location of the air density in relation to the lesion. Air that is trapped between a lesion and the colon wall will be located only in the periphery (see Figure 6.42). Centrally located air within a lesion is a feature of stool. Homogeneous adherent stool particularly if it is spherical or ovoid in shape may be impossible to differentiate from a true polyp on both 2D and 3D views.

Pills and Seeds

Focal lesions in the colon that exhibit attenuation values higher than that of soft tissue are not polyps and may represent residual barium from a recent imaging test (residual barium is often present in diverticula if present) or ingested radiopaque pills (see Figures 6.43 and 6.44). Residual ingested material including food, seeds, pills, or pill fragments may be polypoid in shape and a source of false-positive CTC examinations.[1,2] Undigested food, particularly corn and seeds, may be present anywhere in the colon and may or may not exhibit mobility (see Figure 6.45). Pills and undigested medication may be radiopaque on 2D views. Iron, calcium carbonate, iodinated compounds, acetazolamide, busulfan, and potassium preparations have been found to be radiopaque.[28] Ingested foreign bodies have been described on barium enema, and although rare, may also resemble polyps on 3D endoluminal view; however, unless round or elliptical, they likely would exhibit odd shapes or edges.[29]

Internal Hemorrhoids

Hemorrhoids are very common and the prevalence increases with age. The exact prevalence is not known

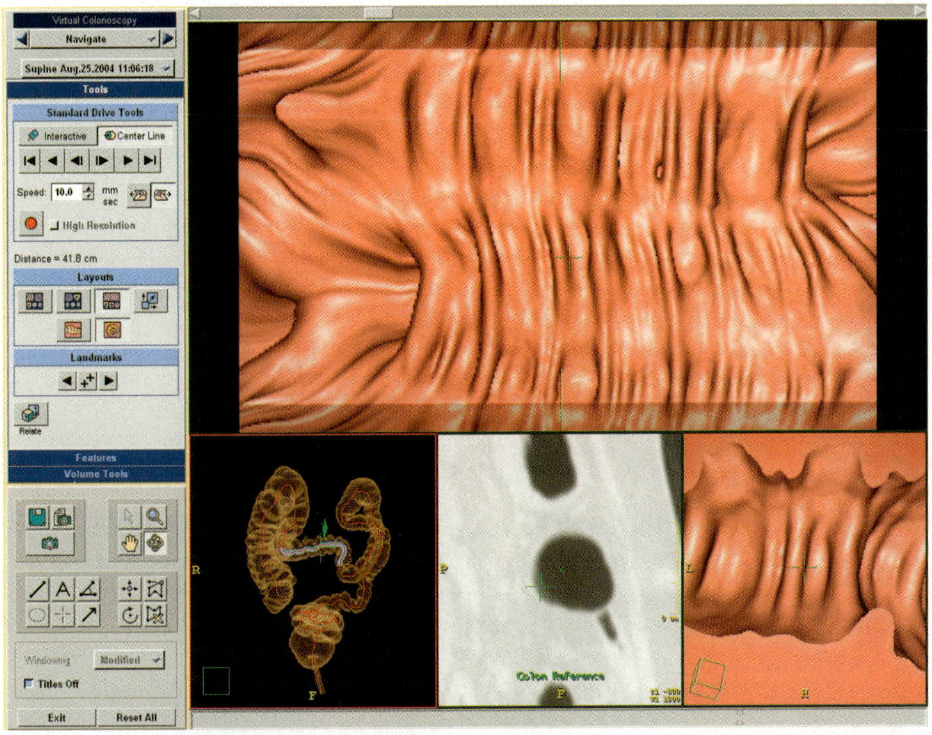

Figure 4-21. Display format that includes the dissection view as the largest window with smaller windows for a colon overview, 2D axial view and 3D view. Distortion of folds and lesions may occur particularly in areas of acute curvature.

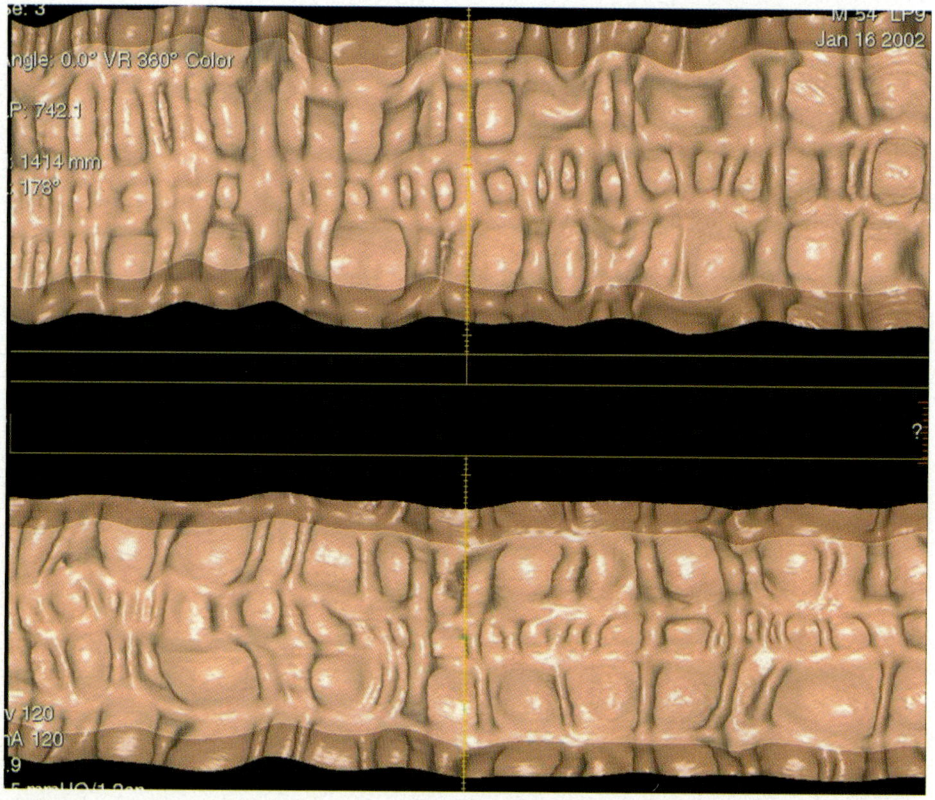

Figure 4-22. Excellent demonstration of normal haustral folds on this 360-degree dissection view using volume rendering.

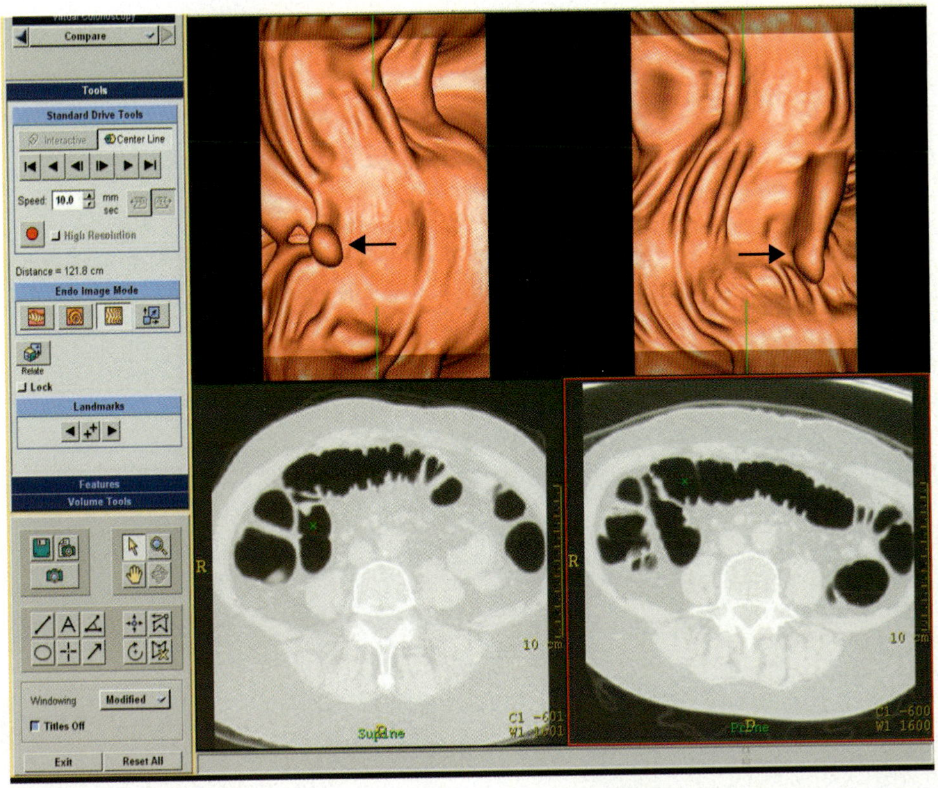

Figure 4-23. Supine and prone CTC datasets may be viewed together with the dissection views on top and the corresponding 2D axial images below. Note a small polyp more easily identifiable on the dissection view.

C

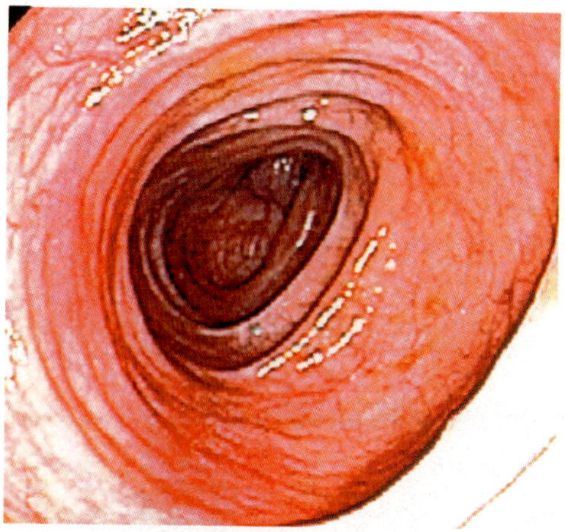

Figure 4-29(C). Endoscopic view of the sigmoid colon shows that the lumen of the normal sigmoid is typically rounded or ovoid.

C

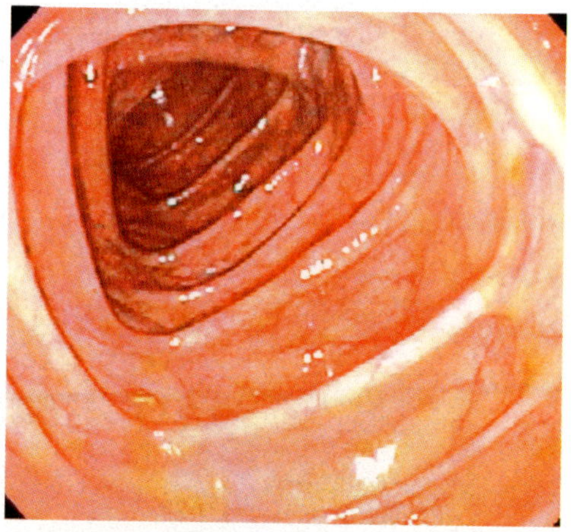

Figure 4-32(C). The transverse colon tends to be better distended in the supine position. The endoscopic view demonstrates the typical triangular appearance of the haustral folds in the transverse colon due to arrangement of the taeniae coli.

D

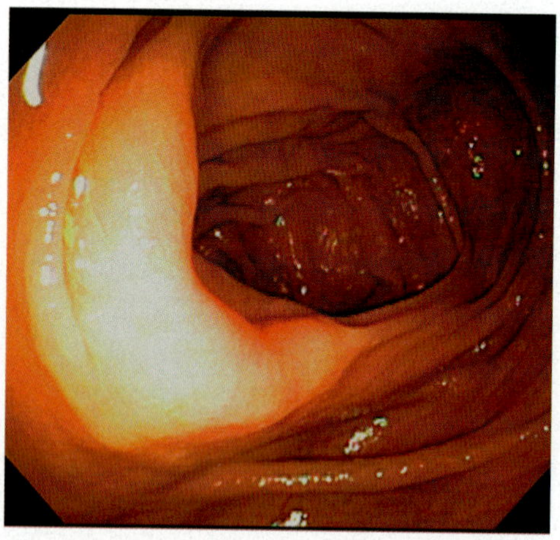

Figure 4-35(D). Papillary IC valve: endoscopic image.

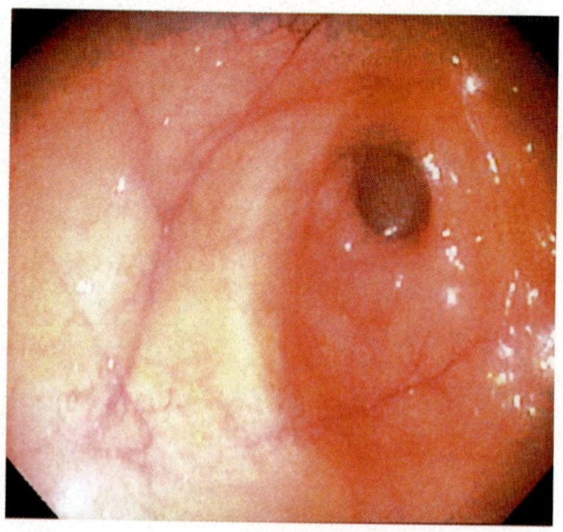

D

Figure 4-39(D). Endoscopic image of the appendiceal orifice.

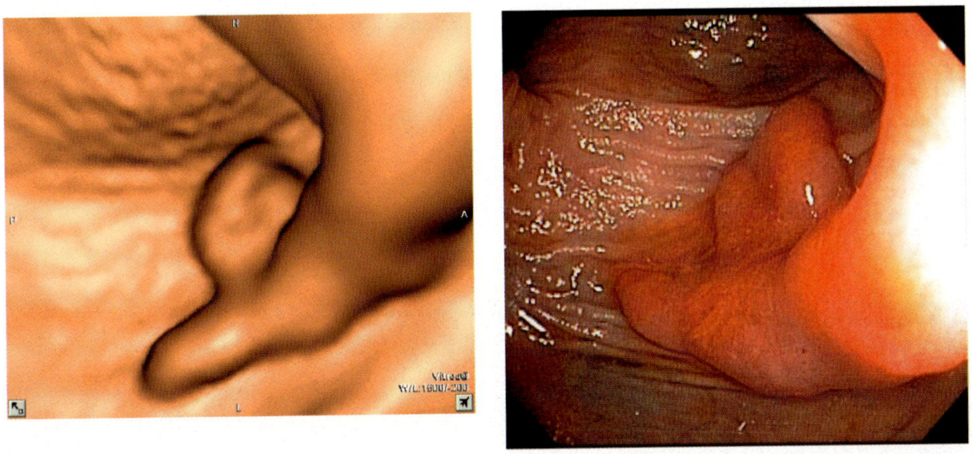

C D

Figure 5-34. Atypical adenocarcinoma. **C:** 3D endoluminal view demonstrates a thickened fold with a sessile broad-based lesion. **D:** Biopsies revealed adenocarcinoma involving both the thickened fold and the polypoid component.

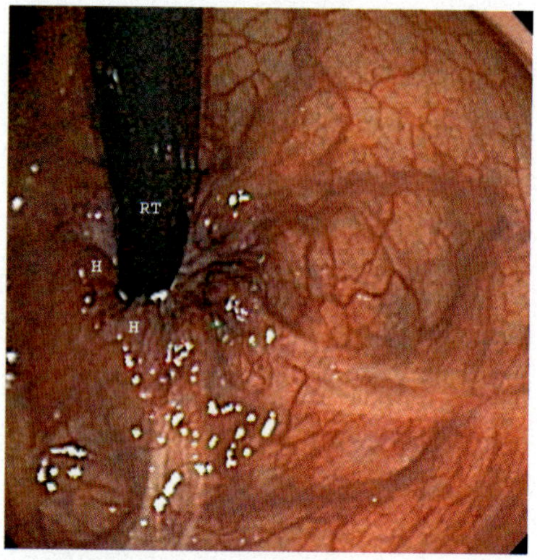

D

Figure 6-46(D). Colonoscopy image shows the rectal tube (RT) and focal protrusions encircling the tube representing internal hemorrhoids (H).

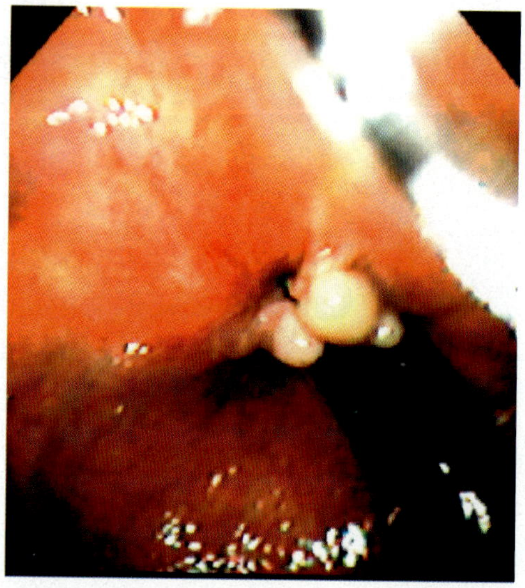

D

Figure 6-50(D). Colonoscopy image showing well-defined small hypertrophied anal papillae.

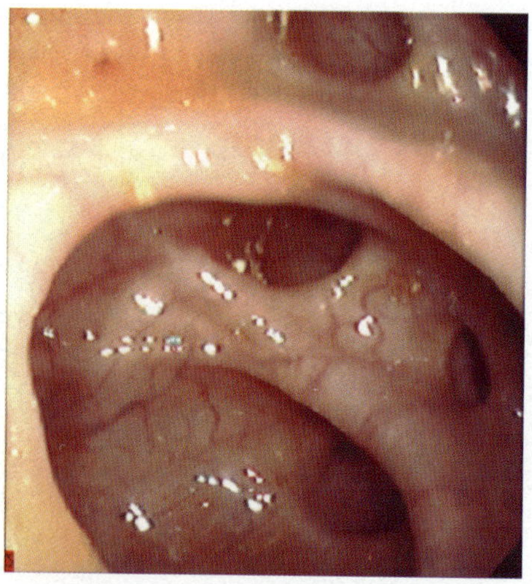

Figure 6-67(B). Diverticulosis: Multiple diverticula are seen on the colonoscopic image.

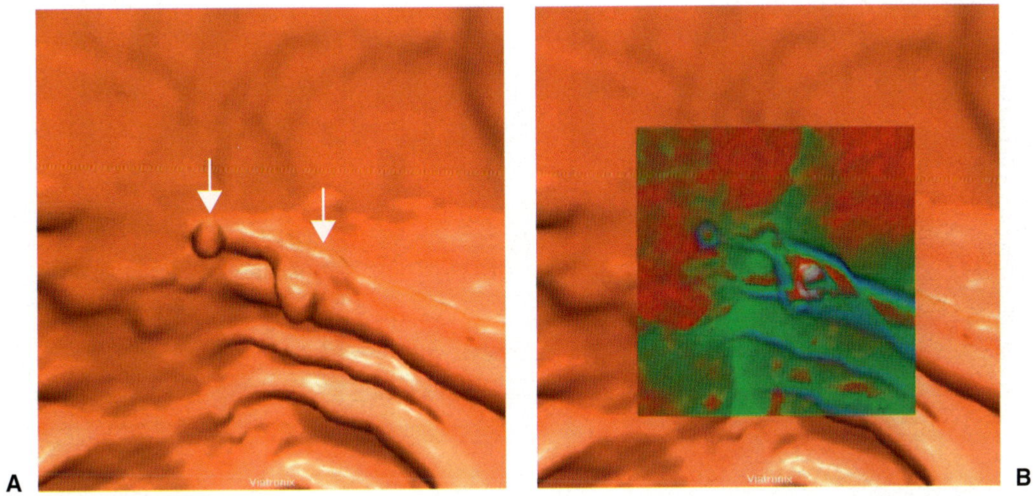

Figure 10-3. Polyp and tagged stool. 3D endoluminal view **(A)** shows two polypoid lesions on a fold. When the translucency view is employed **(B)**, the central white core in the larger lesion demonstrates it to be tagged stool. The color pattern of the smaller lesion with gradual change in the colors red, green and blue suggest a polyp.

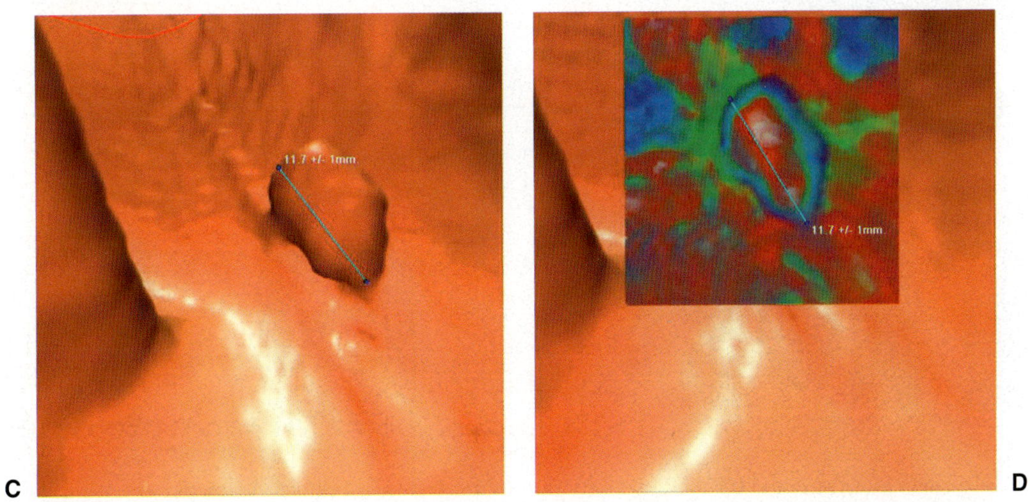

Figure 10-4. Partially tagged stool simulates a polyp on the 3D endoluminal view **(C)**. When the translucency view is applied **(D)**, the color pattern shows white centrally indicating that this lesion is tagged stool.

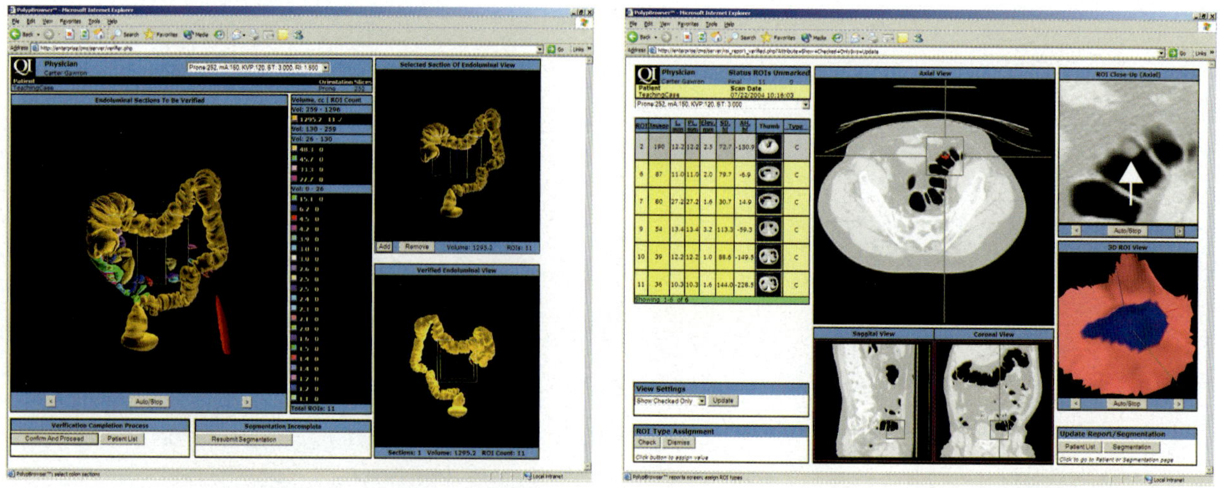

Figure 11-1. CAD for CT colonography first segments the colon from the 3D data set **(A)**. The CAD system then automatically identifies, measures, and characterizes polyp candidates and they are organized into a list of decreasing order of likelihood. **(B)** The display also includes axial, magnified axial, sagittal and coronal multiplanar images, and 3D view of the polyp candidate.

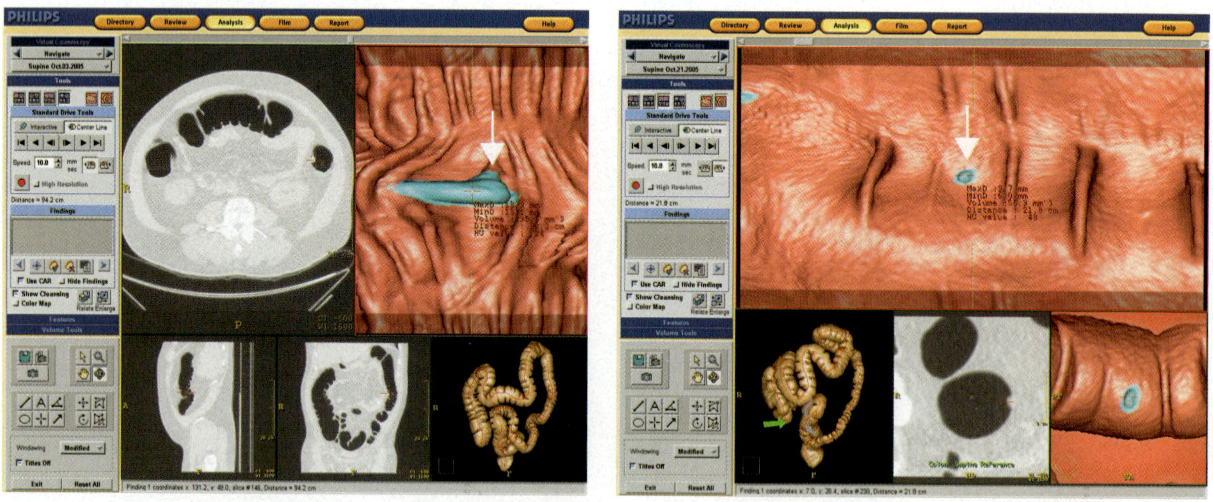

Figure 11-2. CAD algorithm integrated into CTC software with various image display options. A large polyp is identified in the descending colon of the first patient using a display that includes the axial image, dissection view, sagittal and coronal multiplanar reformats, and colon overview. **A:** A small polyp is detected in the sigmoid colon of the second patient using a display that includes dissection views, magnified axial view and the colon overview. **B:** Note that the CAD system provides measurements of polyp candidates automatically.

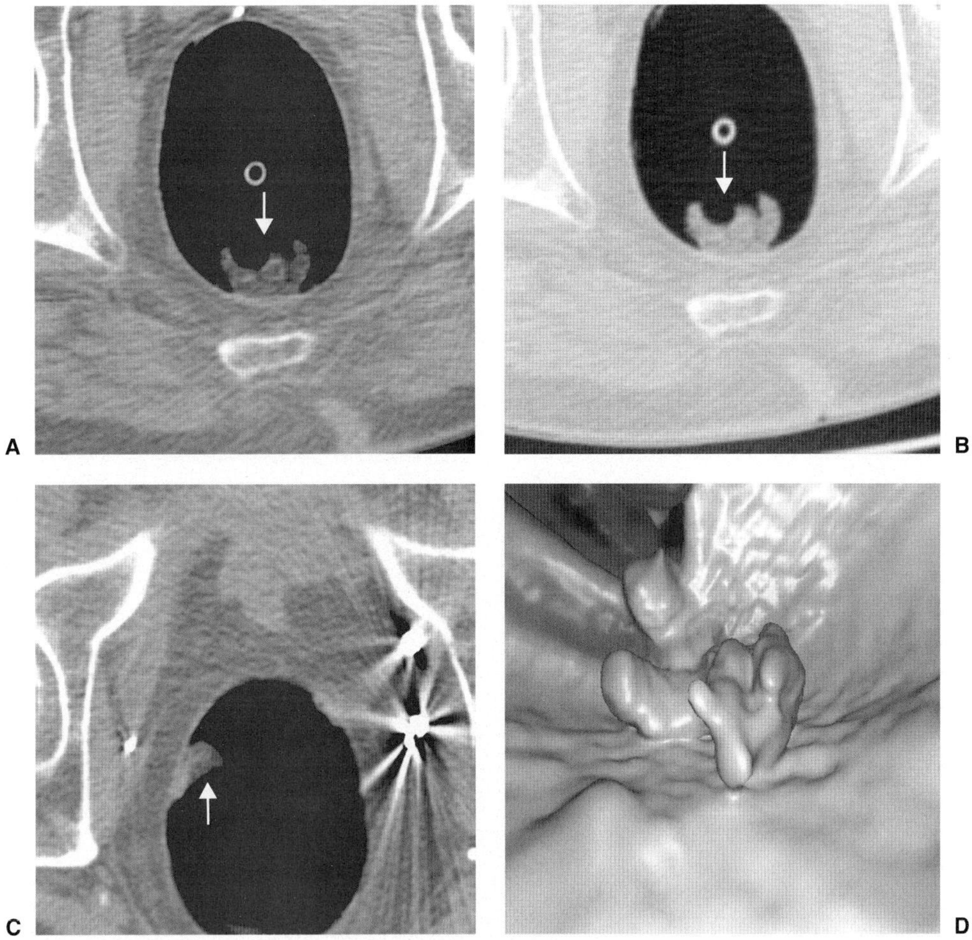

FIGURE 6.31 Heterogeneous Mobile Stool: Supine axial image in abdominal window **(A)** and colon window **(B)** shows large heterogeneous residual stool which shifts to a dependent location on the prone view **(C)**. 3D endoluminal image **(D)** shows typical appearance of stool with irregular surface and angulated appearance.

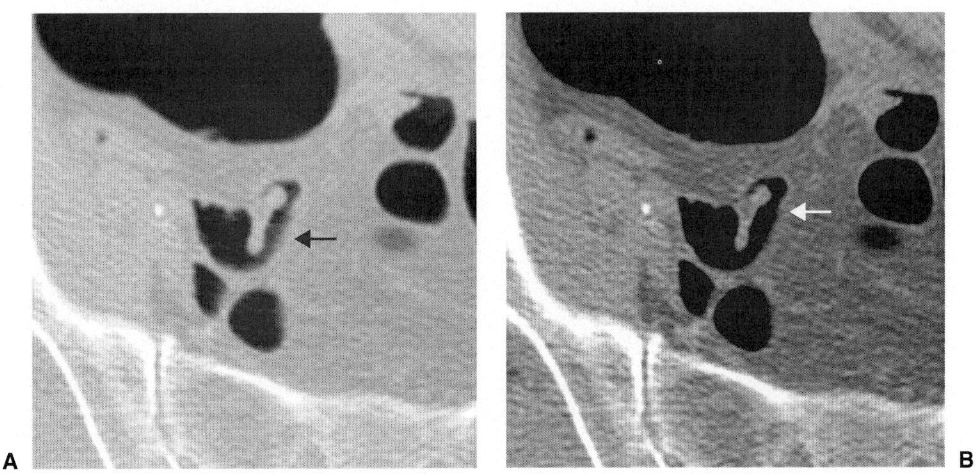

FIGURE 6.32 Vegetable Material: Linear density is seen on the axial image in colon window **(A)** which could simulate the stalk of a pedunculated polyp. The same image using abdominal window **(B)** shows the lesion is heterogeneous and contains low density. This was found to be vegetable material on colonoscopy.

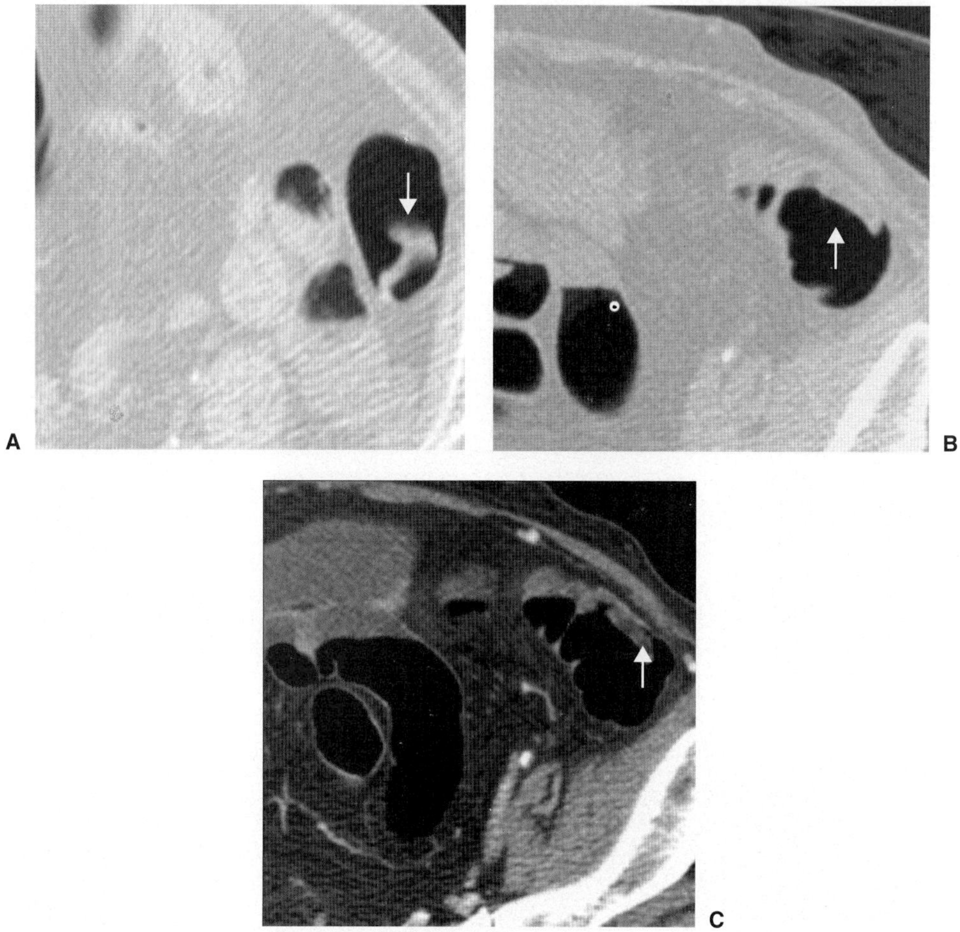

FIGURE 6.33 Vegetable Material: Supine axial image **(A)** shows a lesion with the appearance of a pedunculated polyp. The prone axial image in colon **(B)** and abdominal window **(C)** demonstrate mobility of the lesion to the dependent wall with a change to a linear configuration and a heterogeneous appearance. Vegetable material was found on colonoscopy.

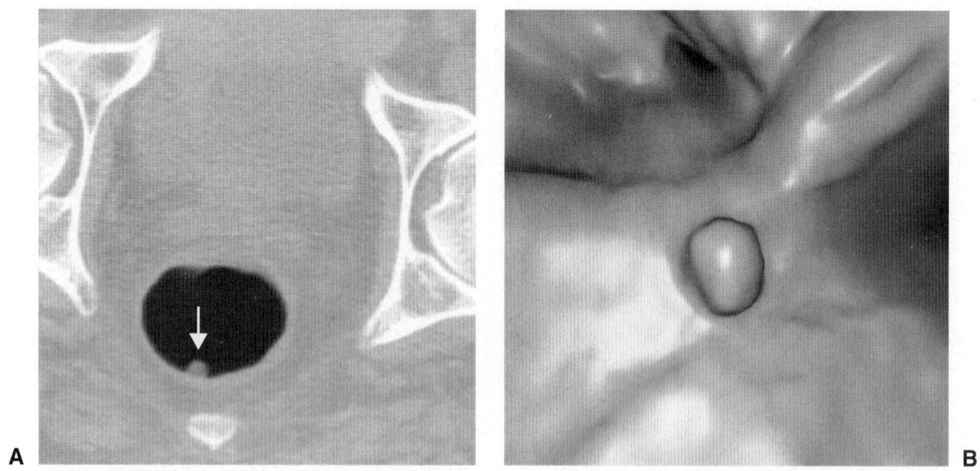

FIGURE 6.34 Heterogeneous Adherent Stool: Supine axial image in colon window **(A)** shows a rounded lesion along the posterior rectal wall that looks like a polyp on the 3D endoluminal view **(B)**. The lesion is in the same location on the prone image in colon window **(C)** and appears heterogeneous on the prone abdominal window **(D),** indicating this is adherent stool.

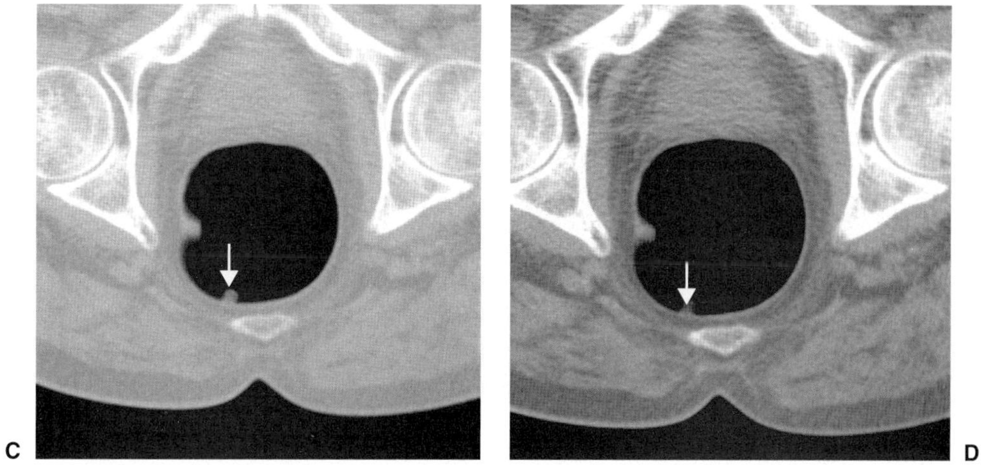

FIGURE 6.34 (*Continued*).

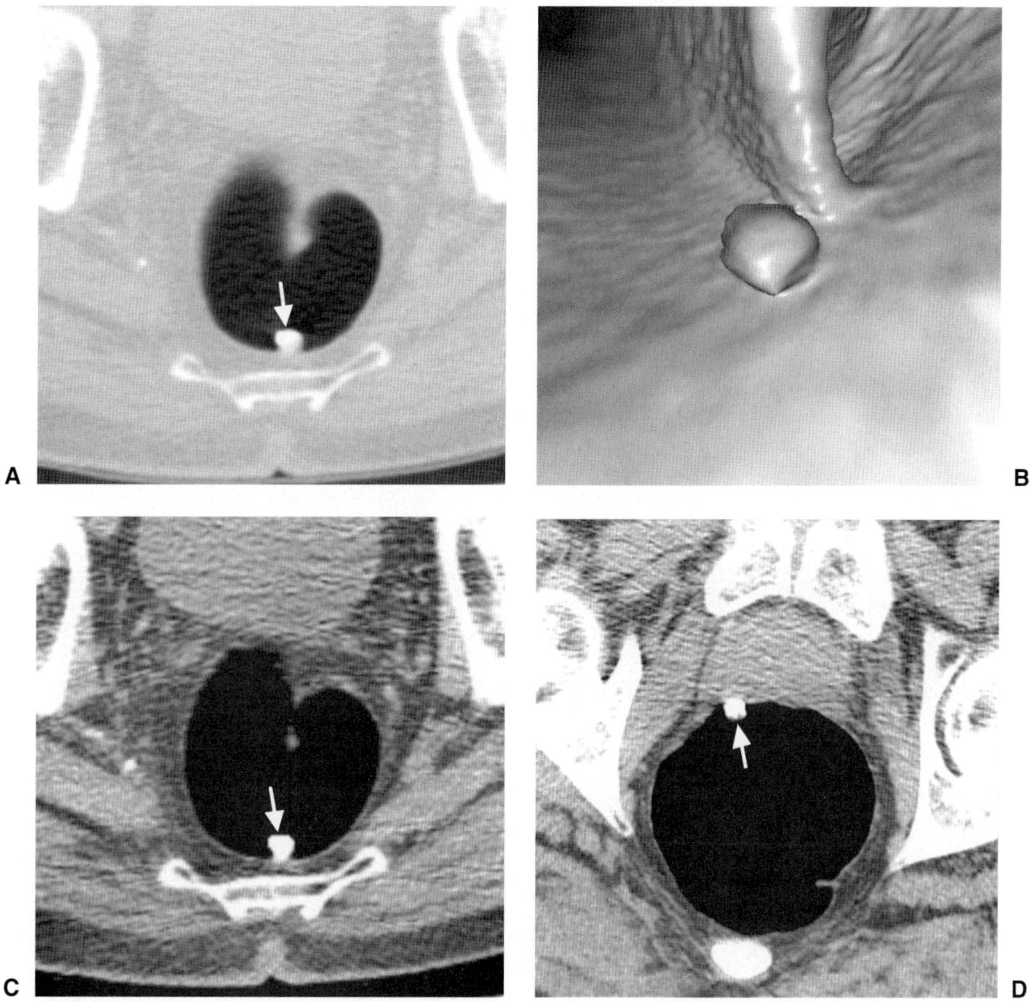

FIGURE 6.35 Homogeneous Mobile Tagged Stool: Supine axial image in colon window **(A)** shows a very dense homogeneous lesion along the posterior rectal wall that looks like a polyp on the 3D endoluminal view **(B)**. Axial images in abdominal window in supine **(C)** and prone **(D)** positions show that this is mobile tagged stool.

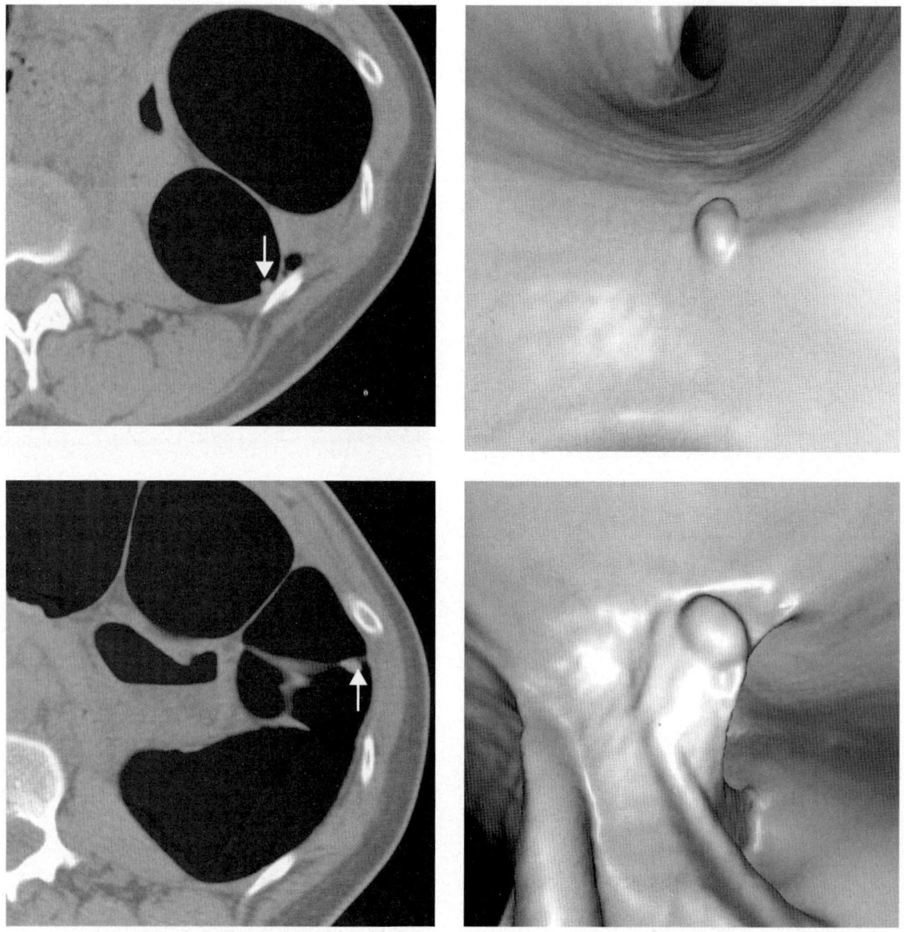

A B C D

FIGURE 6.36 Homogeneous Mobile Stool: Supine axial image **(A)** shows a homogeneous soft tissue density along the posterior colon wall which looks like a polyp on the supine 3D endoluminal view **(B)**. This lesion has moved to the dependent wall on the prone axial image **(C)** and prone 3D endoluminal view consistent with stool.

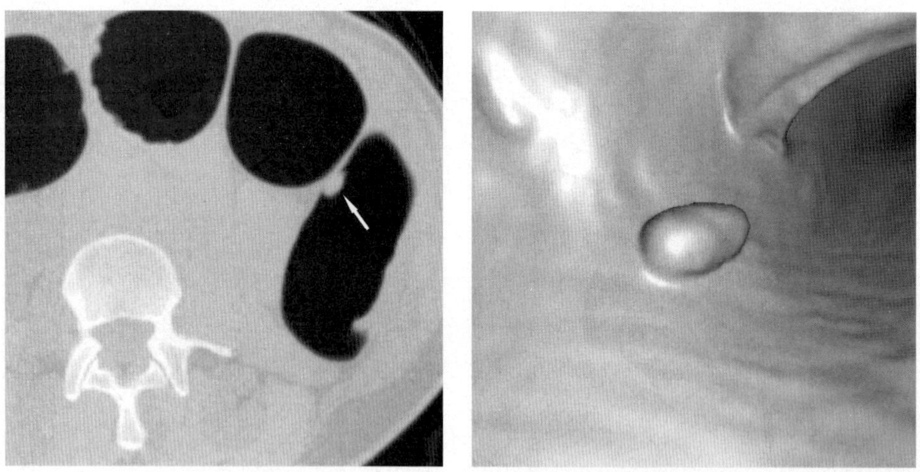

A B

FIGURE 6.37 Homogeneous Adherent Stool: This is one of the most difficult pitfalls on 2D and 3D views. Supine axial image in colon window **(A)** and 3D endoluminal view **(B)** show a polypoid-appearing lesion along the medial colon wall (arrow), which appears to be homogeneous soft tissue density on abdominal window **(C)** and nonmobile on the prone view **(D)**.

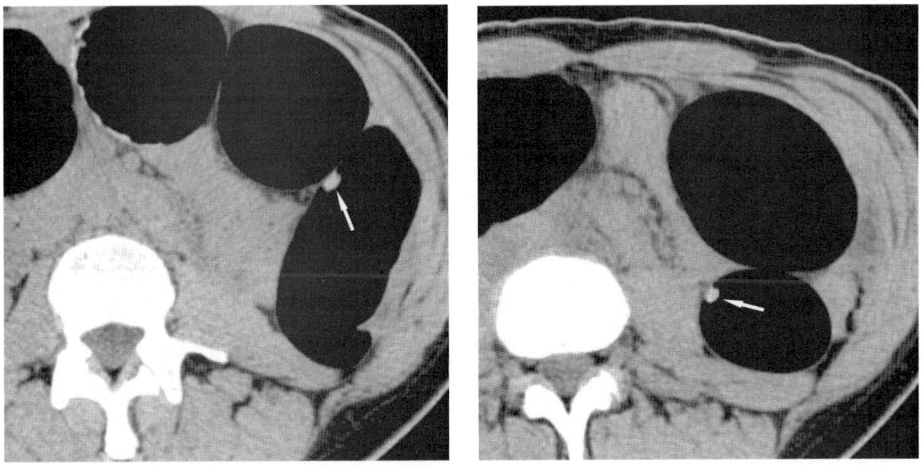

C D

FIGURE 6.37 *(Continued)*.

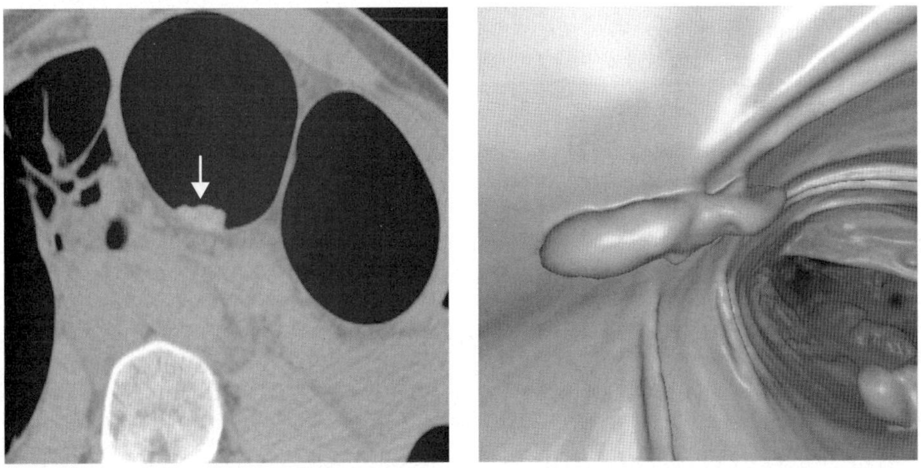

A B

FIGURE 6.38 Linear Stool: A homogeneous lesion is seen on the axial view **(A)** which is seen to represent linear stool on the 3D endoluminal view **(B)**. Other foci of residual stool are seen in the background.

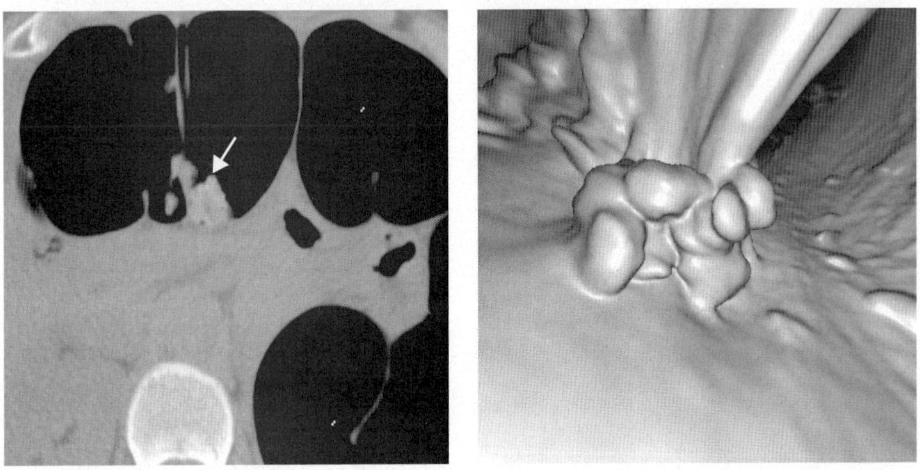

A B

FIGURE 6.39 Lobulated Stool: An irregular, heterogeneous, lobulated lesion on the axial view **(A)** has the typical appearance of stool on the 3D endoluminal view **(B)**. Note the smaller adjacent stool particles.

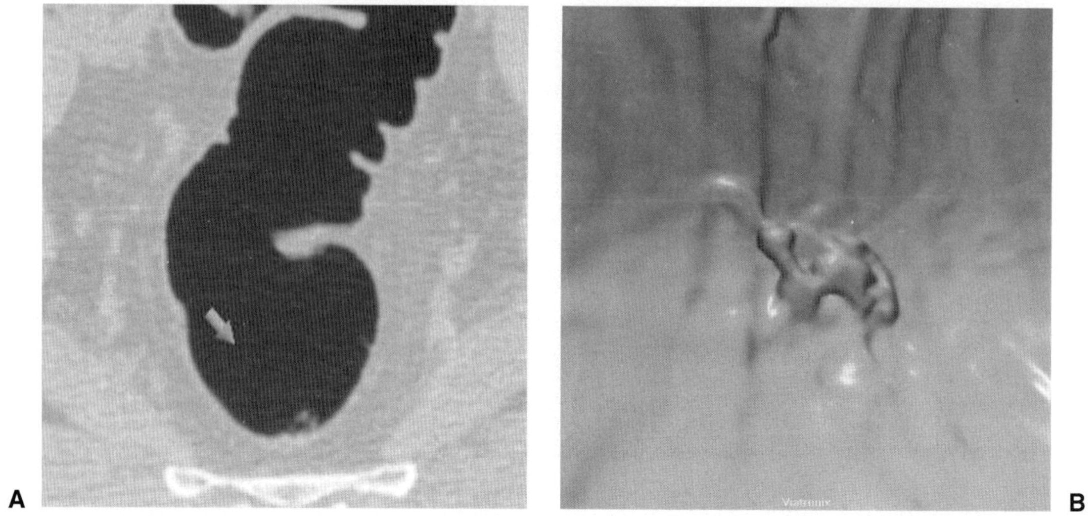

FIGURE 6.40 Angulated Stool on 3D: Axial view **(A)** shows an ill-defined heterogeneous lesion along the posterior rectal wall, which is typical of stool. 3D endoluminal view **(B)** shows the angulated appearance, which is a feature of stool.

because most patients are asymptomatic. They are thought to develop due to vigorous straining, chronic constipation, prolonged sitting, and in pregnancy. Internal hemorrhoids develop above the dentate line whereas external hemorrhoids form below the dentate line. The dentate line divides the squamous epithelium of the anus from the columnar epithelium of the rectum. Mixed hemorrhoids are confluent internal and external hemorrhoids.[30] Internal hemorrhoids become symptomatic (bleeding or pain) when they become enlarged due to dilatation and engorgement of arteriovenous plexuses (between the superior rectal arteries and veins). Prolapsed internal hemorrhoids extend into the anal canal or through the anus. Internal hemorrhoids have been described on barium enema as resembling multiple polyps in the rectum, but may also appear as lobulated folds.[29]

Internal hemorrhoids often appear as small protrusions in the rectal vault extending from the anorectal junction. They typically have a smooth contour and are located in a concentric manner around the rectal tube (see Figure 6.46 and 6.47). Sagittal and coronal multiplanar reformatted views as well as the 3D endoluminal view can easily demonstrate the typical appearance of internal hemorrhoids. Uncommonly, internal hemorrhoids may be difficult to distinguish from rectal polyps and clinical history is necessary. Both internal hemorrhoids and rectal polyps can enhance following intravenous contrast administration.

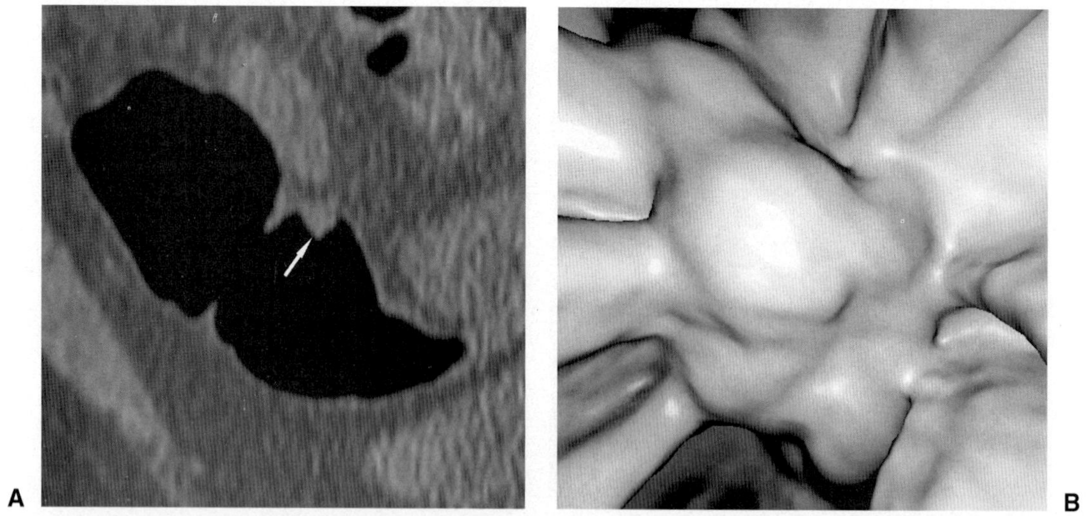

FIGURE 6.41 Angulated Stool on 2D: Coronal multiplanar reformat **(A)** shows angulated appearance of homogeneous stool which is more difficult to see on the 3D endoluminal view **(B)**.

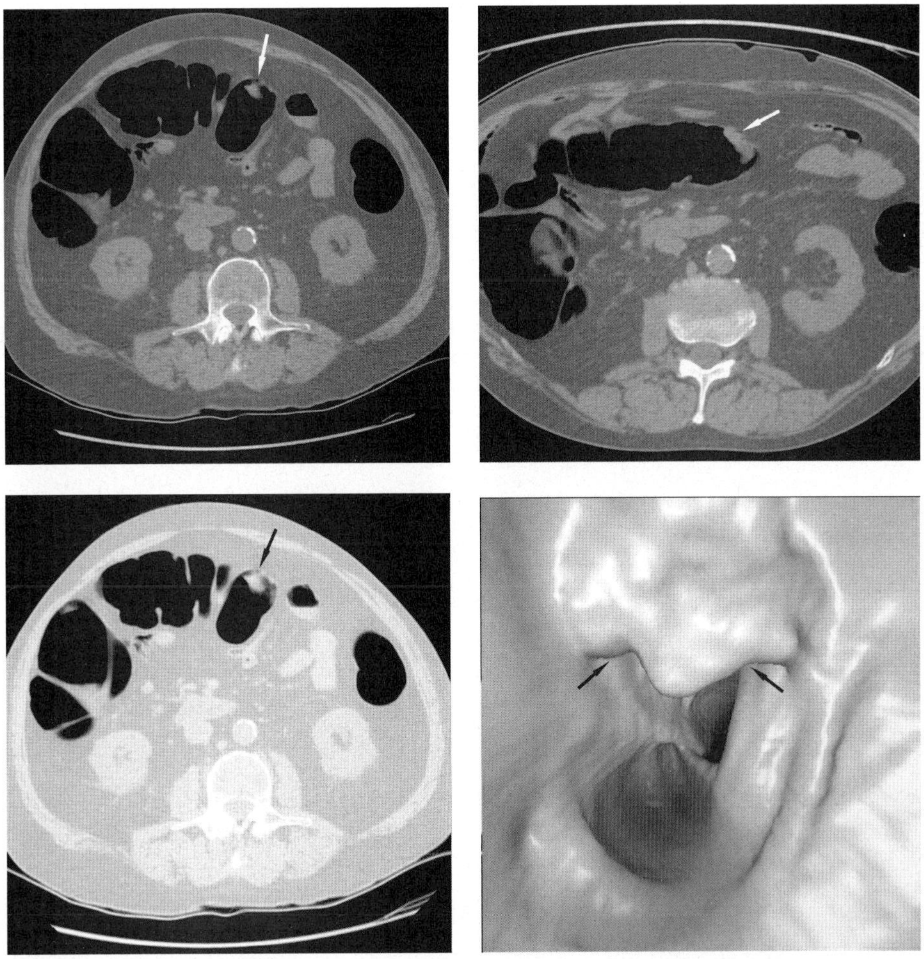

A B C D

FIGURE 6.42 Carcinoma: Air that is trapped between a lesion and the colon wall will be located only in the periphery. Supine axial image in abdominal window **(A)** shows a mass that appears heterogeneous and changes morphology in the prone position **(B)**. Colon window **(C)** shows air that is located around the periphery of the mass. The mass is seen to arise from the wall on the 3D endoluminal view **(D)**.

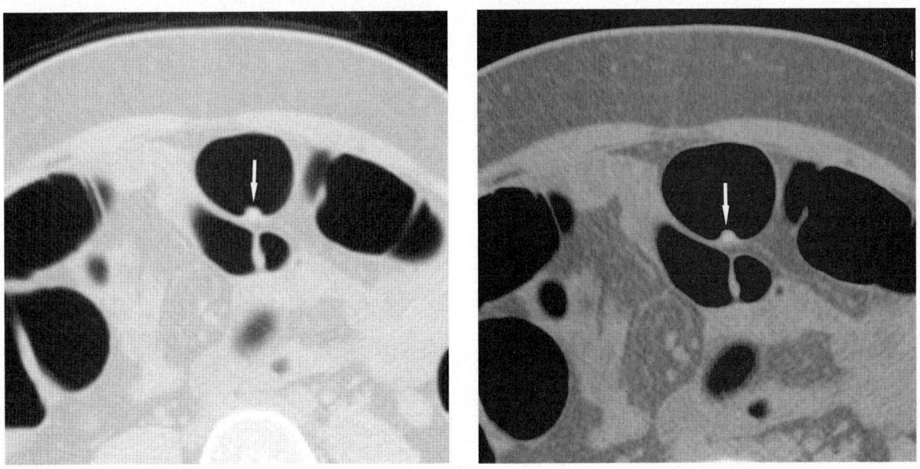

A B

FIGURE 6.43 Radiopaque Pill: Supine axial image in colon **(A)** and abdominal **(B)** windows shows a high density pill (arrow) that shifts to the dependent wall in the prone position **(C)**. The pill is a pitfall on the 3D endoluminal view **(D)** and has the appearance of a polyp. (*Views C and D are on next page.*)

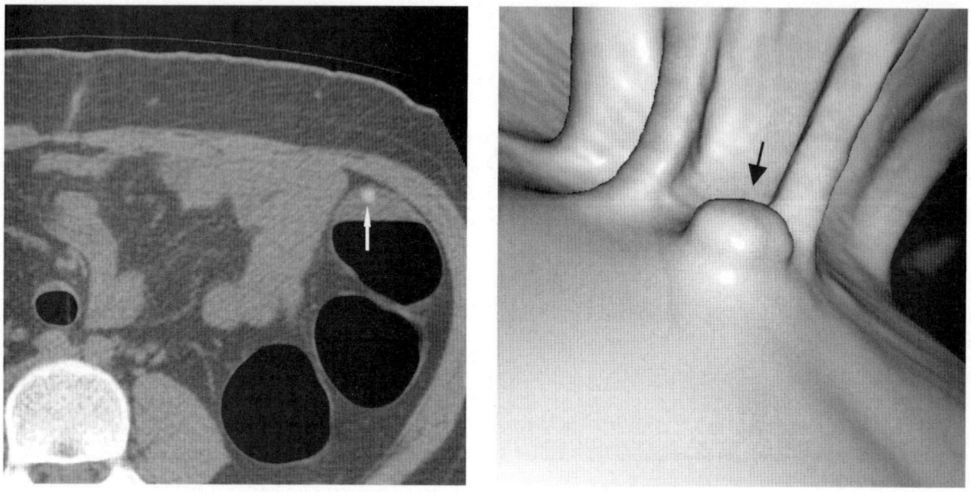

C D

FIGURE 6.43 (*Continued*).

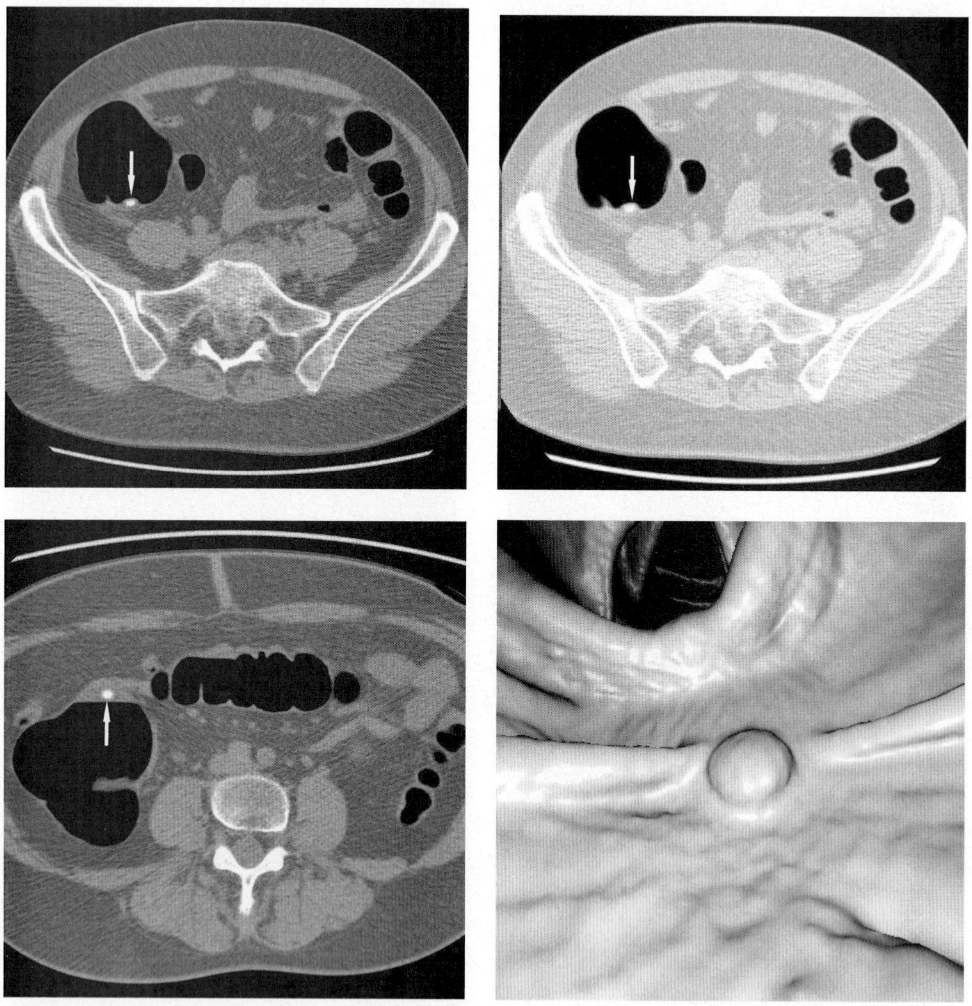

A B

C D

FIGURE 6.44 Radiopaque Pill: Axial image in abdominal **(A)** and colon **(B)** windows shows dependent location of the radiopaque pill in the supine position which moves to the anterior wall in the prone position **(C)**. Note the well-defined spherical shape of the pill on the 3D endoluminal view **(D)** which simulates a polyp.

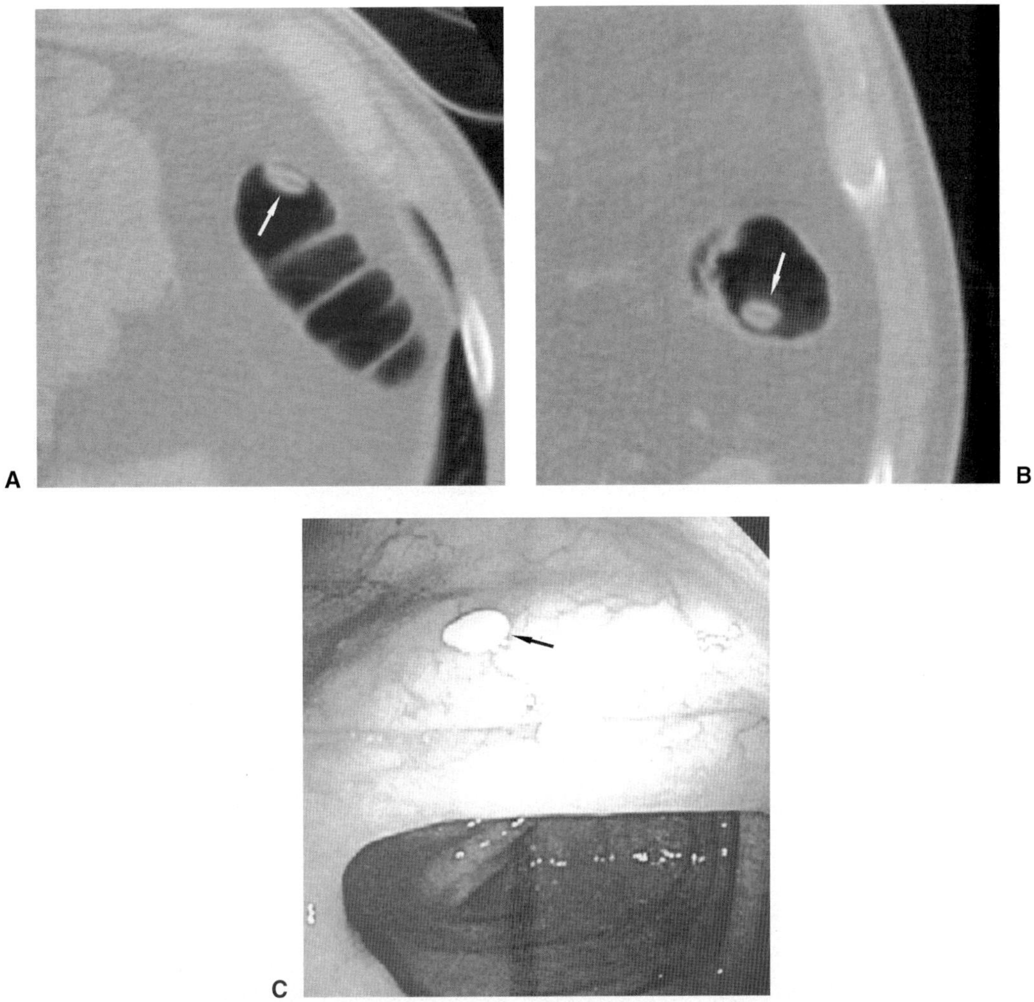

FIGURE 6.45 Seeds: Axial views **(A, B)** shows two different ovoid lesions with central linear low density. Colonoscopy **(C)** revealed several seeds scattered throughout the colon.

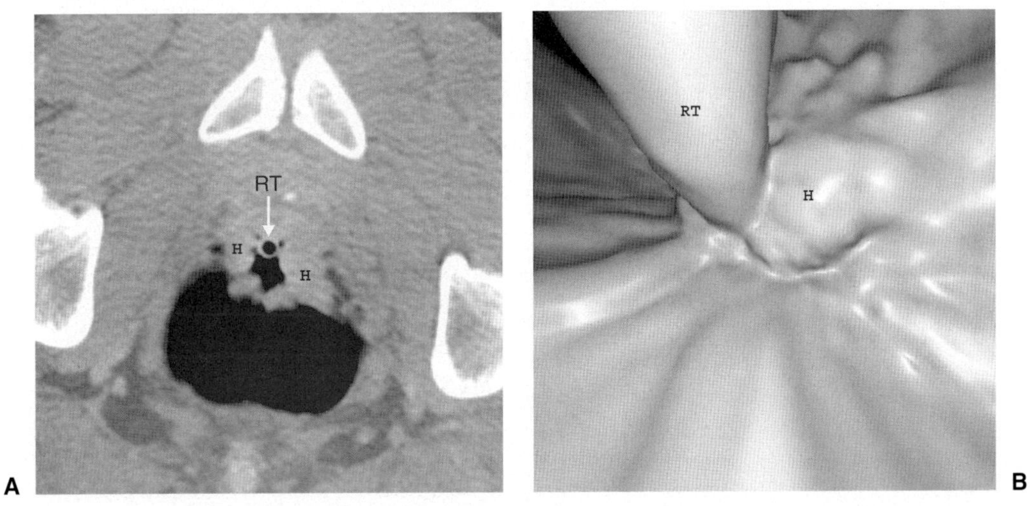

FIGURE 6.46 Internal Hemorrhoids: Axial image **(A)** shows concentric soft tissue surrounding the rectal tube (RT). 3D endoluminal views **(B, C)** and colonoscopy image **(D)** shows the RT and focal protrusions encircling the tube representing internal hemorrhoids (H). (*Views C and D are on next page*; View D: See also color plate.)

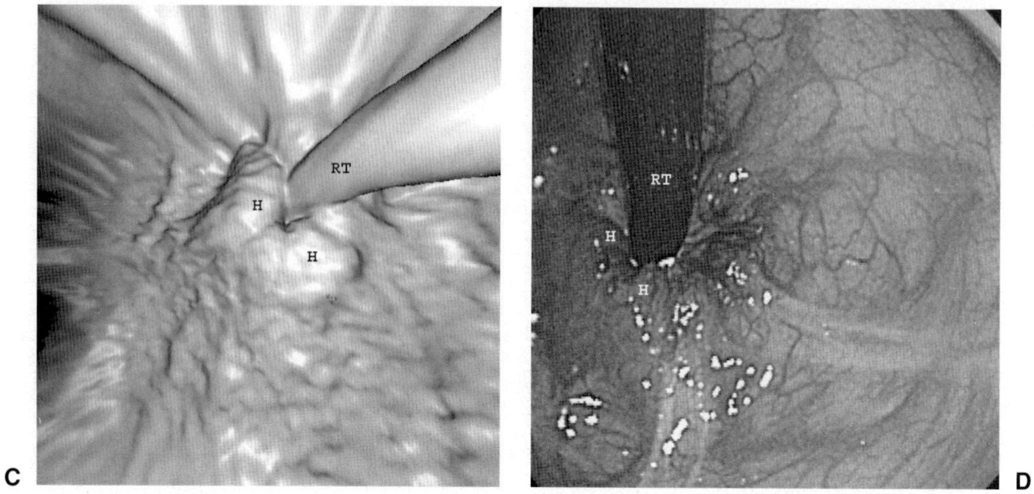

FIGURE 6.46 (*Continued*).

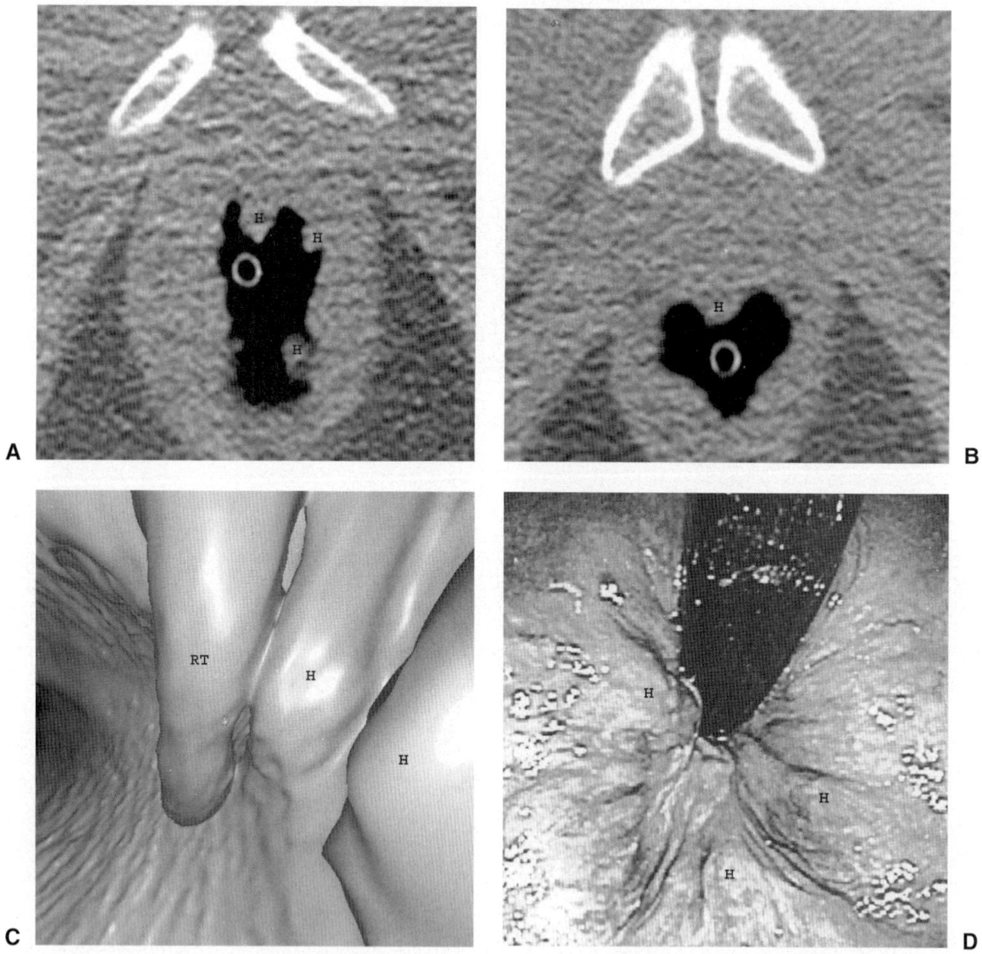

FIGURE 6.47 Internal Hemorrhoids: Axial images in supine **(A)** and prone **(B)** positions shows several focal protrusions along the rectal wall due to hemorrhoids (H) extending from the anorectal junction. These are seen to have a smooth, linear configuration on the 3D endoluminal view **(C)** located adjacent to the rectal tube (RT). Colonoscopy **(D)** demonstrates the enlarged hemorrhoids surrounding the scope.

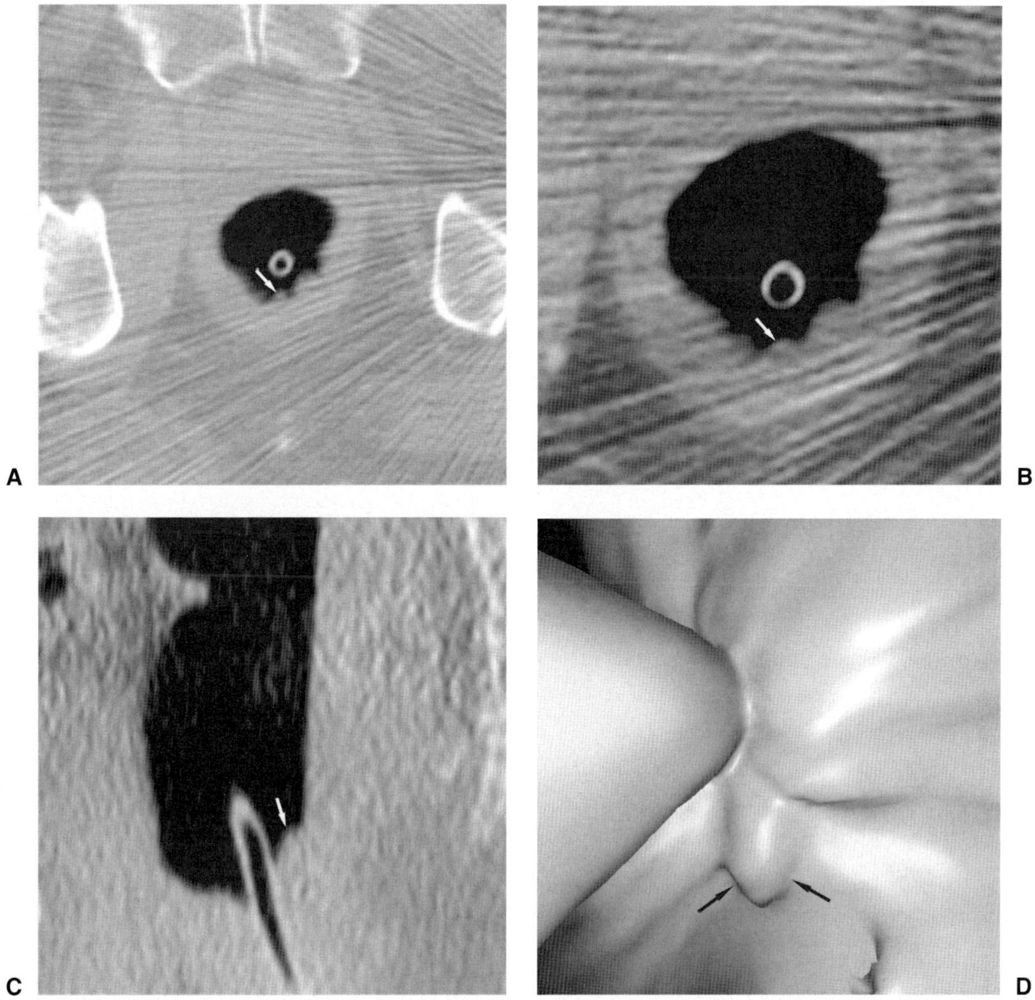

FIGURE 6.48 Hypertrophied Anal Papilla: Supine view in colon **(A)** and abdominal **(B)** windows demonstrates a single protrusion near the anorectal junction (arrow). The sagittal reformat **(C)** and 3D endoluminal view **(D)** also show the polypoid appearing lesion, which was a benign hypertrophied anal papilla on colonoscopy. Differential diagnosis on CTC includes rectal polyp and internal hemorrhoid. CTC, computed tomographic colongraphy.

Hypertrophied Anal Papillae

There are other lesions located at the anal verge that may be indistinguishable from polyps and patients may require further evaluation with digital examination, anoscopy, or sigmoidoscopy. Anal papillae are acquired lesions that arise from the base of the rectal columns of Morgagni at the dentate line. They are covered by stratified squamous epithelium and can become enlarged as a result of congestion, irritation, injury, or infection.[31] These lesions, have been described on barium enema, and although common on proctoscopy, are a relatively rare finding radiographically. They can be single or multiple. In patients with anal papillae, approximately 25% will have one, 45% have two or three and 30% have four or more.[32] A clinical history of chronic anal irritation or inflammation may suggest the diagnosis. These lesions appear as smooth, polypoid lesions at the anal verge with soft tissue attenuation and are indistinguishable from true polyps (see Figures 6.48–6.50). However, the possibility of hypertrophied anal papillae should be included in the differential diagnosis especially if these are the only lesions because anoscopy may demonstrate the classic whitish appearance of these lesions.

Mucous Strand

A mucous strand can sometimes be confused as the stalk of a pedunculated polyp. They are typically thin, linear, and will extend across normal haustral folds (see Figures 6.51 and 6.52). Their appearance is often characteristic but care should be taken to investigate the area completely to exclude the presence of a pedunculated polyp. If fecal and fluid tagging has been performed, the tagging agent may be incorporated into the mucus strand and it will appear high density.

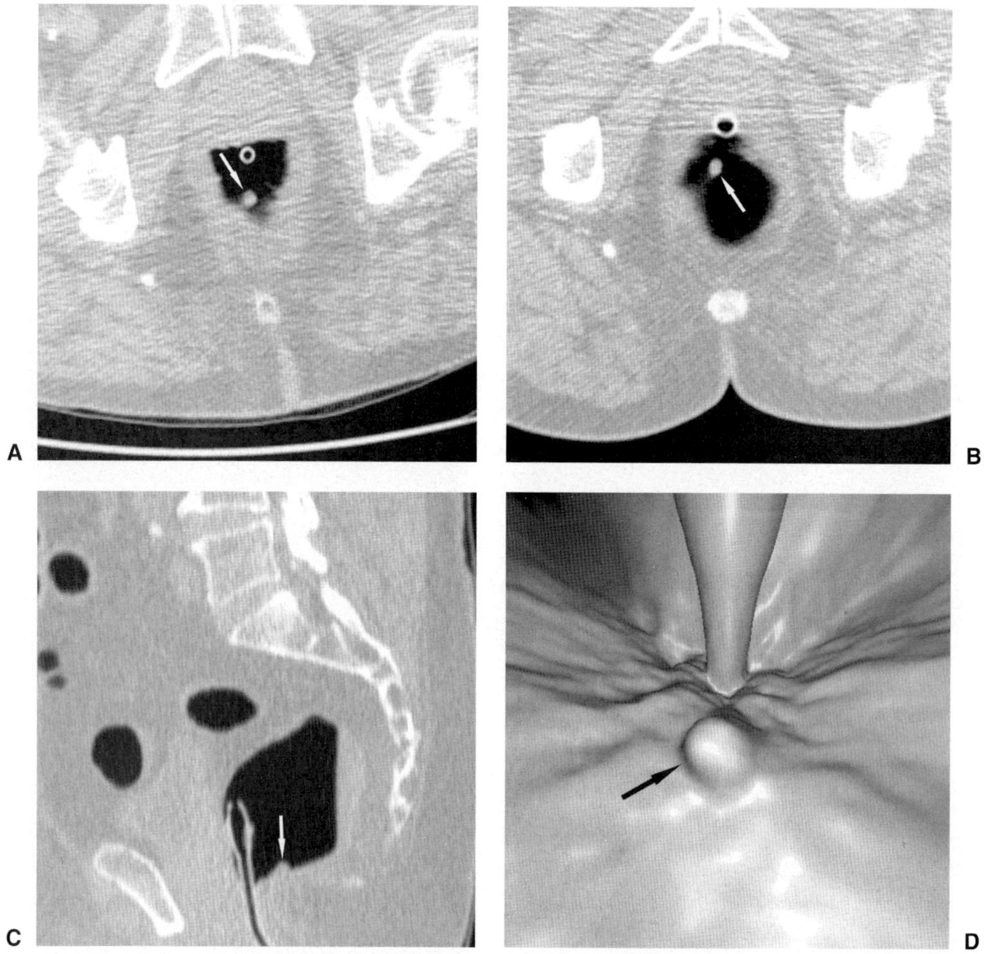

FIGURE 6.49 Hypertrophied Anal Papilla: Supine **(A)** and prone **(B)** axial images shows a small polypoid-appearing lesion adjacent to the anal verge. Sagittal reformat **(C)** and 3D endoluminal image **(D)** shows the hypertrophied anal papilla near the rectal tube.

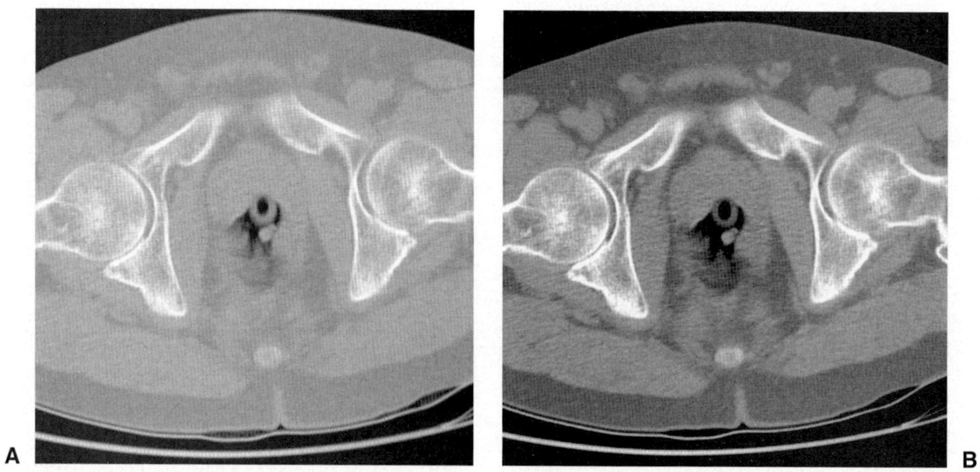

FIGURE 6.50 Multiple Hypertrophied Anal Papillae: Most patients with hypertrophied anal papillae (75%) will have multiple. Axial view in colon **(A)** and abdominal **(B)** windows demonstrates a cluster of small polypoid lesions around the anorectal junction. The 3D endoluminal view **(C)** and the colonoscopy image **(D)** show the well-defined small hypertrophied anal papillae. (View D: See also color plate.)

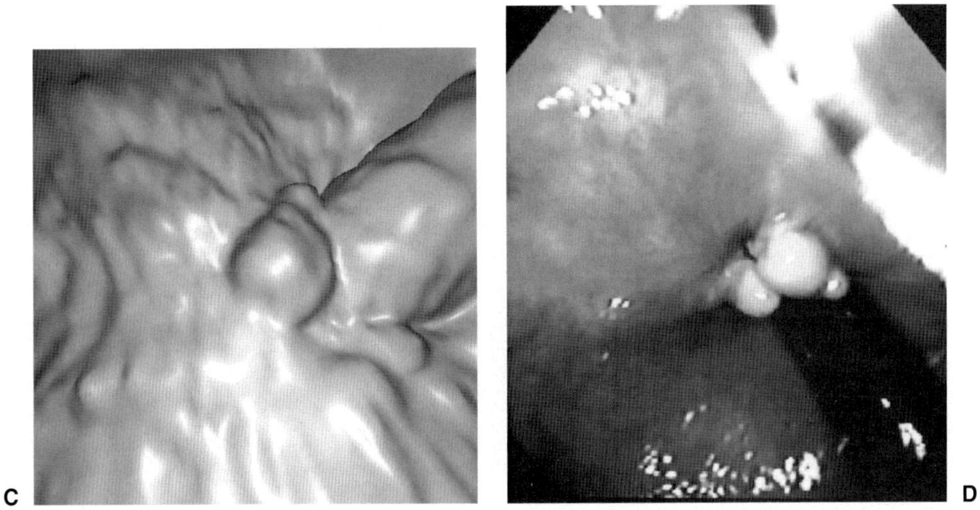

FIGURE 6.50 (*Continued*).

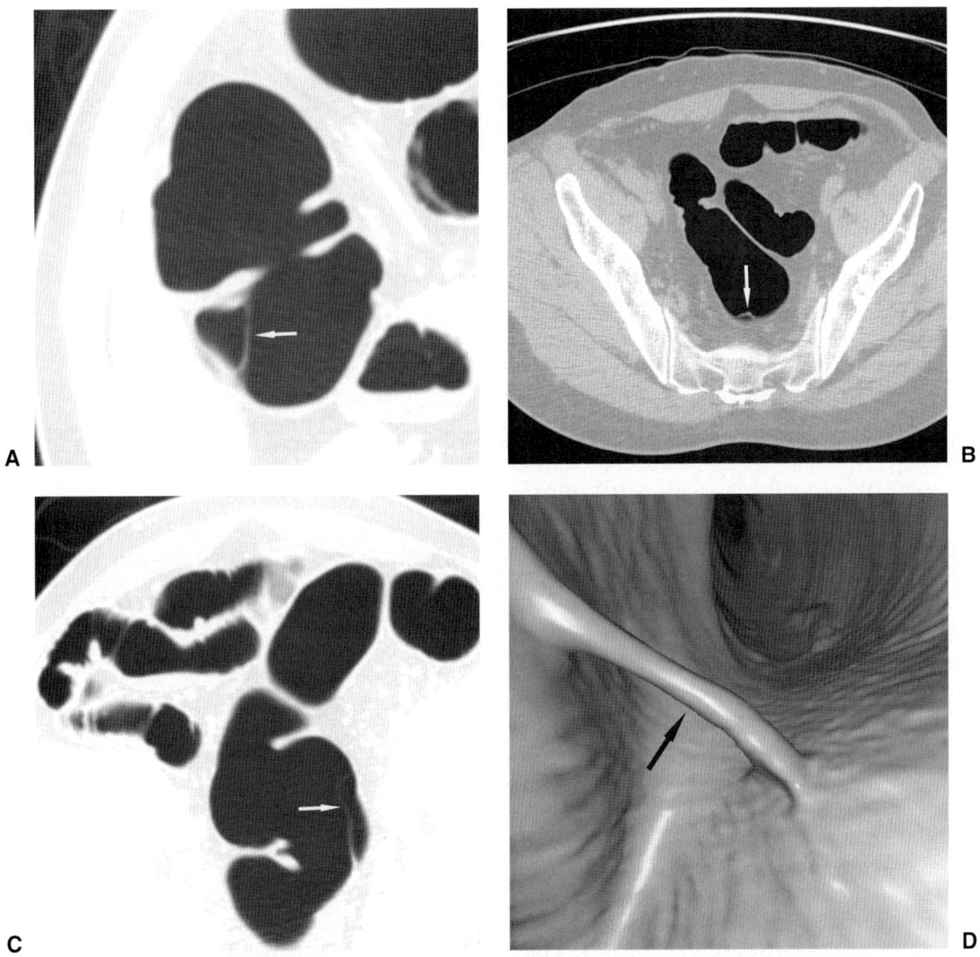

FIGURE 6.51 Mucous Strands: Axial images in lung window **(A, C)** and prone axial image in colon window **(B)** taken from the same patient show multiple mucous strands which appear as thin, linear strands attached to the colon wall in various atypical orientations on the 2D views and on the 3D endoluminal view **(D)**. These can occasionally be mistaken for the stalk of a pedunculated polyp.

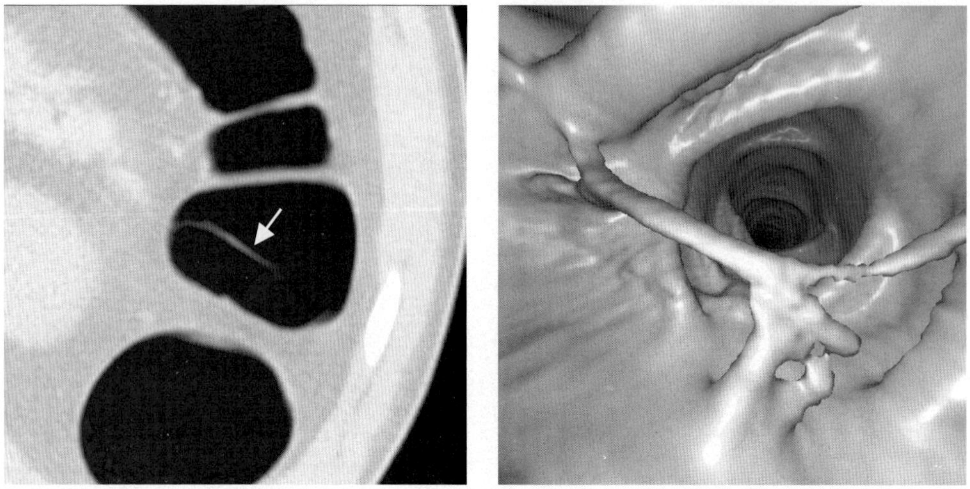

A B

FIGURE 6.52 Mucous Strand: Axial image in colon window shows a mucous strand **(A)** which shows complex bridging to the colon wall on the 3D endoluminal view **(B)**.

Air Bubble

Air bubbles within residual fluid appear as a rounded defect and can sometimes resemble a polyp on 3D endoluminal views. Interactive rotation around the air bubble on 3D views will show that the air bubble is not actually protruding into the lumen. Switching to the 2D views will easily show the air density and the characteristic appearance (see Figures 6.53 and 6.54). These are often located in the rectum and are due to gaseous insufflation of the colon when the tip of the rectal tube may be partially or completely submersed in a liquid pool.

Lipoma

The colon is the most common site of gastrointestinal lipomas and approximately two thirds of all gastrointestinal lipomas are located in the large bowel.[33] Lipomas are the most common benign tumor of the colon except for adenomas. These lesions are typically smaller than 3 cm and located in the right colon.[34] Most colonic lipomas originate in the submucosa and many are pedunculated with a short broad-based stalk. Patients are often asymptomatic and lipomas are typically incidental findings on CTC. However, when colonic lipomas become large they may cause bleeding, alterations in bowel habit, obstruction and colocolic intussusception.[35] Therefore, large lipomas should be reported, particularly if there is associated significant luminal compromise. Intussuscepted lipomas have been reported to have an atypical appearance with loss of fat attenuation on CT scan.[36]

Lipomas appear as round or ovoid polypoid lesions on 3D endoluminal views (see Figures 6.55–6.57). They typically have a smooth or mildly lobulated contour. 2D views using abdominal windows are necessary to identify the intrinsic uniform fat density (−50 to −150 HU) of these lesions. Large lipomas may contain high density due to hemorrhage. Additionally, intussuscepted lipomas have been reported to have an atypical appearance with loss of fat attenuation on CT scan.[36] These lesions may appear to change morphology with a change in position and depending upon the degree of luminal distention. They can often still be identified on 2D views even in areas of poor distention or collapse because of their fat density.

Gastrointestinal Stromal Tumor

Most gastrointestinal stromal tumors (GISTs) occur in the stomach (60%–70%) and small bowel (25%–35%).[37] Only 5% of GISTs occur in the colon. Most GISTs are undifferentiated spindle cell or epithelioid neoplasms. Some tumors thought to be leiomyomas or leiomyosarcomas in the past are now classified as stromal tumors because many have been found to not originate from true muscle cells. Colonic stromal tumors are very uncommon and tend to occur in the rectum.

Small GISTs are often benign and appear as small polypoid lesions in the rectum that may be sessile or pedunculated. It is usually not possible to differentiate small GISTs from adenomatous or other types of polyps. Large GISTs are typically malignant and can have a variety of appearances. They may present as large polypoid or cavitary masses as well as annular lesions simulating colonic adenocarcinoma (see Figure 6.58).

Rare Entities

Other etiologies that may resemble polyps or masses have also been described on barium enema, including pneumatosis cystoides coli, bezoar, amyloidosis, and pseudotumors caused by adhesions.[29] These findings are rare on CTC and may mimic polyps or masses on the 3D endoluminal view. The 2D views are often more helpful in differentiating these entities from true polyps or cancers. In particular, the air density of the cysts due to pneumatosis cystoides coli is easily identified on the 2D views.

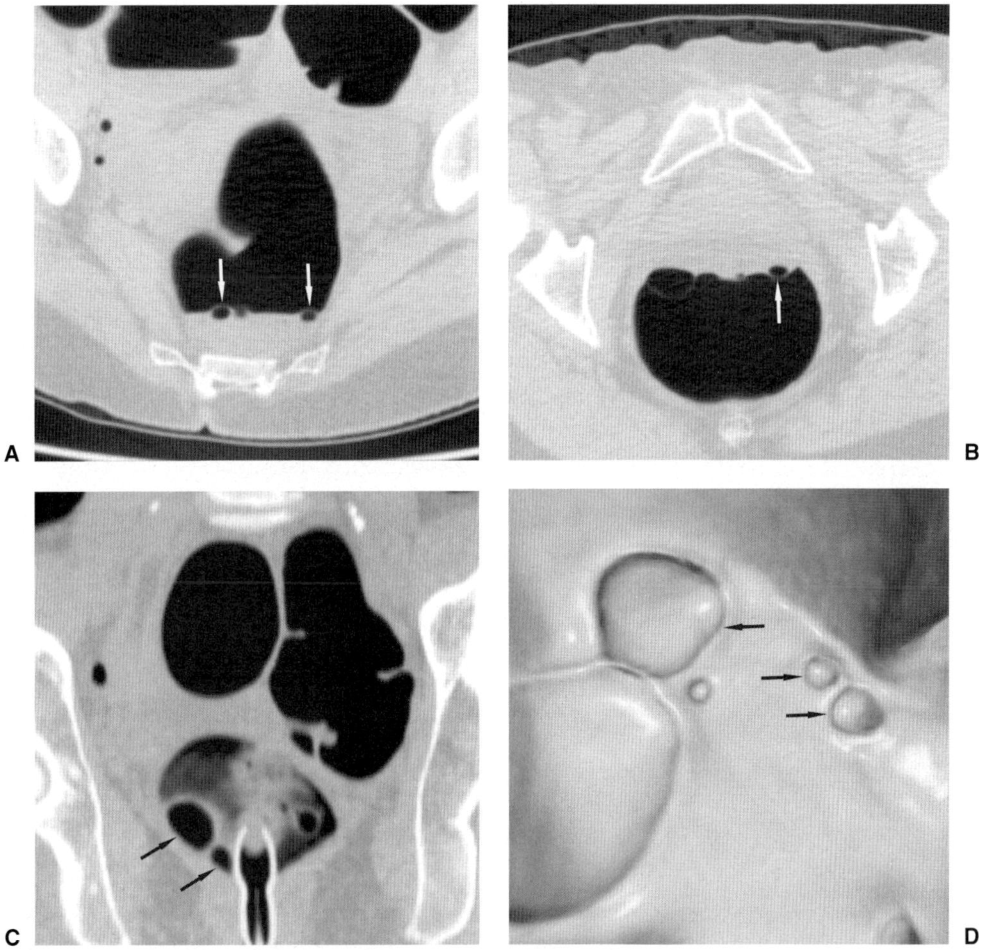

FIGURE 6.53 Rectal Air Bubbles: Axial views in supine **(A)** and prone **(B)** positions show multiple air bubbles in the rectum at the top of a fluid pool. Coronal reformat **(C)** demonstrates the typical well-defined air densities adjacent to the rectal tip. The air bubbles may simulate polyps on the 3D endoluminal view **(D)** although interactive rotation will demonstrate that these do not protrude into the lumen.

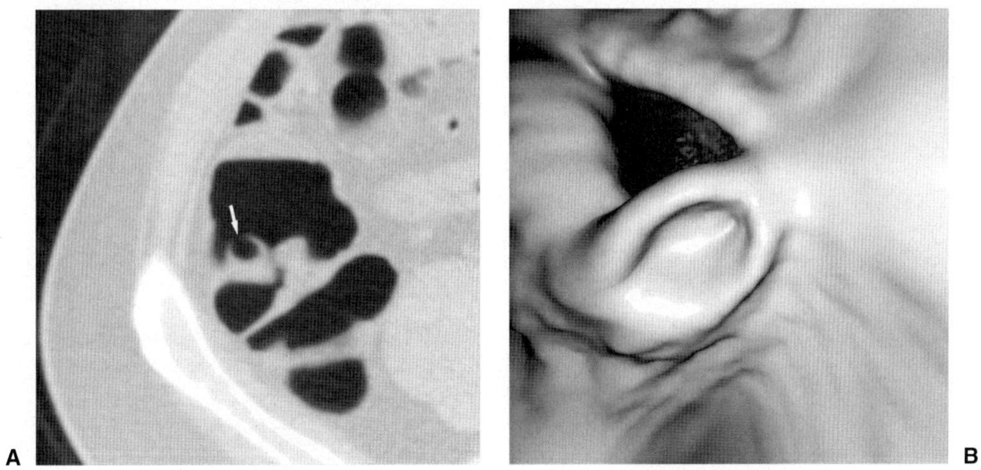

FIGURE 6.54 Air Bubble: Axial view **(A)** shows an air bubble on a fold which appears as an ovoid lesion with a large central hole on the 3D endoluminal view **(B)**.

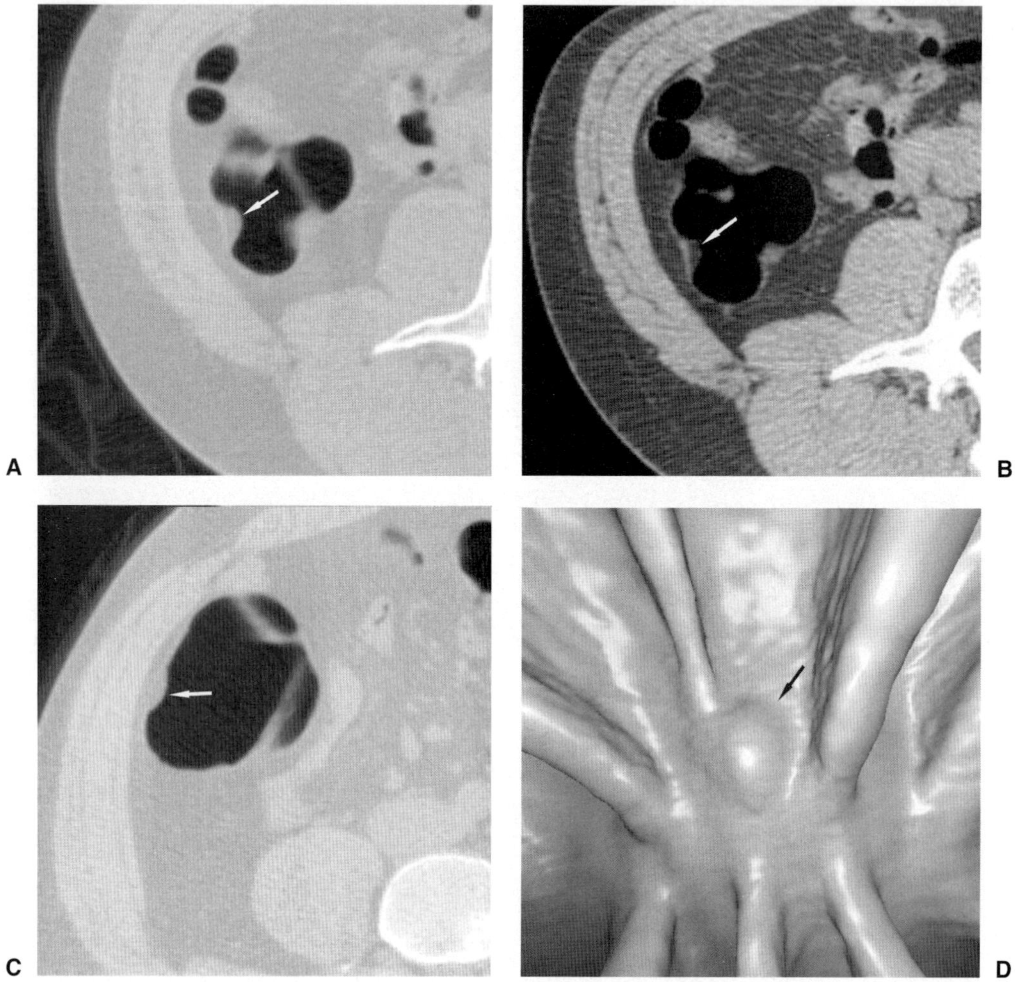

FIGURE 6.55 Lipoma: Supine axial image in colon window **(A)** shows a polypoid lesion that is clearly fat density on the abdominal window **(B)**. The lesion is also seen on the prone view **(C)** and is nonmobile. The polypoid appearance on the 3D endoluminal view **(D)** is not specific.

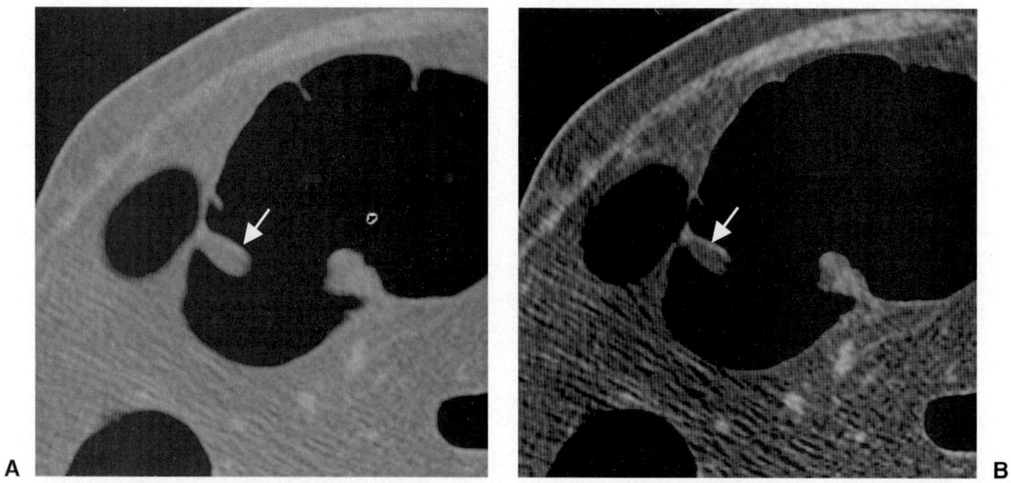

FIGURE 6.56 Lipoma: Axial image in colon **(A)** and abdominal **(B)** window shows a lipoma on a fold which appears as a polyp on the 3D endoluminal view **(C)**.

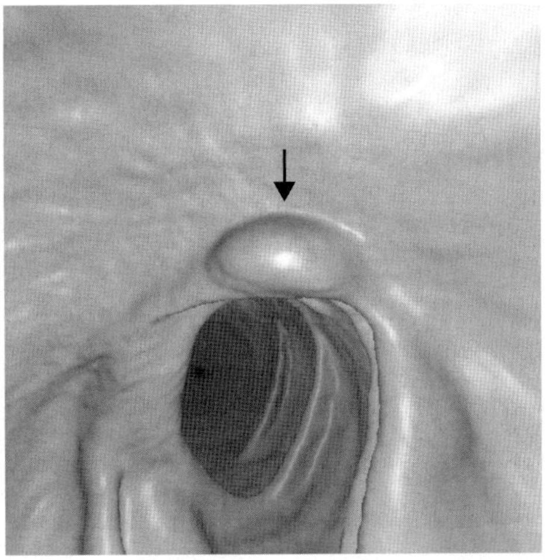

C

FIGURE 6.56 (*Continued*).

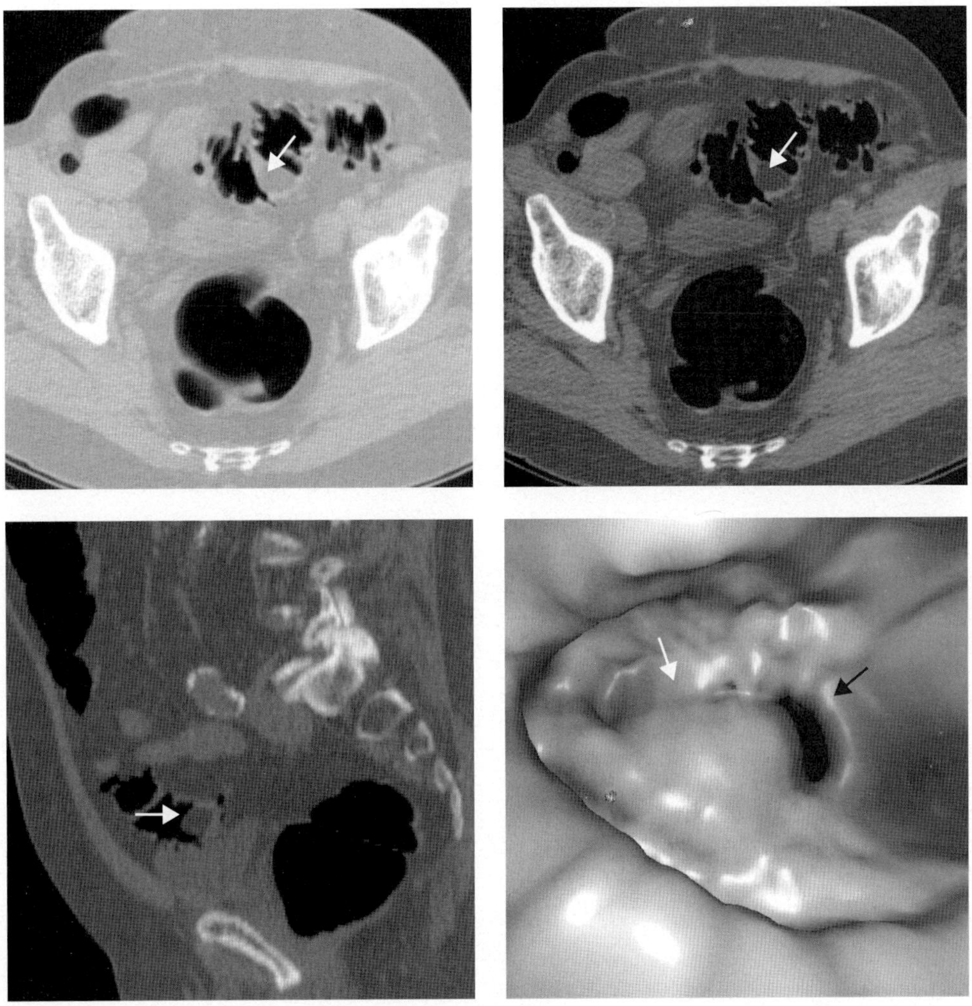

A B C D

FIGURE 6.57 Sigmoid Lipoma: A large lesion is identified in the sigmoid on the axial view in colon window **(A)**. The axial image **(B)** and sagittal reformat **(C)** in abdominal window shows the uniform fat density of this benign lipoma. The 3D endoluminal view **(D)** shows a nonspecific mass partially occluding the lumen.

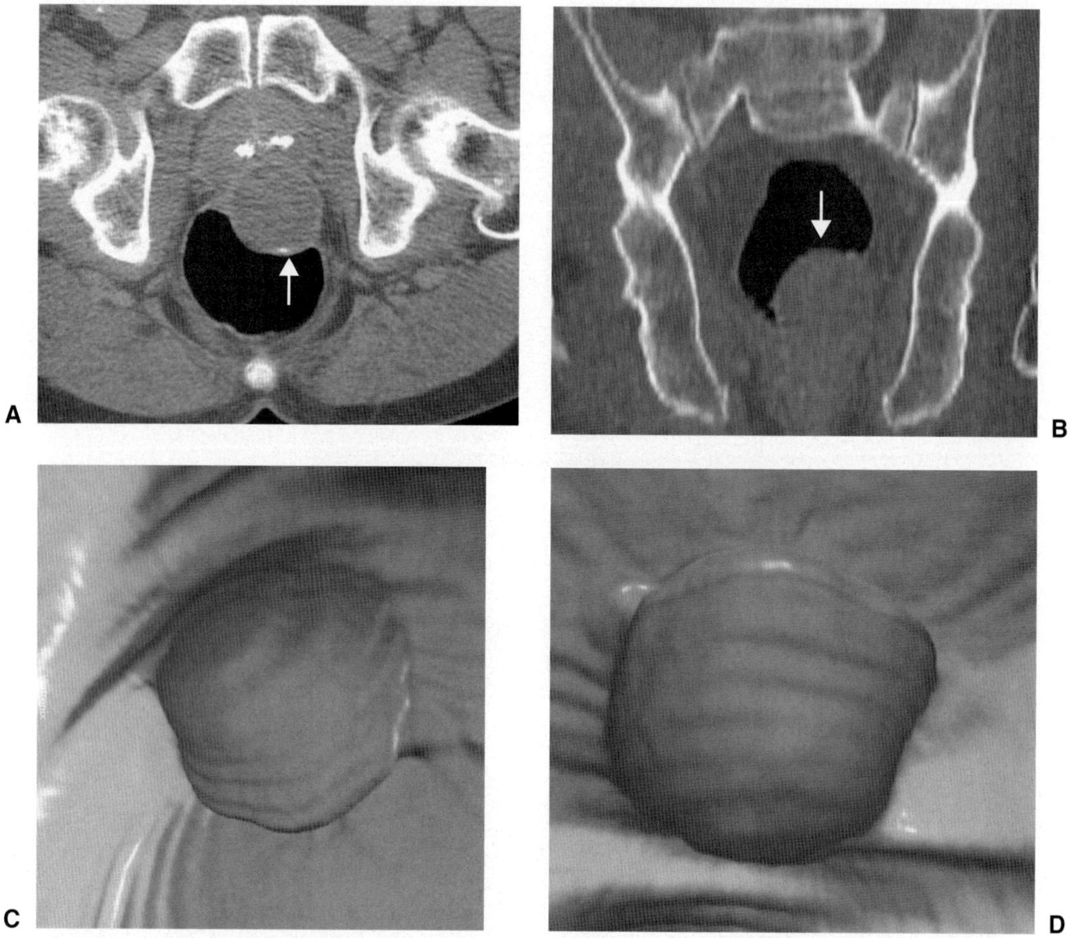

FIGURE 6.58 Rectal Gastrointestinal Stromal Tumor (GIST): A large polypoid mass is identified in the anterior rectum containing peripheral calcification on the axial **(A)** and coronal multiplanar reformat **(B)** views. Note that a significant portion of the mass extends outside of the lumen. The 3D endoluminal views **(C, D)** demonstrate a nonspecific appearing large rounded polypoid mass.

Intestinal implants due to endometriosis occur in approximately 4% of women.[38,39] Symptoms of pain (pelvic or rectal) often wax and wane with the menstrual cycle similar to other endometriomas in the pelvis. Endometriomas tend to involve specific sites within the colon: (a) superior rectal wall near the rectosigmoid junction; (b) superior margin of the sigmoid at the attachment of the sigmoid mesentery.[39] The implants typically invade the mucosa and submucosal layers of the bowel wall and appear as smooth, eccentric submucosal lesions.[38] If a clinical history of endometriosis is given, or if the patient is a woman of child-bearing age with an unusual appearing intracolonic mass at the specific sites, this diagnosis should be considered.

Colitis cystica profunda is a rare, benign process that causes pseudopolypoid lesions most often encountered in the rectum or descending colon. They consist of dilated, epithelial-lined mucous cysts located within the muscularis mucosae of the wall.[40] These lesions can resemble single or multiple polyps and often occur in association with inflammatory colitis or following surgery.

PSEUDOANNULAR LESIONS

Poor Distention or Collapse

Collapsed or underdistended colonic segments make it difficult or impossible to detect lesions on both 2D and 3D views. Collapsed colon present in the same segment on both supine and prone positions should be reported as nondiagnostic for that segment. Alternative positioning, such as the decubitus position, can assist in achieving adequate distention in collapsed segments. However, this requires review of acquired images for detection of underdistended segments on routine supine and prone views when the patient is still on the CT table.

Collapsed segments are impossible to navigate through on 3D imaging, but it is also difficult to track the lumen on 2D views particularly if there are small bowel segments adjacent to the collapsed colon or if there is a lack of mesenteric fat. Isolated collapsed segments within abundant mesenteric fat may be easy to track on 2D views. Switching to abdominal windows to highlight the collapsed, opposed higher attenuation bowel wall can

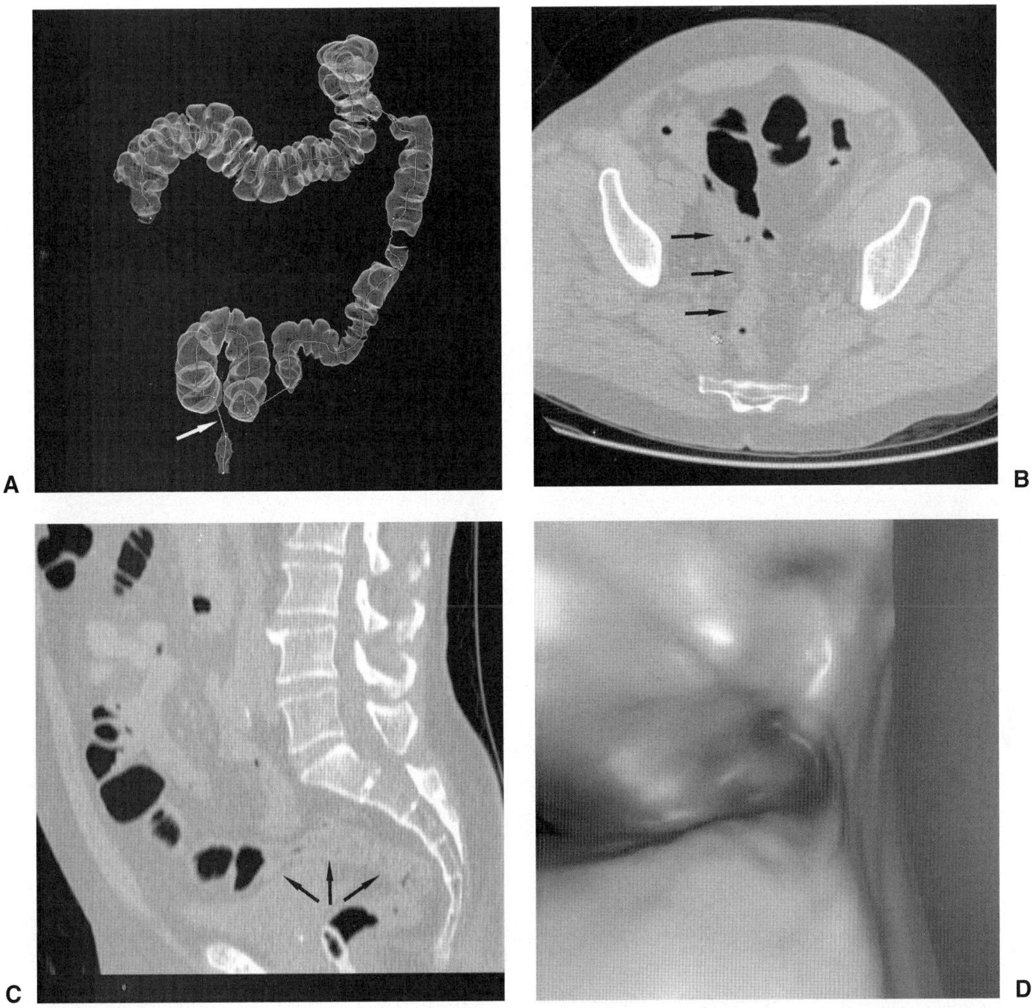

FIGURE 6.59 Collapsed Sigmoid: 3D transparency view shows multiple areas of collapse throughout the colon. **(A)** There is a long length of collapse involving the sigmoid (*arrow*) also seen on the axial image **(B)** and sagittal reformat **(C)**. Navigation is impossible on the 3D endoluminal view **(D)**, which shows a blind end to the lumen due to complete collapse.

be helpful to assist in tracking. Haustral folds may appear polypoid on axial views when there is poor distension and should be evaluated using multiplanar reformats or 3D views. The sigmoid colon is the segment that is most commonly collapsed or underdistended, particularly in elderly patients[27,41] (see Figure 6.59). Poor distention may mask true lesions, especially if residual stool is present (see Figures 6.60 and 6.61). Diverticular disease can predispose the sigmoid colon to collapse or poor distention. If a collapsed segment is present, the reader should evaluate the segment in the opposing position to attempt to clear the segment on one view only. If a suspicious lesion is present on one view but cannot be detected because of collapse on the opposing view, a decision must be made as to whether the lesion has characteristics of a true polyp based on the single view. If this occurs in the sigmoid with a large lesion and there are no other findings identified in the rest of the colon, referral for sigmoidoscopy may be necessary.

Colorectal adenocarcinoma with an annular or apple-core morphology simulates poor distention or collapse on 3D views. The 2D views are essential for the diagnosis of malignancy and must be reviewed. Extension through the colon wall with infiltration of the adjacent fat and pericolonic adenopathy may be detected on the 2D views. The sagittal and coronal multiplanar reformats are particularly helpful for demonstrating the overall morphology of an annular malignancy and often provide more accurate measurements of length of involvement and size of the tumor. The 3D transparency view can also provide an overview of the size and location of an apple-core malignancy.

Wall Thickening

Wall thickening of the colon may be due to infection or inflammation versus malignancy. Various causes of infectious colitis include Escherichia coli,

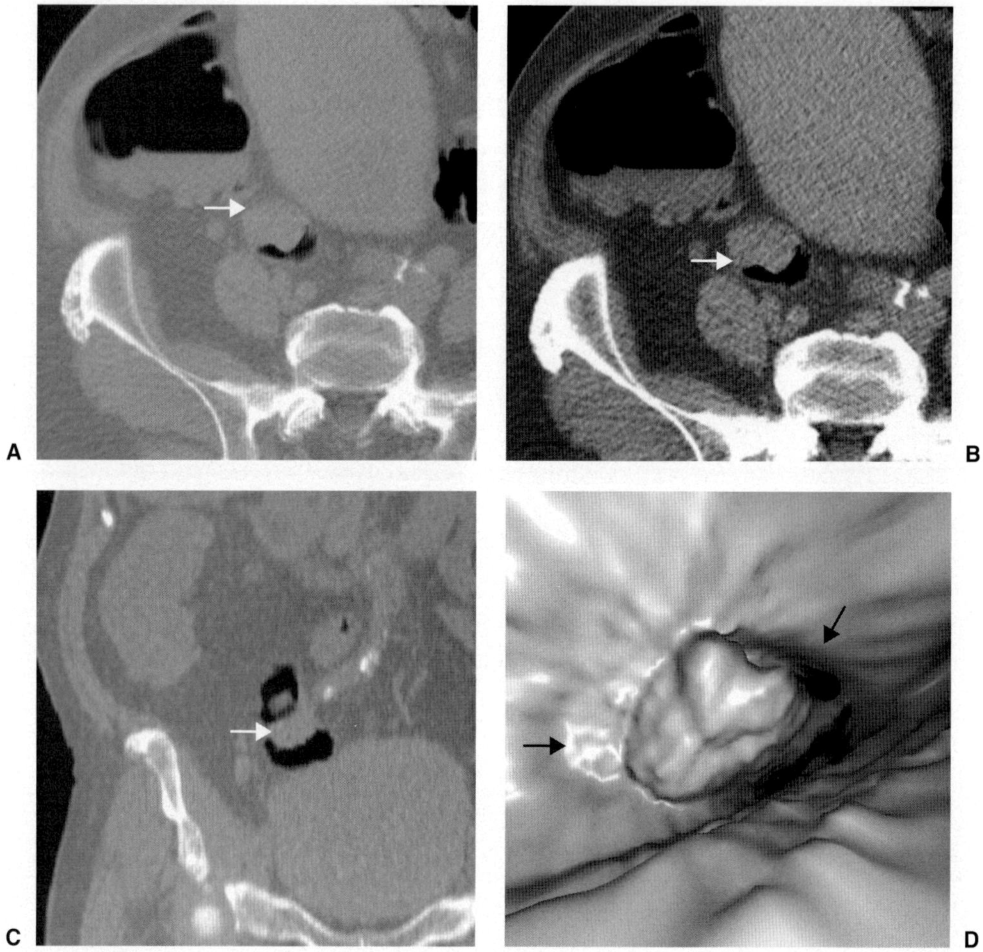

FIGURE 6.60 Poor Distention and Carcinoma: Axial view in colon **(A)** and abdominal **(B)** windows shows suboptimal distention of a portion of the sigmoid. The lumen appears filled with a large mass, which is also seen on the coronal reformat **(C)**. The large irregular mass is seen narrowing the lumen on the 3D endoluminal view **(D)**.

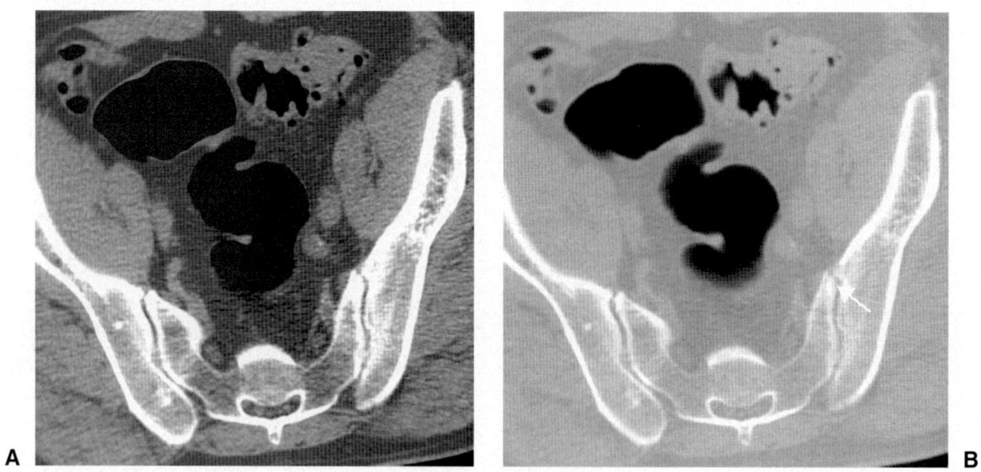

FIGURE 6.61 Poor Distention and Polyp: Supine axial view in abdominal **(A)** and colon **(B)** windows shows sigmoid diverticulosis with poor distention. In the prone axial view **(C)** and 3D endoluminal view **(D)** there is improved sigmoid distention allowing detection of a large polyp.

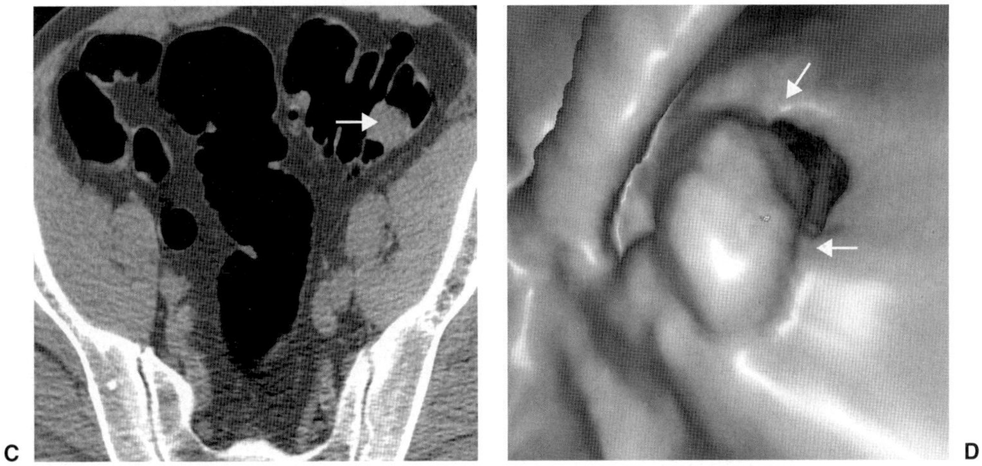

FIGURE 6.61 (*Continued*).

campylobacter, shigella, salmonella, Clostridium difficile (pseudomembranous colitis), amebiasis, and viruses such as cytomegalovirus, which often occurs in immunocompromised patients (see Figure 6.62). Inflammatory disorders that involve the colon include diverticulitis, inflammatory bowel disease, radiation injury, caustic colitis, and ischemic colitis (see Figure 6.63). In general, CTC is not indicated or performed for infectious or inflammatory disorders of the colon.

CTC may be valuable for the evaluation of Crohn's colitis when stenotic lesions are present. Ota et al. evaluated 33 patients with Crohn's disease and found that CTC allowed identification of significant lesions in the colon proximal to a stenosis and was superior to both barium enema and colonoscopy. Ulcerated lesions were less well visualized on CTC.[42] Biancone et al. evaluated 16 patients with ileocolonic anastomosis for Crohn's disease and found that CTC showed perianastomotic recurrence of disease in 15 of 16 subjects.[43] However, perforation of the colon has been reported to occur in patients with ulcerative colitis or Crohn's disease who undergo CTC.[21,44,45] Therefore, CTC should only be performed in patients with inflammatory bowel disease when there is clear indication and only with appropriate caution when distending the colon. However, if the patient is asymptomatic or previously undiagnosed, CTC may detect wall thickening due to infection or inflammation incidentally.

Malignant lesions can also cause colonic wall thickening. In addition to colorectal adenocarcinoma other tumors that may cause thickening of the colon wall include metastases, lymphoma, and GISTs. It is often

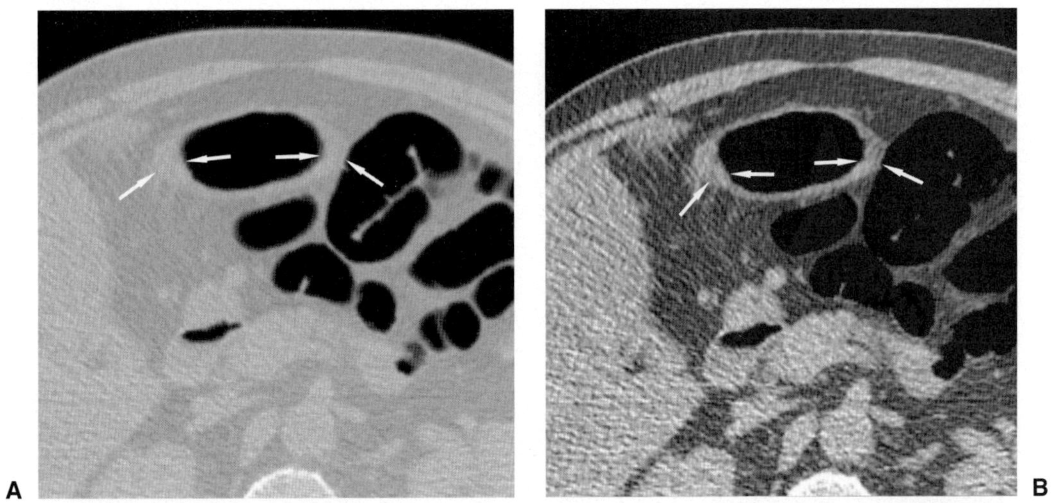

FIGURE 6.62 Infectious Colitis: Axial view in colon **(A)** and abdominal **(B)** windows show mild diffuse thickening of the wall of the transverse colon. The sagittal reformat also **(C)** shows the circumferential thickening of the colon wall. 3D endoluminal view **(D)** reveals an irregular wall contour. Campylobacter was identified on stool culture. (*Views C and D are on next page.*)

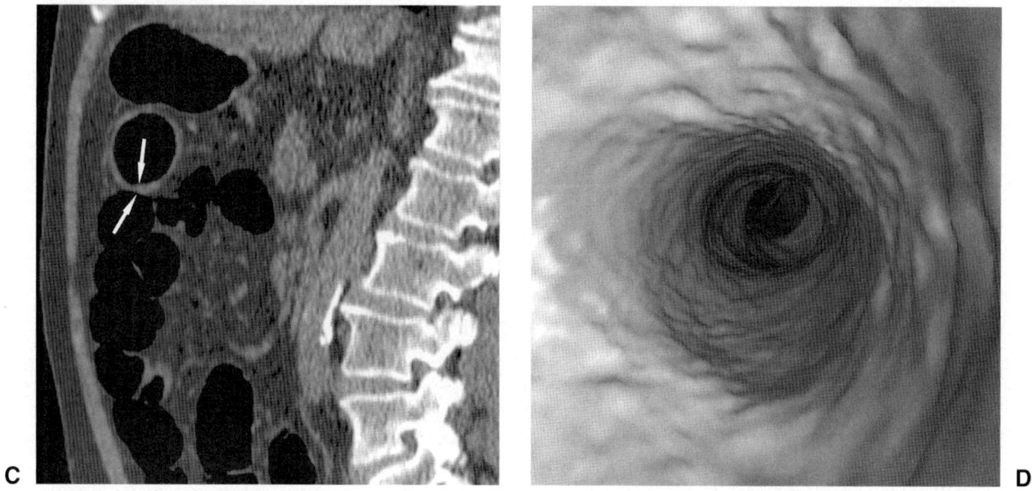

FIGURE 6.62 *(Continued).*

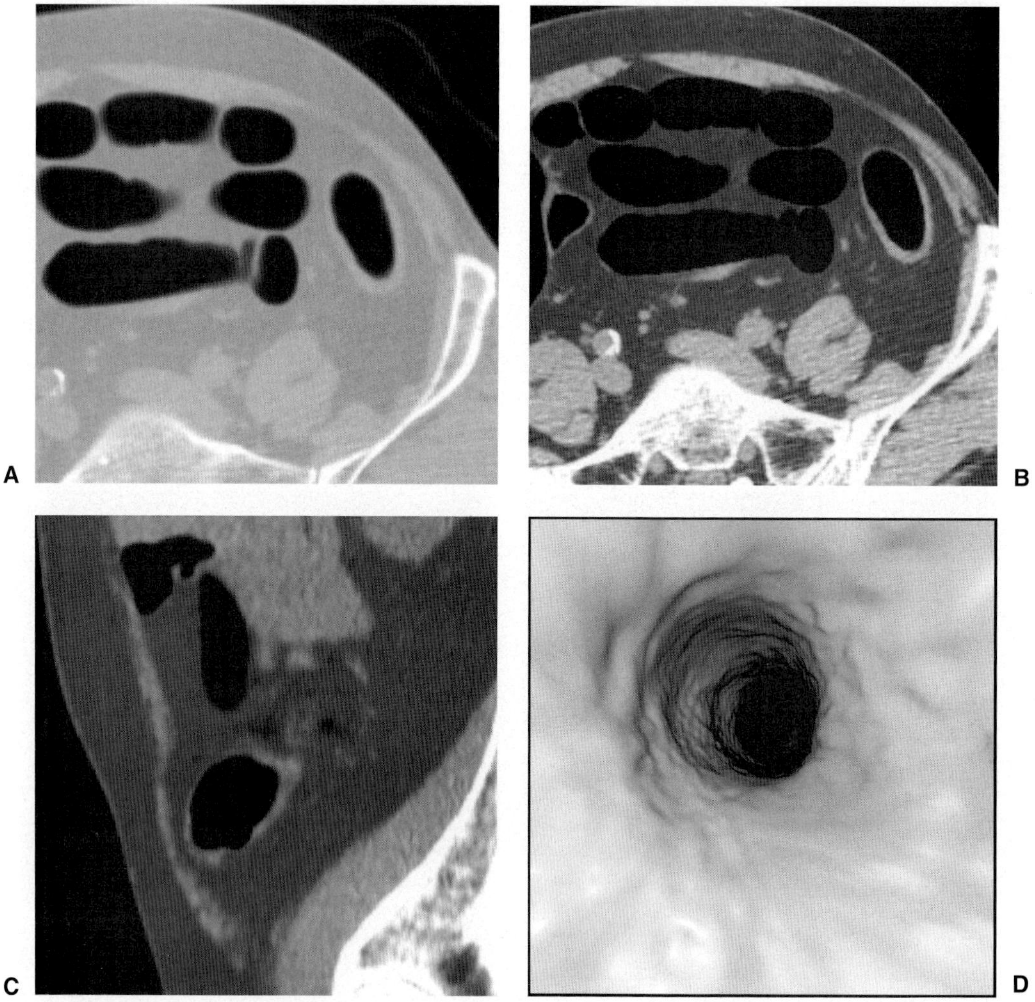

FIGURE 6.63 Crohn's Colitis: Mild wall thickening of the descending colon is seen on the axial images **(A, B)** and on the sagittal reformat **(C)**. 3D endoluminal view **(D)** shows loss of normal haustra and mild nodularity of the wall surface. Patient was asymptomatic.

difficult to differentiate a particular malignancy based on the CTC appearance unless ancillary findings are present on the 2D views. Metastases to the colon occur through three main routes—direct invasion, peritoneal seeding, and hematogenous spread. Direct invasion of adjacent colon segments may be from renal cell carcinoma (ascending, descending, or transverse colon), prostate (rectum) and ovary or uterus (rectosigmoid). Additionally, gastric carcinoma can extend along the gastrocolic ligament to involve the superior transverse colon and pancreatic carcinoma can spread along the transverse mesocolon to involve the inferior transverse colon. Intraperitoneal seeding may occur with any malignancy once there is extension into the peritoneal cavity. Common locations to evaluate for intraperitoneal metastases include the pouch of Douglas, which involves the anterior rectosigmoid, right lower quadrant involving the cecum, and the pelvis involving the superior sigmoid. Hematogenous metastases to the colon are most commonly due to breast carcinoma but may be seen with bronchogenic carcinoma and melanoma.

CARPET LESION

Carpet lesions are flat, lobulated villous tumors which are typically large at the time of presentation (average size of 4 × 6 cm) and can undergo malignant degeneration.[46,47] Approximately 20% of carpet lesions encircle the entire lumen. They usually occur in the cecum, ascending colon, or rectum, and appear as nodular, irregularly thickened wall or fold with little protrusion into the lumen (see Figure 6.64). Carpet lesions are often difficult to distinguish from adherent residual stool on the colon wall or on a fold[5] (see Figure 6.65). Other clinical entities may have an appearance similar to carpet lesions on barium enema and potentially on CTC. Endometriosis, rectal varices, and proctitis can appear

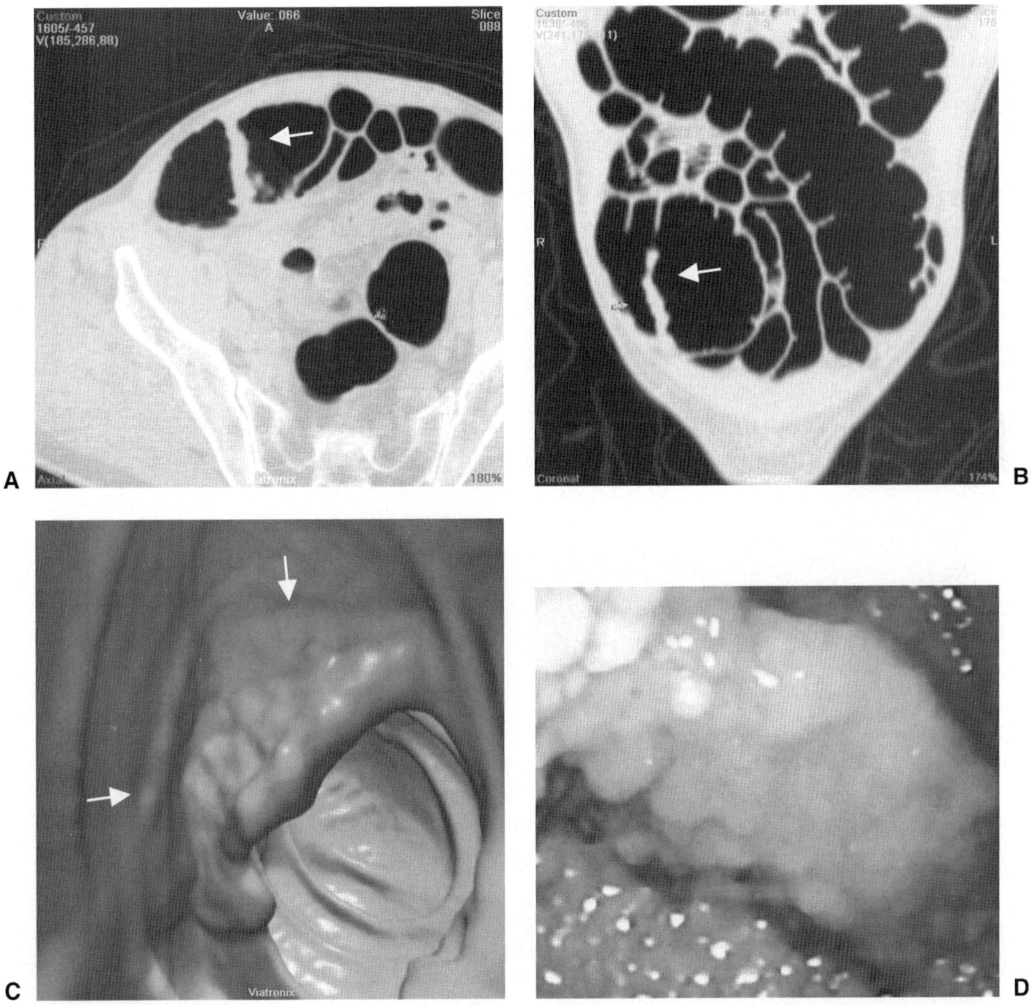

FIGURE 6.64 Carpet Lesion: Thickened nodular haustral fold is seen on the axial and coronal views **(A, B)**. The 3D endoluminal view **(C)** shows the irregular, nodular surface of the lesion. Colonoscopy **(D)** revealed a large carpet lesion in the cecum. These lesions also occur in the ascending colon and rectum.

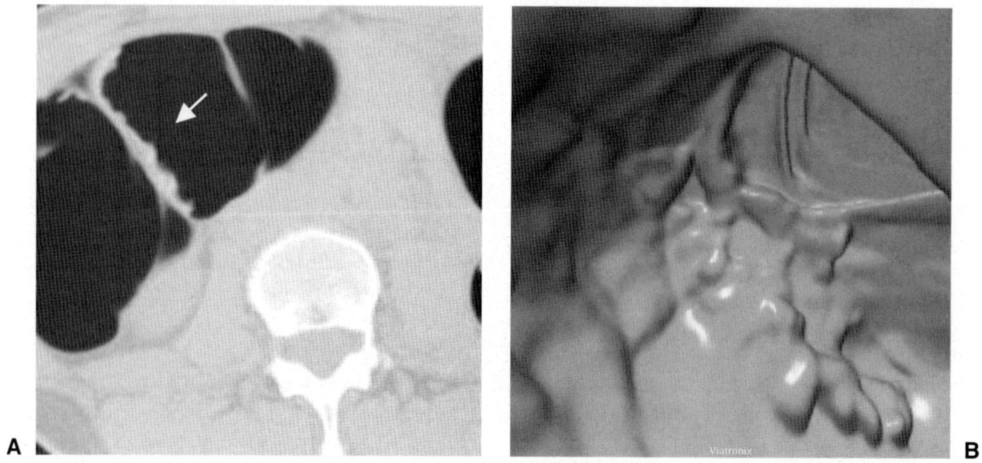

FIGURE 6.65 Pseudocarpet Lesion: Axial view **(A)** demonstrates an irregularly thickened fold. The 3D endoluminal view **(B)** shows a large area with surface nodularity. Colonoscopy found only adherent stool in this area.

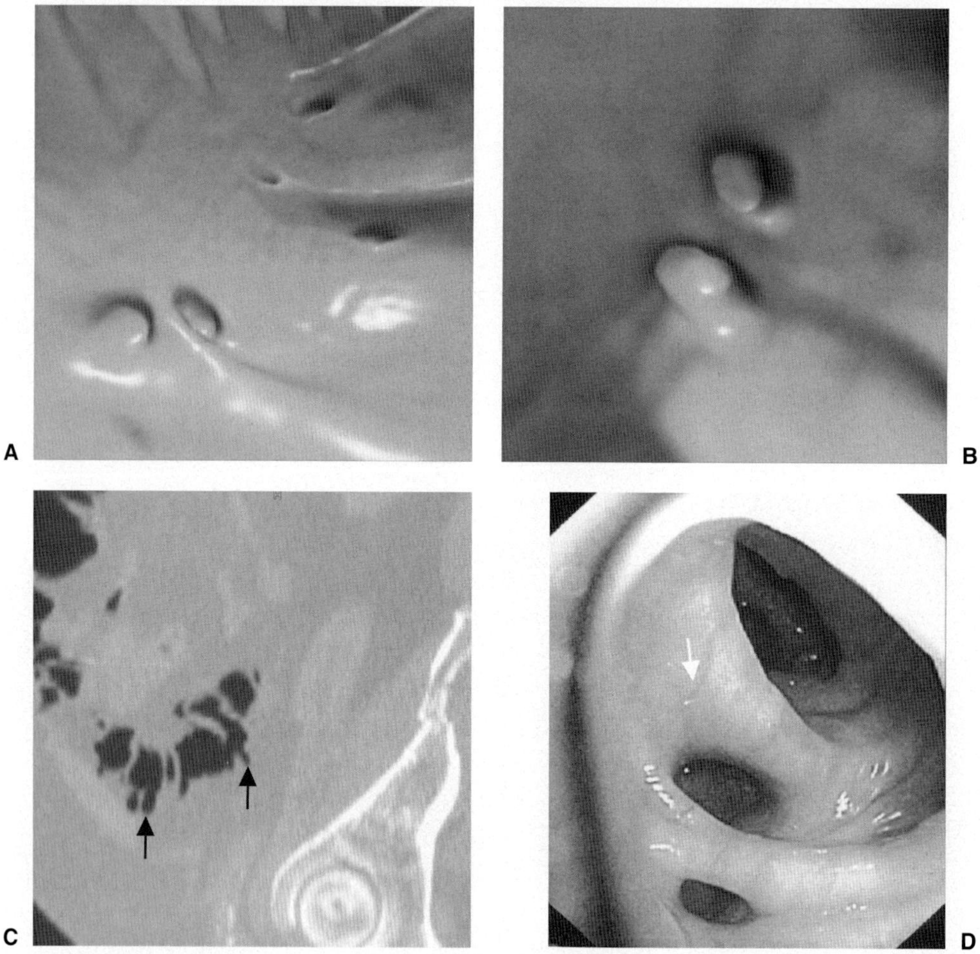

FIGURE 6.66 Diverticulosis: Rounded or ovoid appearance of diverticula which will often display a complete dark ring at the orifice on the 3D endoluminal views **(A, B)**. These may be a pitfall on 3D views, but are easily identified as outpouchings extending outside the colonic lumen on 2D views such as the sagittal reformat **(C)**. Endoscopic appearance of diverticula show clearly defined openings **(D)**.

as contour deformities with a nodular appearance and wall thickening. Submucosal spread of tumor and an area of prior biopsy can also simulate a flat irregularly thickened wall. Familial polyposis can simulate a carpet lesion although involvement is usually much more diffuse. Uncommonly, colonic urticaria due to submucosal edema can resemble a carpet lesion.[47] Some carpet lesions are so flat that they may not be detected on colonoscopy. Histologically, these lesions may be found to have only tubular adenomatous components although most carpet lesions contain some villous change. It may be difficult to detect the villous histology because of the large size of these lesions. The exact prevalence of these lesions is uncertain, but surgical resection is recommended given the large size at presentation and the suspected higher incidence of malignant degeneration.

DIVERTICULOSIS

Colonic diverticula represent herniations of mucosa and submucosa through the muscularis propria.[48] They are considered to be false diverticula because they do not contain muscle and tend to develop in areas of weakness where nutrient arteries extend through the submucosa. In Western countries, colonic diverticulosis increases in prevalence with age and is found in 5% of individuals by age 40 and in 33% to 50% of the population after age 50.[49] Contributing factors for the development of diverticula include a low-fiber diet, high red meat and fat consumption and frequent use of anti-inflammatory drugs. The sigmoid colon is involved in 95% of patients whereas the cecum is involved in only 5% of cases.[49]

Most sigmoid diverticula are associated with thickening of the circular muscle layer and shortened taeniae (myochosis) that can cause luminal narrowing and an "accordion-like" appearance.[49] Thickened folds due to muscular hypertrophy present in diverticular disease, particularly with a narrowed lumen, can mimic polyps or masses on both 2D and 3D endoluminal views.[1–4,6] Attempts should be made to achieve adequate distension if possible in the sigmoid to avoid this pitfall. Limited rescanning in a decubitus position may be performed through the sigmoid to help problem-solve an area with a possible lesion. Gollub et al. evaluated 97 patients who underwent CTC and found that the minimum sigmoid diameter in patients without muscular hypertrophy irrespective of the presence of diverticula was 8.76 mm compared with a minimum sigmoid diameter of 3.88 mm in patients with muscular hypertrophy which was significantly smaller.[50] In a study of 160 patients, Lefere et al. found diverticular disease in 56% with diffuse wall thickening, focal wall thickening in 4%, diverticula in 52%, impacted diverticula in 39%, and inverted diverticula in 1%.[51] A difficult pitfall described in this study was a pseudopolypoid lesion due to mucosal prolapse causing for a redundant thickened fold that may be impossible to differentiate from a true polyp.

Diverticula appear as air-filled outpouchings that extend beyond the colon wall into the pericolonic fat on 2D views and are easily recognizable. They typically range in size from 5 to 10 mm. Diverticula in the left colon often demonstrate a narrow ostia whereas diverticula in the right colon commonly have a wide ostia. If focal thickening of the colonic wall is present with associated stranding of the pericolonic fat, diverticulitis should be considered especially if in the correct clinical setting. Carcinoma may also be a cause of focal wall thickening and should be excluded. An interval abdomen and pelvis CT as a follow-up study may be performed to assess for improvement or resolution.

Diverticula often have a well-defined, complete dark ring at the orifice which is seen on 3D endoluminal views[1–3] (see Figures 6.66 and 6.67). This appearance is in contrast to the raised appearance of polyps which often have an incomplete or ill-defined dark ring surrounding their base on 3D endoluminal views.[1,2] However, a sessile polyp viewed *en face* on the 3D endoluminal view can also have a continuous dark ring at its base. Additionally, a diverticulum may have an ill-defined dark ring (see Figure 6.68). Switching to the 2D views allows for easy diagnosis of diverticula. The 3D cube view, which allows interactive rotation of the data volume, can be used to rapidly differentiate diverticula from polyps as well.

Diverticula that are impacted with stool or barium often have a rounded polypoid shape on 3D endoluminal views that mimic polyps, and often require 2D views for definitive evaluation (see Figures 6.69–6.73). Diverticula filled with residual stool have a heterogeneous appearance on 2D views as a result of air trapped within the stool. Diverticula impacted with barium exhibit characteristic high attenuation on 2D views. A less commonly encountered entity, inverted diverticula, can have the appearance of a polyp on both 2D and 3D views. An inverted diverticulum develops when the head of the diverticulum prolapses into the lumen of the diverticulum and extends into the colonic lumen. The base of the diverticulum may also invaginate into the lumen.[52] The 2D views are helpful for diagnosis when the inverted diverticulum contains air or fat density due to inclusion of pericolonic fat[1,51] (see Figure 6.74).

ARTIFACTS

Artifacts may be a source of both false-positive and false-negative findings on CTC. Types of artifacts encountered on CTC include motion artifact due to breathing or peristalsis, beam hardening from metallic objects such as prostheses or clips, stair-step artifact and digital subtraction artifact if tagging is performed.

Motion artifact on CTC is due to breathing, peristalsis, or actual movement of the patient during the data acquisition period. Motion will cause misregistration of the data, which can make it difficult to detect polyps and even large masses on both 2D and 3D endoluminal views (see Figures 6.75–6.77). Additionally truncated or focally thickened folds can appear as pseudopolypoid lesions. Fortunately motion artifacts are not frequently encountered following the introduction of multislice CT scanners which have rapid acquisition times of <15 seconds. Motion artifacts are often more

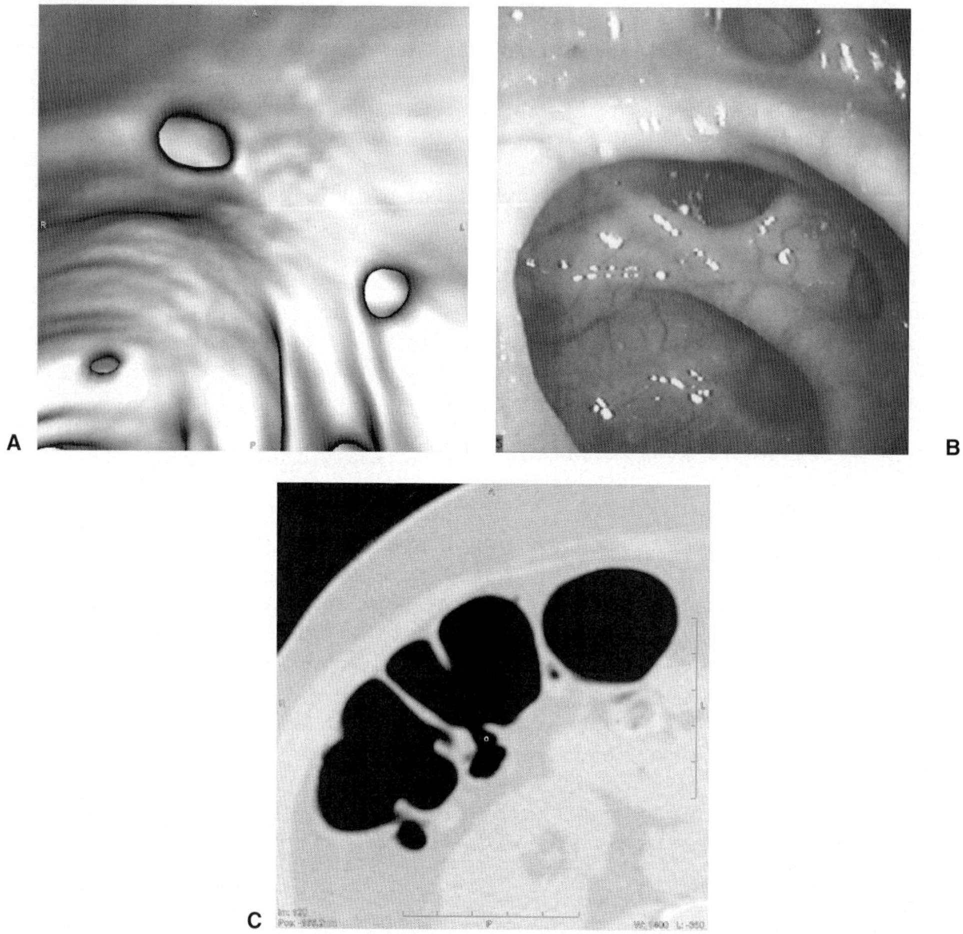

FIGURE 6.67 Diverticulosis: Well-defined dark rings are seen at the openings of these diverticula on the 3D endoluminal view **(A)**. Multiple diverticula are seen on the colonoscopic image **(B)** with an appearance similar to the 3D view. Switching to the 2D axial view **(C)** is a way to easily determine that these are outpouchings rather than polyps. (View C: See also color plate.)

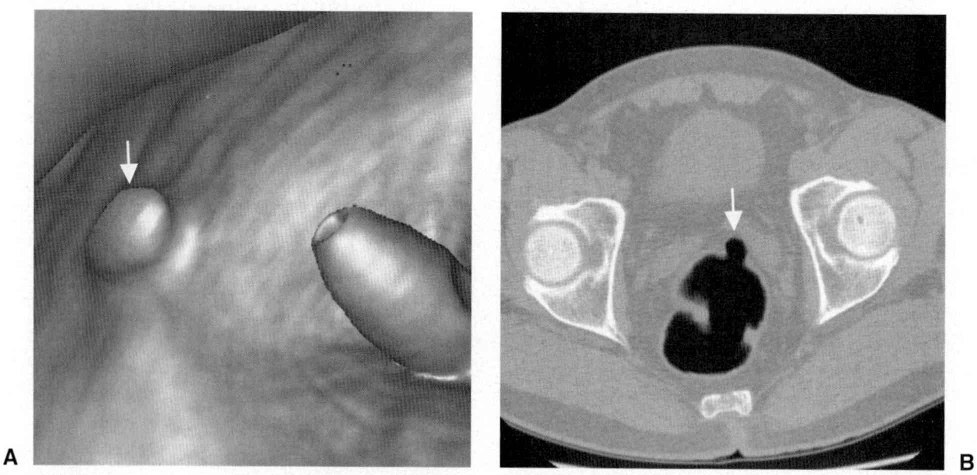

FIGURE 6.68 Rectal Diverticulum: 3D endoluminal view **(A)** shows a diverticulum in the rectal vault near the rectal tube. It has a dark ring at the orifice, which is partly ill defined. Switching to the axial image **(B)** shows the outpouching extending from the anterior rectal wall. The 3D transparency view **(C)** and the barium enema **(D)** show the rare finding of a large rectal diverticulum which almost always is associated with sigmoid diverticula such as in this case.

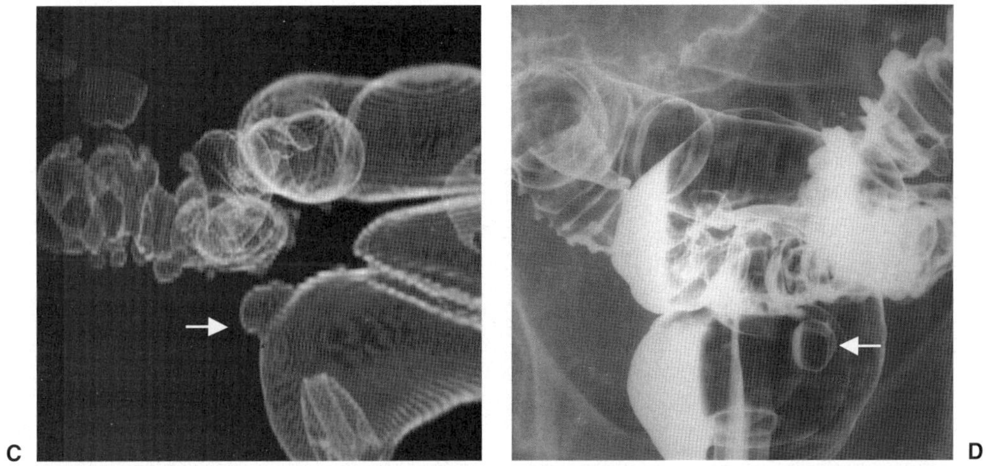

FIGURE 6.68 (*Continued*).

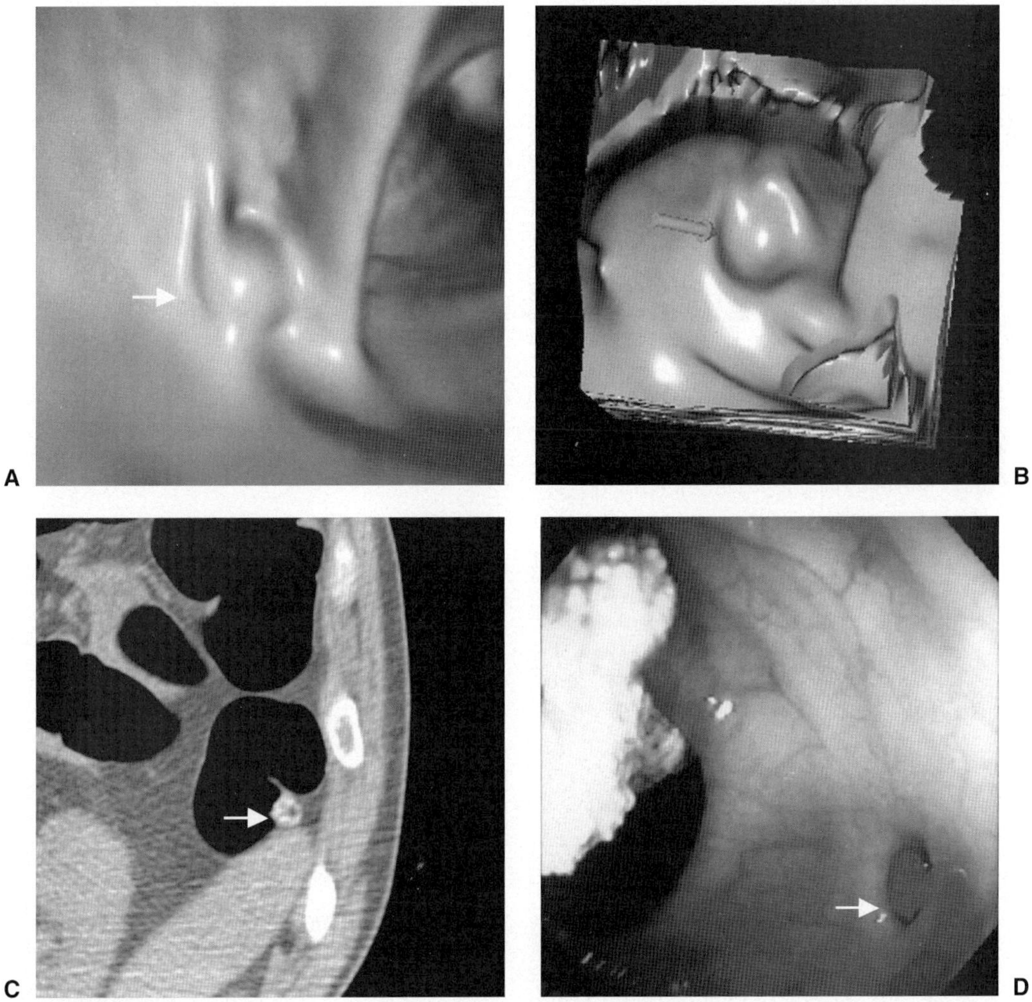

FIGURE 6.69 Impacted Diverticulum: A pseudopolypoid lesion is seen adjacent to a fold on the 3D endoluminal **(A)** and cube **(B)** views. The axial image **(C)** shows a diverticulum filled with stool and dense contrast material protruding into the lumen. The colonoscopic image **(D)** shows a large amount of residual stool in the lumen as well as some located in a diverticulum.

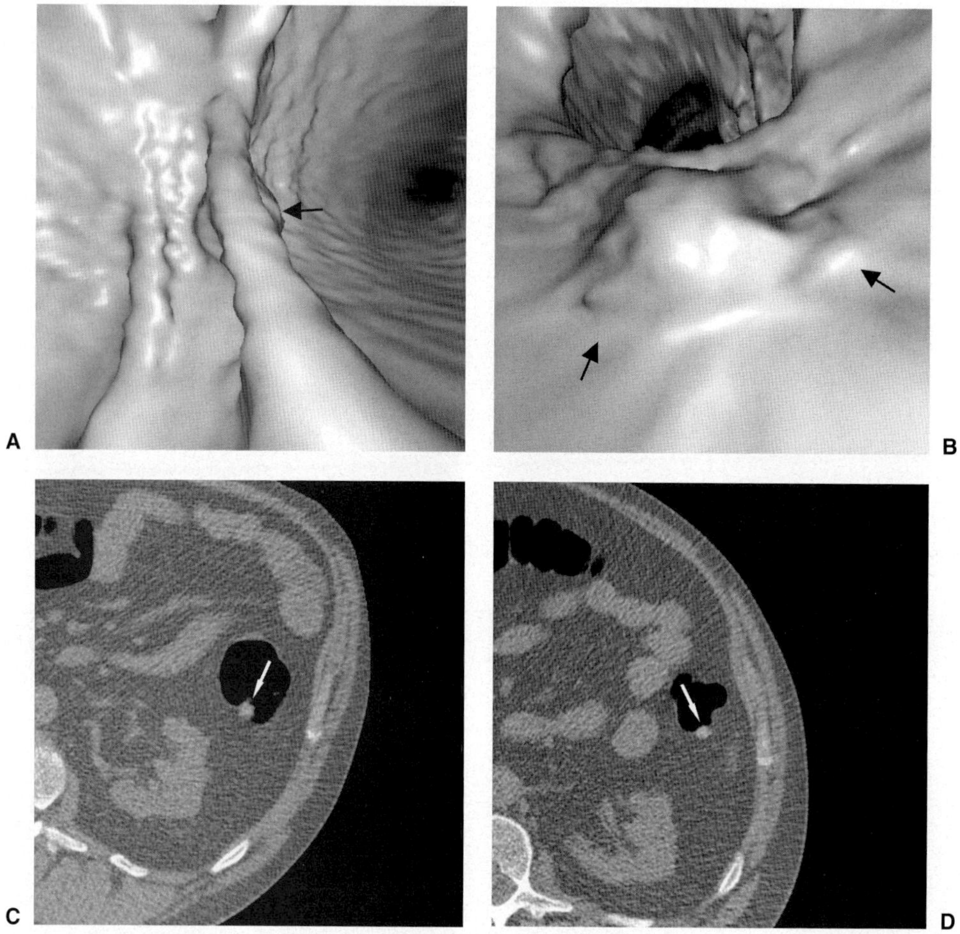

FIGURE 6.70 Impacted Diverticulum: A protrusion is seen hiding behind a fold on the 3D endoluminal view **(A)**. Viewed from another angle **(B)**, there is a pseudopolypoid lesion extending into the lumen. Prone axial image **(C)** shows a hyperdense lesion protruding into the lumen, which is seen to represent a diverticulum actually extending outside the lumen filled with residual contrast and stool on the supine axial view **(D)**.

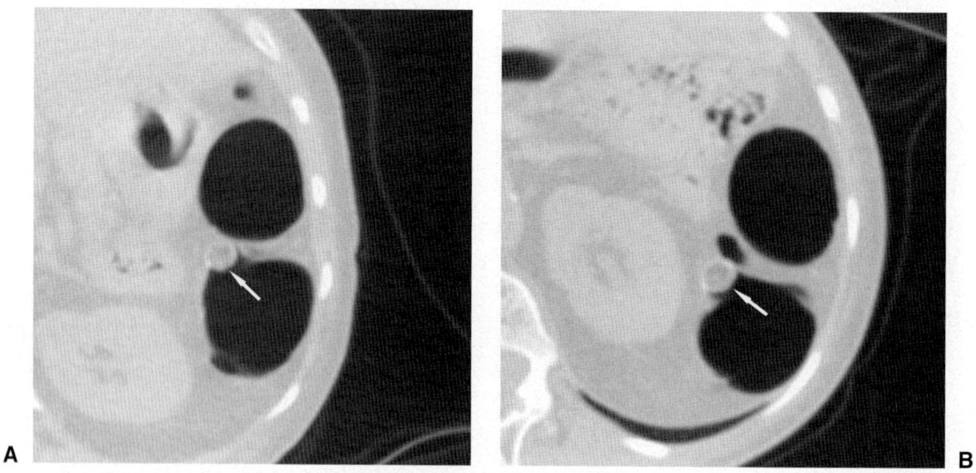

FIGURE 6.71 Impacted Diverticulum: Supine **(A)** and prone **(B)** axial images shows a diverticulum in the same location filled with heterogeneous stool protruding into the colonic lumen. This is seen to simulate a polyp on the 3D endoluminal view **(C)**.

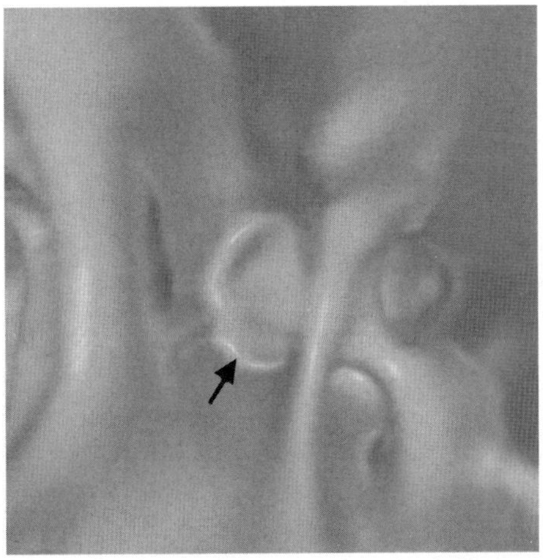

C

FIGURE 6.71 (*Continued*).

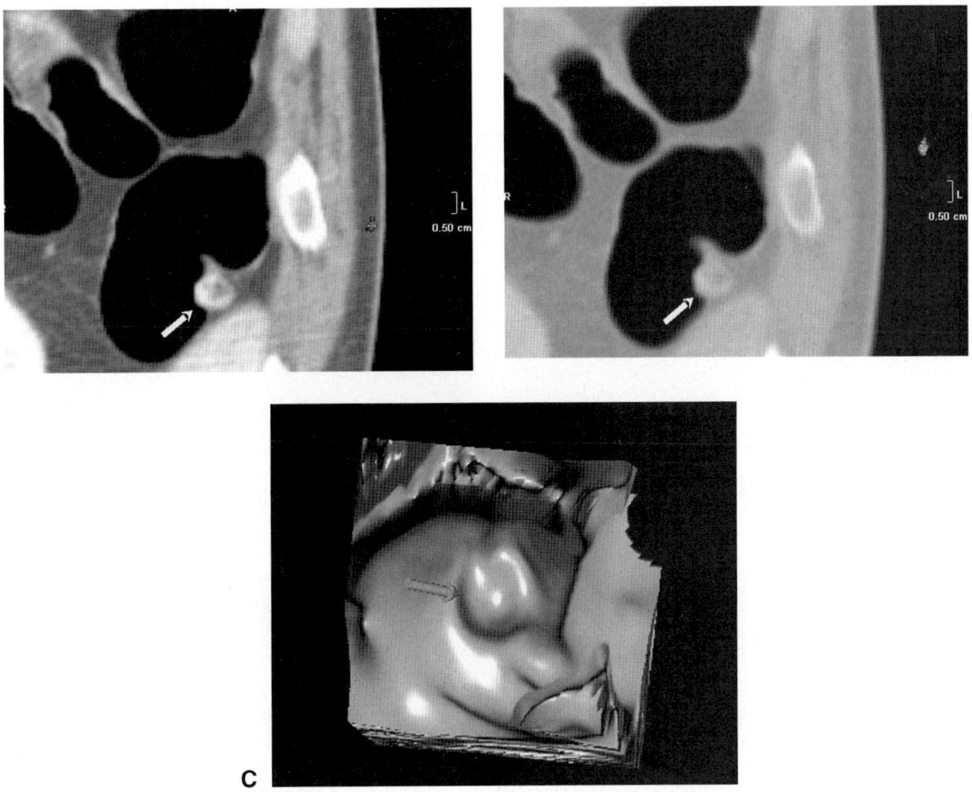

A B C

FIGURE 6.72 Impacted Diverticulum: Supine axial image in abdominal **(A)** and colon **(B)** windows show residual contrast and stool in an impacted diverticulum which appears polypoid on the 3D cube view **(C)**.

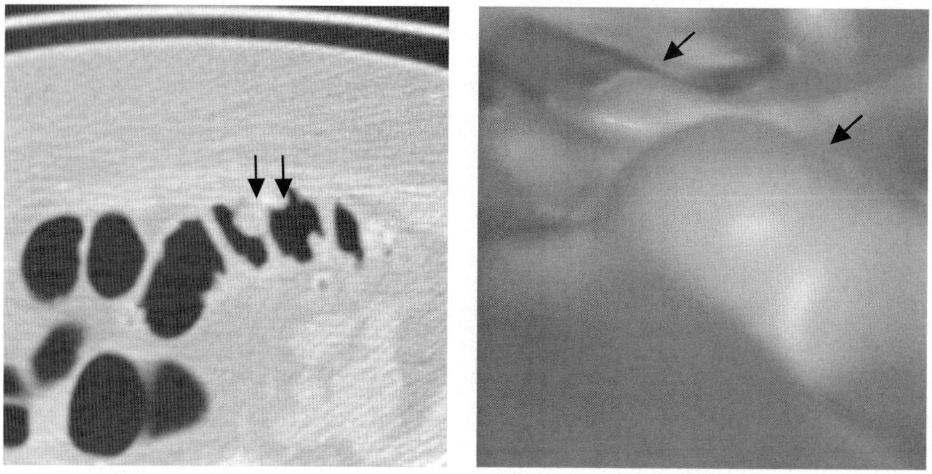

A B

FIGURE 6.73 Impacted Diverticula: Axial image **(A)** shows two impacted diverticula, the larger one filled with homogeneous stool and the other with high density material. The 3D endoluminal view **(B)** shows the two pseudopolypoid lesions. No polyps were found at colonoscopy.

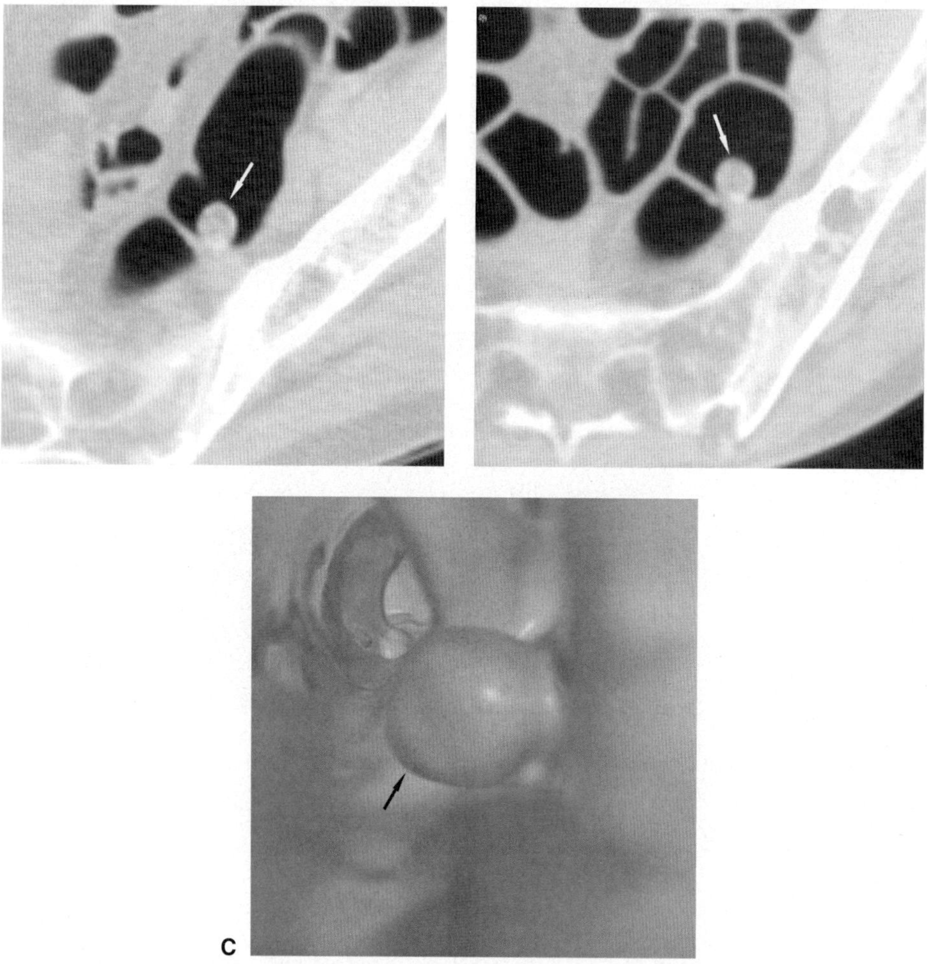

A B C

FIGURE 6.74 Inverted Diverticulum: Supine **(A)** and prone **(B)** axial images shows a fixed heterogeneous lesion along the posterior wall of the sigmoid. The 3D endoluminal view **(C)** shows a well-defined polypoid lesion, which was found to be an inverted diverticulum at colonoscopy.

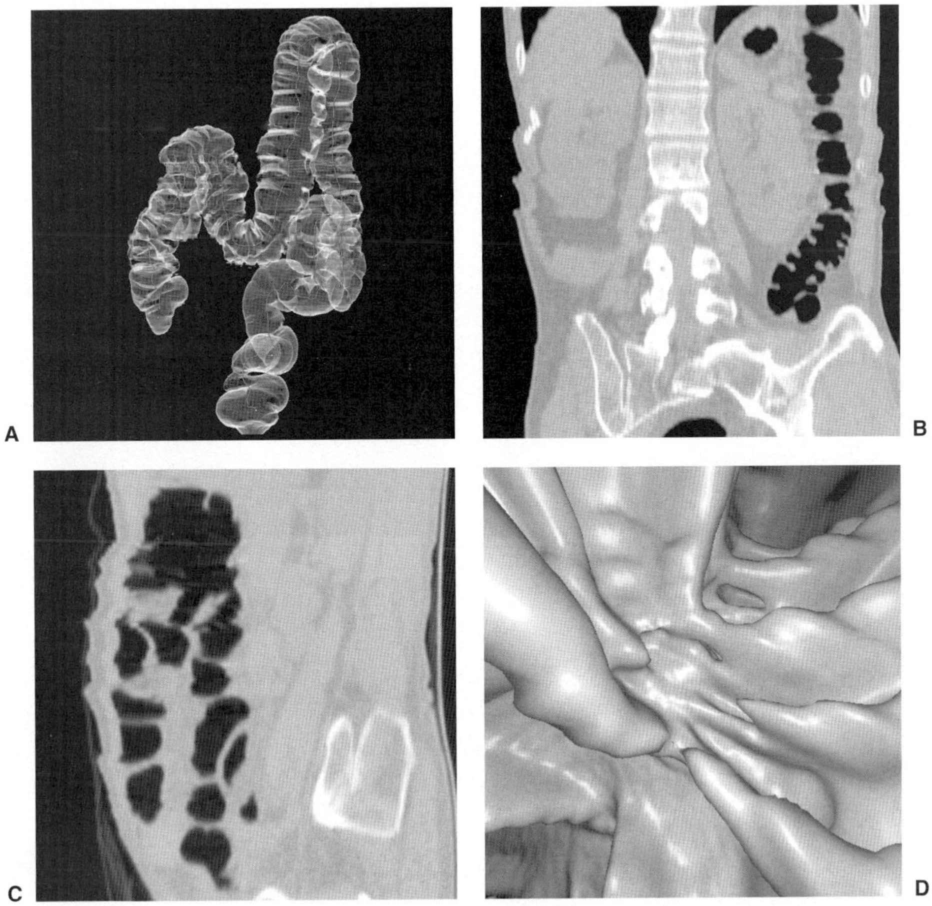

FIGURE 6.75 Motion Artifact: Respiration, peristalsis, or patient movement on the scanner table are causes of motion artifact. 3D transparency view **(A)** shows a rippled appearance throughout most of the colon above the pelvis due to breathing in this patient. The coronal **(B)** and sagittal **(C)** reformats show the typical jagged appearance of the abdominal wall and colon at the levels where the patient was breathing. Bizarre truncated and lobulated folds are observed on the 3D endoluminal view **(D)**.

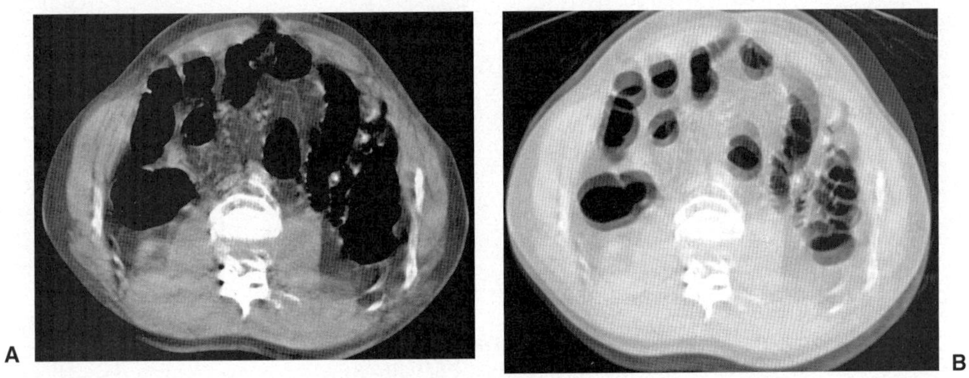

FIGURE 6.76 Motion Artifact: Axial images in abdominal **(A)** and colon **(B)** windows show severe motion artifact in this patient who moved on the CT table during data acquisition. Areas of data loss, truncated folds as well as pseudopolypoid lesions are seen on the 3D endoluminal views **(C, D)**. CT, computed tomography. (*Views C and D are on next page.*)

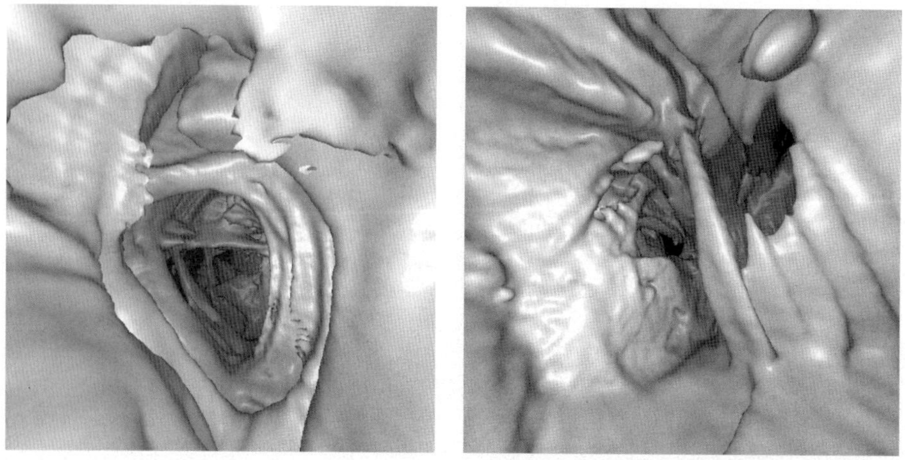

C D

FIGURE 6.76 (*Continued*).

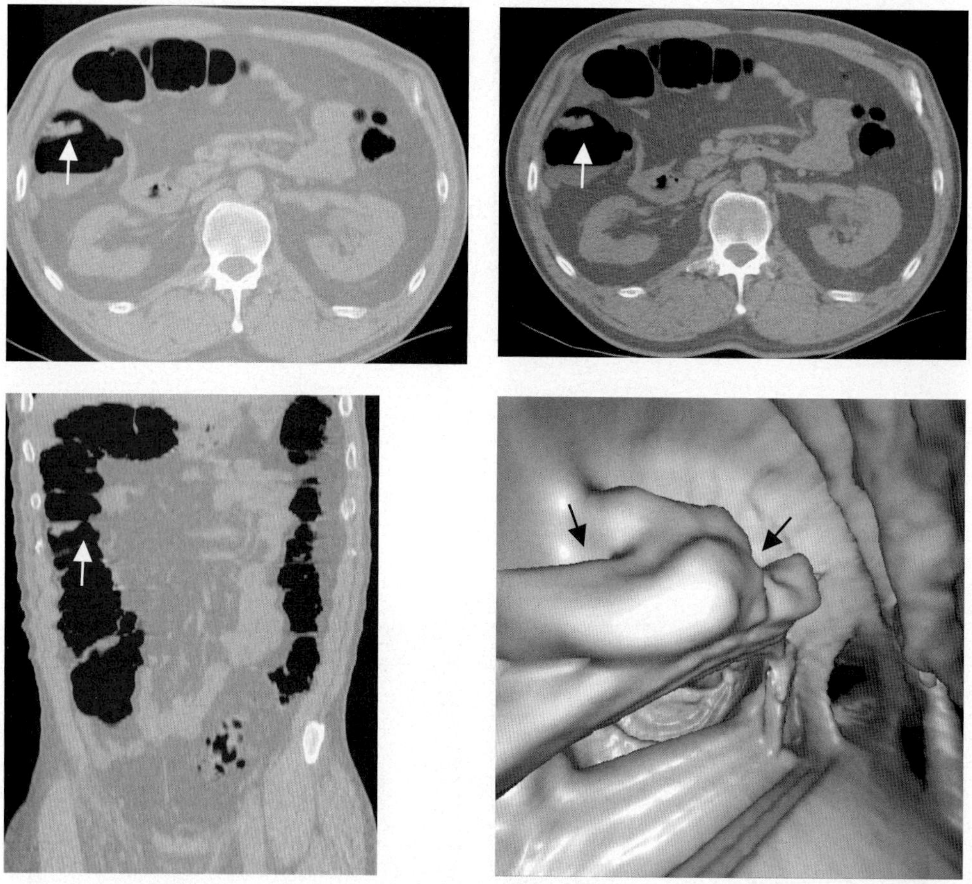

A B C D

FIGURE 6.77 Motion Obscuring Carcinoma: Axial images in colon **(A)** and abdominal **(B)** windows show a thickened fold with angular borders in the ascending colon which could be mistaken for stool. Coronal reformat **(C)** shows the same lesion along with extensive motion artifact throughout most of the colon. The 3D endoluminal view **(D)** could not be used to problem-solve this area because of motion artifact. The lesion is visualized but appears to be angulated and is easily mistaken as a truncated fold or stool. This proved to be a carcinoma at colonoscopy.

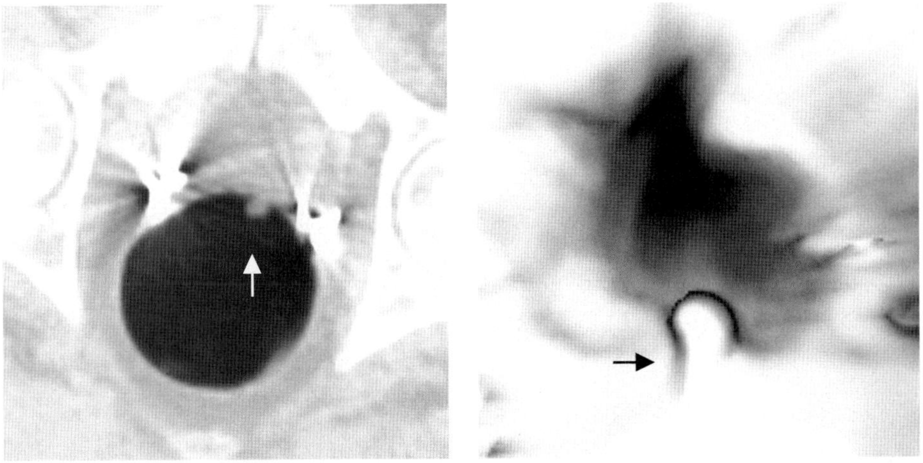

FIGURE 6.78 Surgical Clip Artifact: Metallic clips from prior radical prostatectomy produce local beam hardening artifact that extends across the rectum as seen on the axial view **(A)**. Note the polyp located between the clips. There is distortion of the colon wall on the 3D endoluminal view **(B)** although the polyp can still be identified.

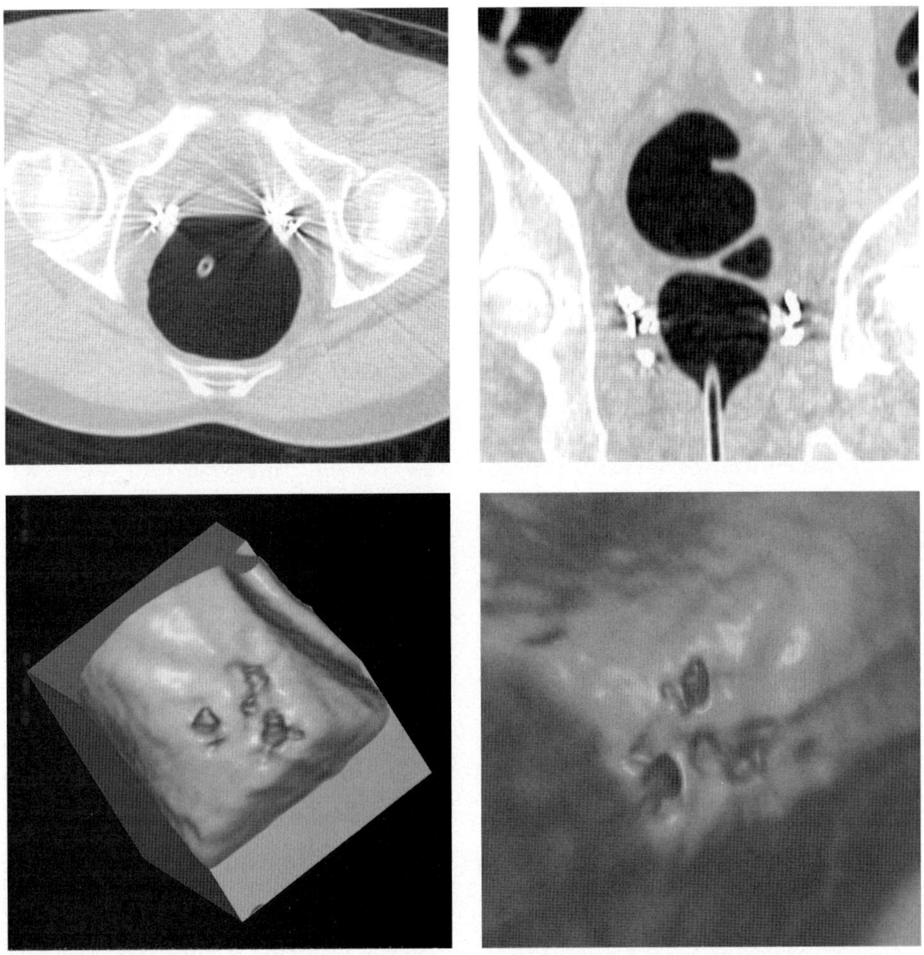

FIGURE 6.79 Surgical Clip Artifact: Clusters of metallic clips cause beam-hardening artifact through the rectum on the axial **(A)** and coronal reformat views **(B)** in this patient who had a prostatectomy. The 3D cube view **(C)** and endoluminal view **(D)** show multiple small surface protrusions which are artifactual.

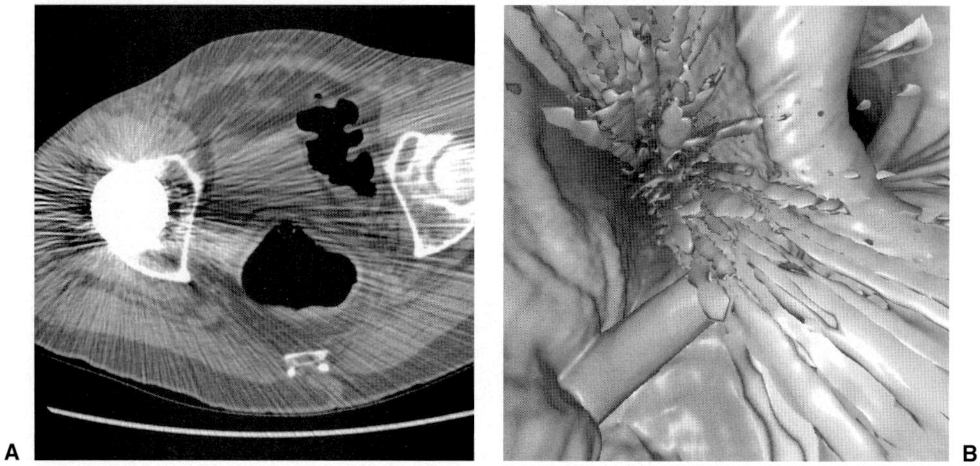

FIGURE 6.80 Metallic Artifact: Hip prostheses typically produce extensive beam-hardening artifact which can affect the rectum and sigmoid. Right hip prosthesis causes significant streak artifact across the lower pelvis on the axial image **(A)**. The top of the rectal tube is obscured by the linear artifacts on the 3D endoluminal view **(B)**.

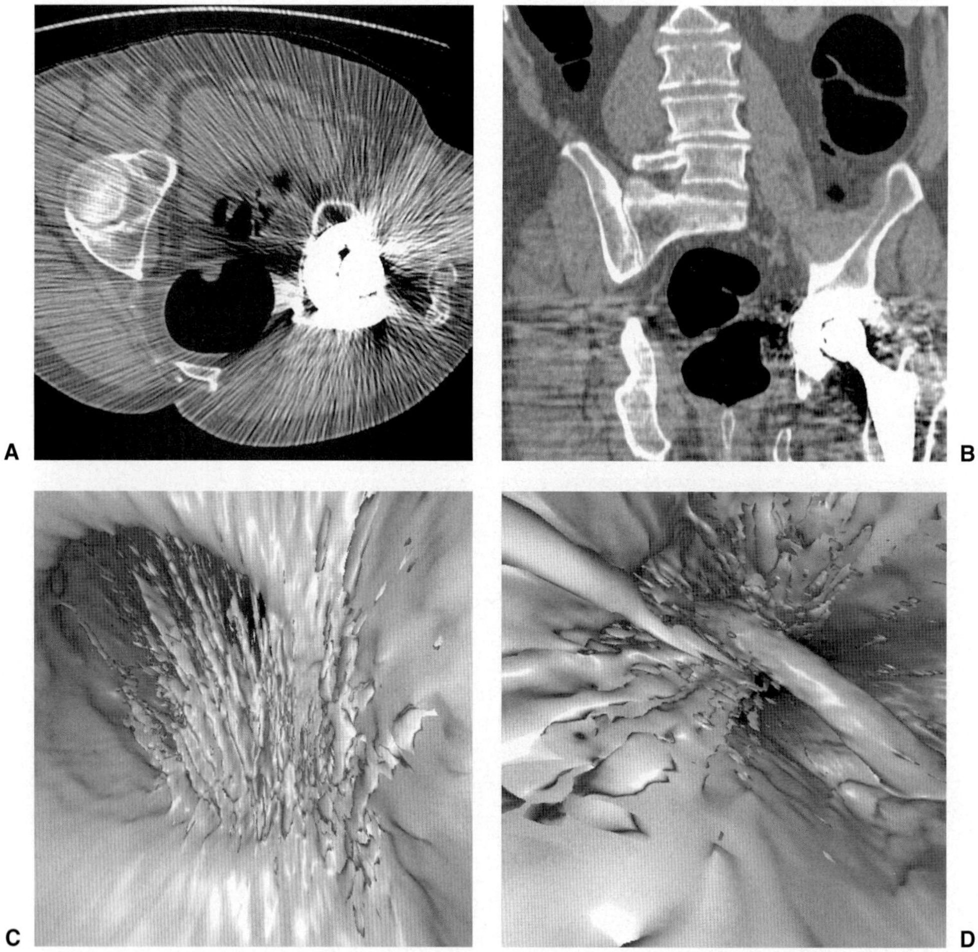

FIGURE 6.81 Metallic Artifact: Axial image **(A)** and coronal reformat **(B)** show severe beam-hardening artifact due to the patient's left total hip replacement. The 3D endoluminal views **(C, D)** show the characteristic linear artifacts produced which may obscure polyps and masses.

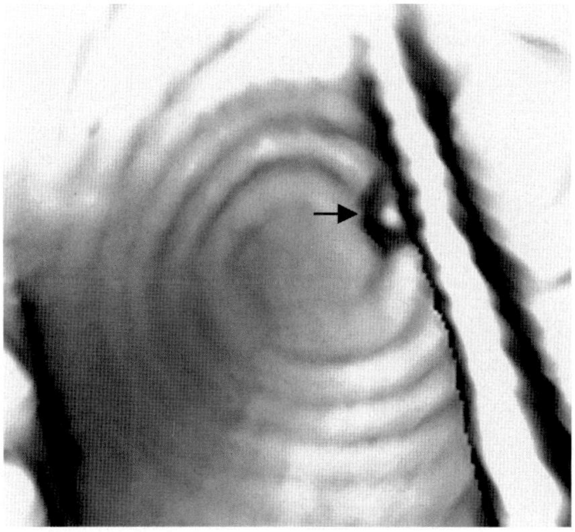

FIGURE 6.82 Stair-Step Artifact: This is an artifact seen only on the 3D endoluminal view due to the helical acquisition of the data. Multiple concentric rings are present on the wall in the cecum along with a small polyp adjacent to a fold. Minimizing collimation and table increment as well as using a smooth reconstruction algorithm can help to reduce stair-step artifact.

pronounced on the multiplanar reformatted views and the 3D endoluminal views when compared to the axial view.

Beam-hardening artifact is due to metallic objects such as hip prostheses or surgical clips (see Figures 6.78 and 6.79). Large streaks of data loss or gaps can extend across and obscure the colon wall. The 2D and 3D views are both degraded and may cause missed lesions. Hip prostheses often cause beam-hardening artifact that involves the rectum (see Figures 6.80 and 6.81).

Stair-step artifact is due to the helical acquisition of data and is seen only on the 3D endoluminal view. The artifact appears as multiple rings around the colonic lumen and are most noticeable in the cecum and the rectum near the anal verge where there is a change is bowel contour (see Figure 6.82). Adequate distention of the segment is necessary to visualize this artifact. Minimizing collimation and table increment as well as using a smooth reconstruction algorithm can help to reduce stair-step artifact.[4,53]

If tagging is performed in conjunction with digital subtraction, artifacts are commonly present at the border of the fluid–air interface, which may resemble polyps on the 3D endoluminal view. This "bath tub"–like ring artifact is nearly always present following digital subtraction of layering fluid (see Figure 6.83). This artifact has a high attenuation border on 2D images, which is an indication that residual tagged fluid was digitally subtracted. Following digital subtraction, a portion of a haustral fold at the fluid–air interface may remain that was partially submerged in fluid and may be mistaken for a polyp.

EXTERNAL COMPRESSION

External structures can compress or indent the colon and appear as a mass on the 3D views.[1–3] Structures that indent the colon often cause a broad bulge into the lumen,

A

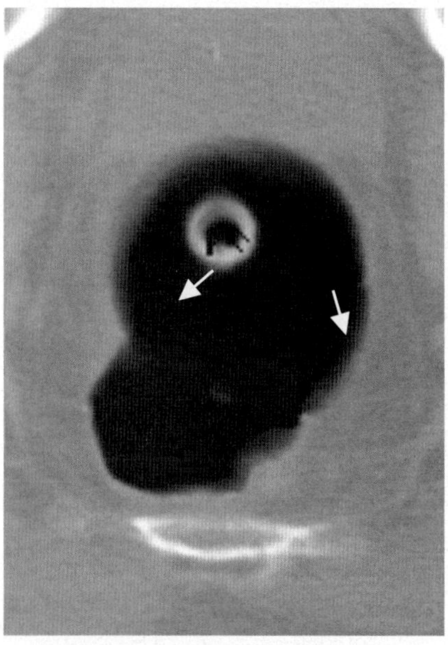

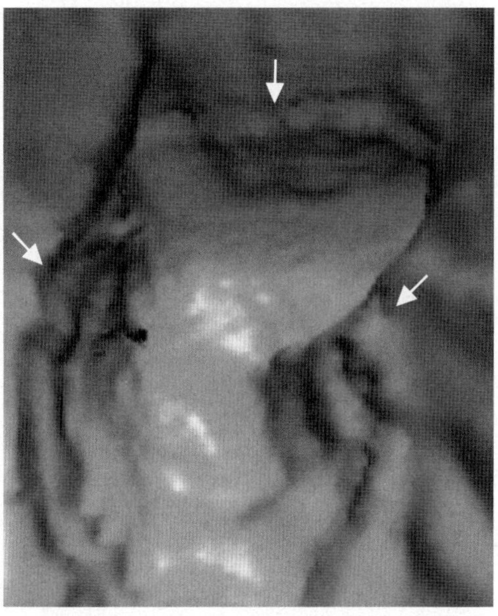

B

FIGURE 6.83 Digital Subtraction Artifact: If tagging is performed in conjunction with digital subtraction artifacts are commonly present at the fluid–air interface. The axial image **(A)** shows mild irregularity of the colon wall at the border of where the tagged fluid was subtracted. This is seen as the "ring around the tub" effect on the 3D endoluminal view **(B)**.

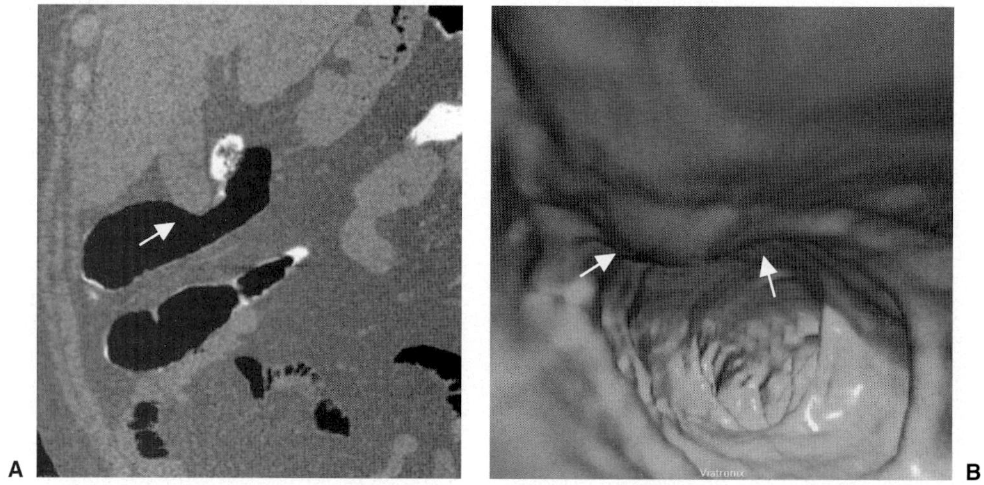

FIGURE 6.84 Gallbladder: The gallbladder can normally indent the superior surface of the transverse colon as seen on the coronal reformat **(A)**. This may produce a broad bulge that may be mistaken for a mass on the 3D endoluminal view **(B)**.

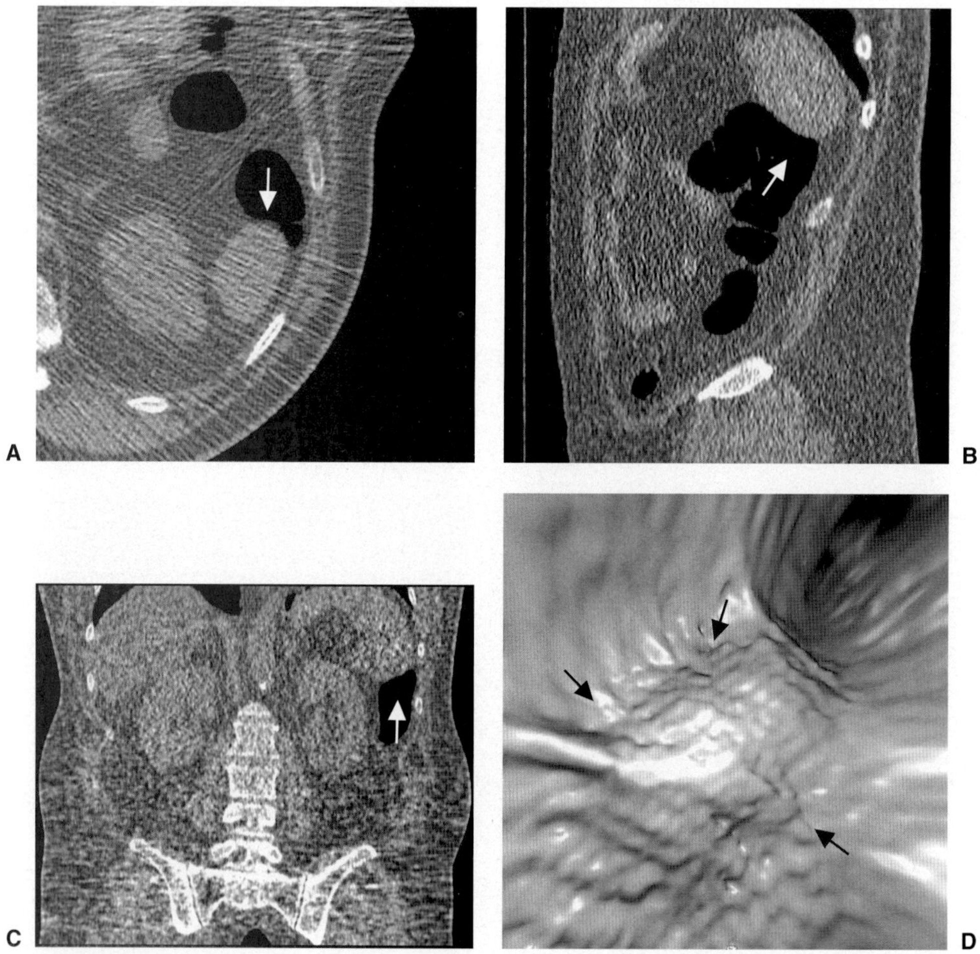

FIGURE 6.85 Spleen: Axial image **(A)**, sagittal **(B)** and coronal reformat **(C)** views show compression of the superior surface of the splenic flexure by a normal spleen. 3D endoluminal view **(D)** reveals a bulge that simulates a large flat lesion.

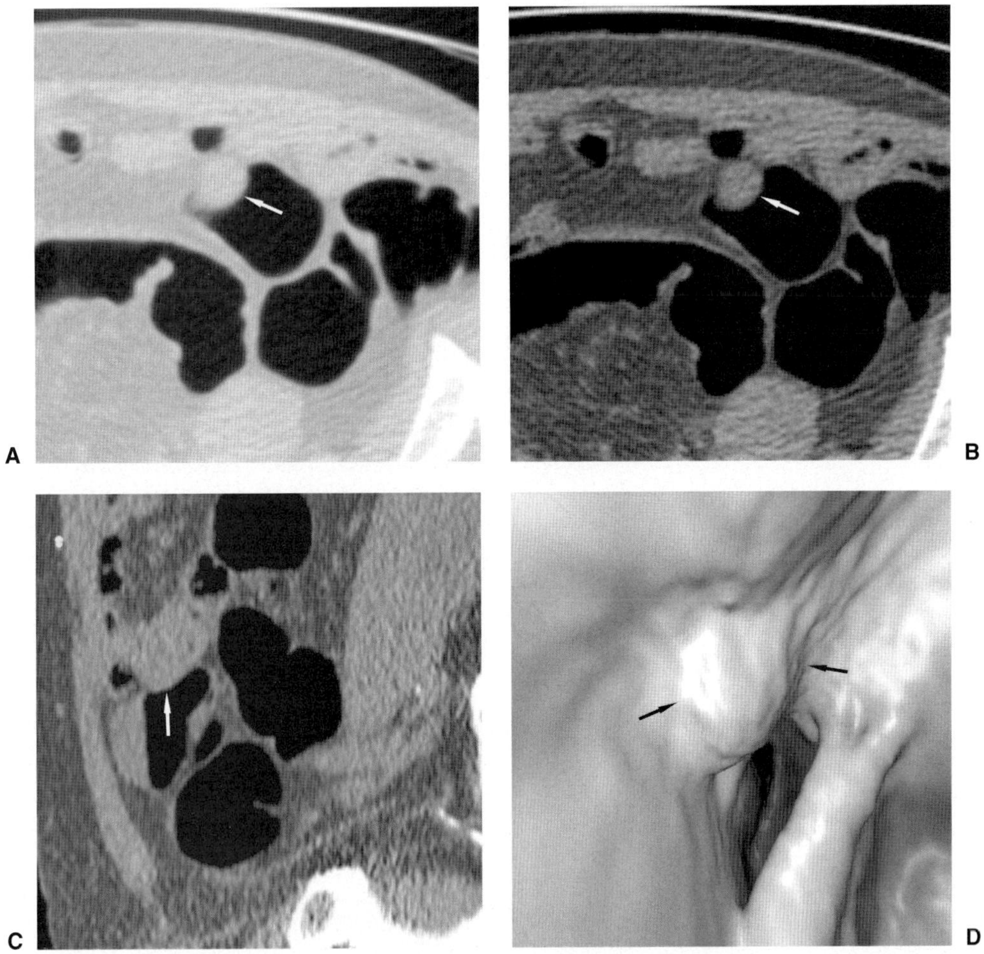

FIGURE 6.86 Small Bowel: Collapsed or distended bowel loops can compress portions of the colon. Axial image in colon **(A)** and abdominal **(B)** windows show a rounded polypoid lesion in the sigmoid. The sagittal reformat **(C)** shows the tubular nature of this pseudopolyp representing a collapsed small bowel loop. 3D endoluminal view **(D)** shows obtuse angles of the protrusion with the colon wall due to external compression.

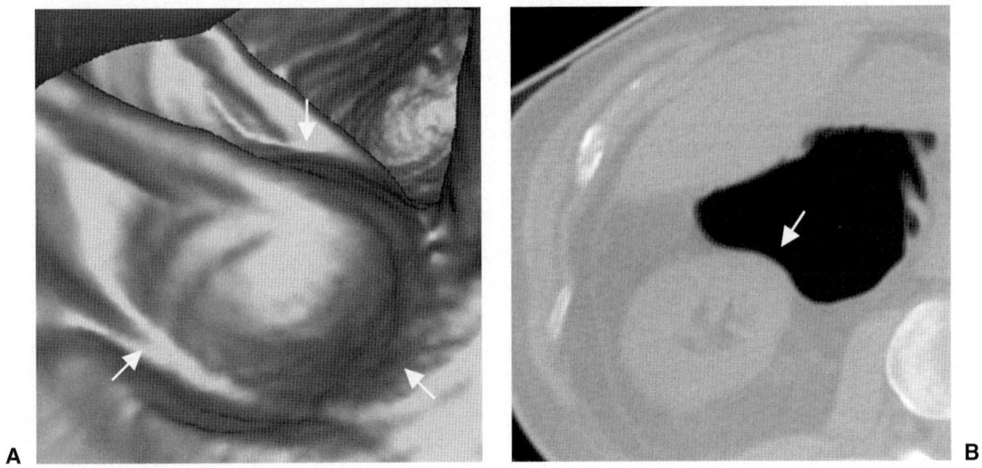

FIGURE 6.87 Kidney: Large broad-based bulge in the hepatic flexure is seen located between folds on the 3D endoluminal view **(A)**. The axial view **(B)** shows external compression of the colon due to the right kidney.

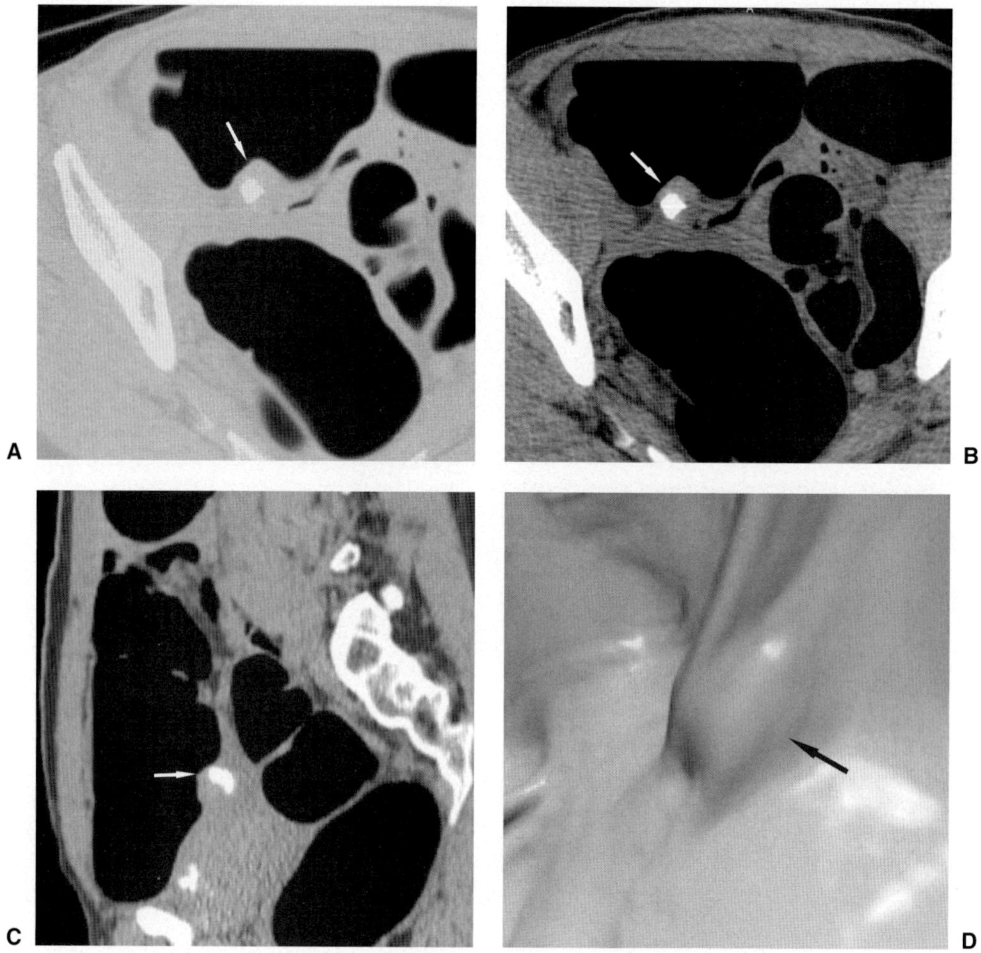

FIGURE 6.88 Uterine Fibroid: Axial image in colon **(A)** and abdominal **(B)** windows show a focal lesion with central calcification protruding into the cecal lumen. The sagittal reformat **(C)** shows that this is caused by one of two calcified uterine fibroids. This may be mistaken for a polyp on the 3D endoluminal view **(D)**.

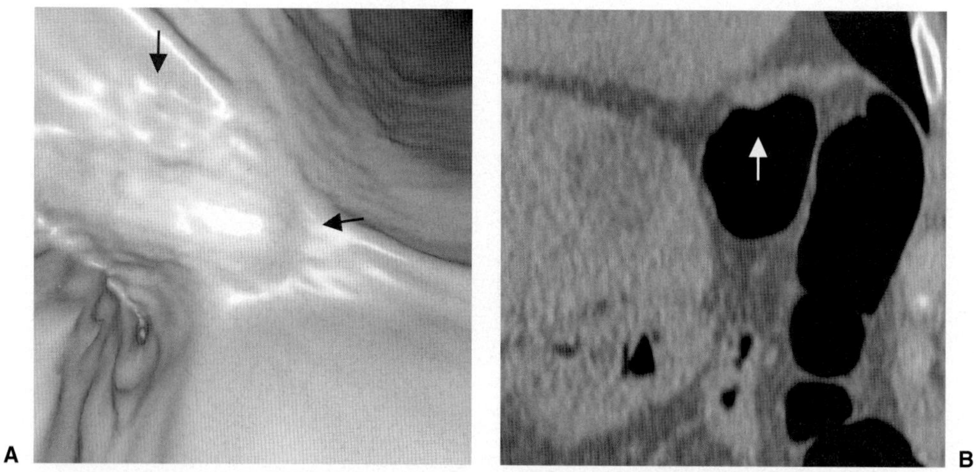

FIGURE 6.89 Diaphragmatic Crus: A mild bulge is seen in the colonic lumen interrupting a haustral fold on the 3D endoluminal view **(A)**. The coronal reformat **(B)** shows indentation of the superior surface of the distal transverse colon by the left diaphragmatic crus.

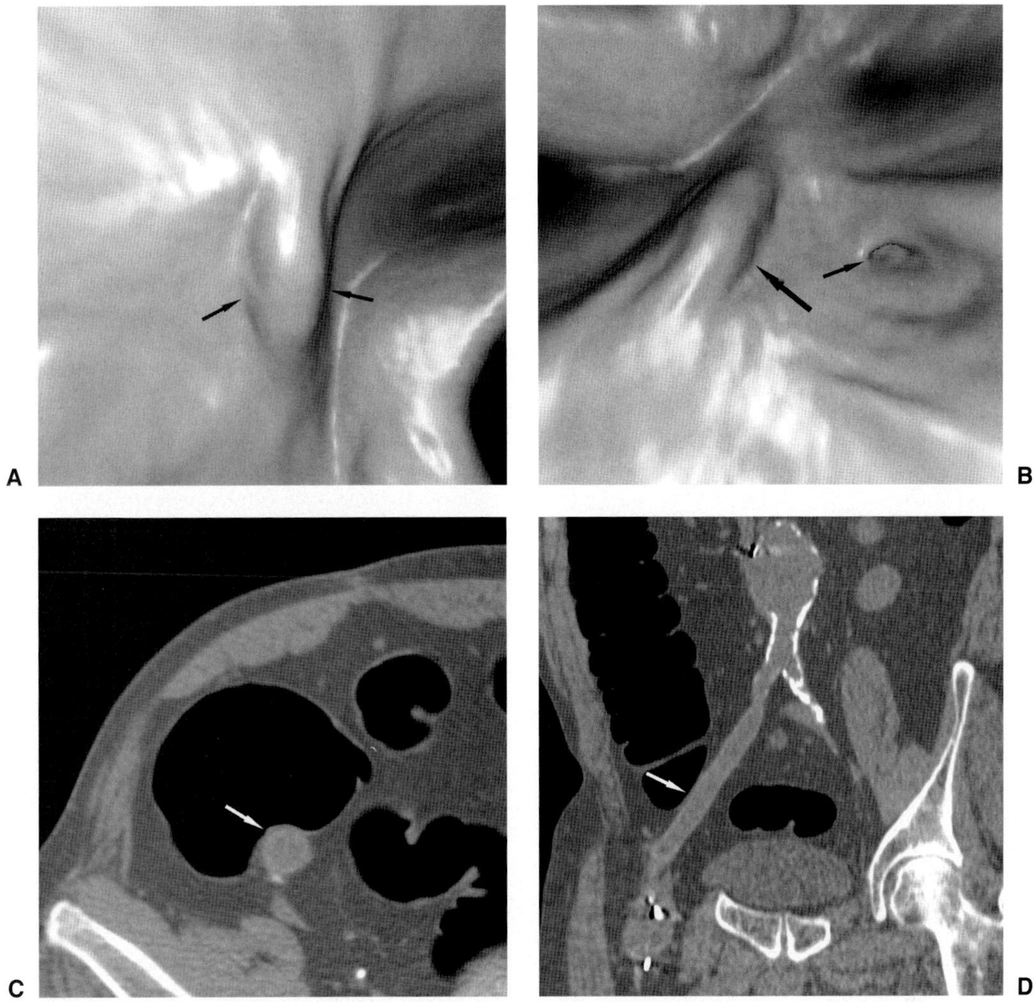

FIGURE 6.90 Aortofemoral Bypass Graft: Focal ovoid protrusion is seen at the cecal tip near the appendiceal orifice on the 3D endoluminal views **(A, B)**. Axial image **(C)** and coronal reformat **(D)** show that this is caused by an aortofemoral bypass graft.

simulating a submucosal lesion with obtuse rather than acute angles to the colon mucosa. External compression of the colon does not typically appear as an occlusive lesion. Many structures and masses arising from adjacent organs can cause compression of the colon, including the liver, spleen, gallbladder, kidney, other bowel loops, uterus (and fibroids), psoas muscle, and diaphragmatic crus[1–3] (see Figures 6.84–6.89). Vascular structures may also indent the colon such as the aorta, common iliac arteries, and vascular grafts (see Figure 6.90). These pseudomasses occur more commonly in thin patients.[1] Structures causing compression of the colonic lumen are usually readily identified on 2D views.

REFERENCES

1. Fenlon HM. CT colonography: pitfalls and interpretation. *Abdom Imaging*. 2002;27:284–291.
2. Macari M, Megibow AJ. Pitfalls of using three-dimensional CT colonography with two-dimensional imaging correlation. *Am J Roentgenol*. 2001;176:137–143.
3. Macari M, Bini E, Jacobs SL, et al. Filling defects at CT colonography: pseudo and diminutive lesions (the good), polyps (the bad), flat lesions, masses, and carcinomas (the ugly). *Radiographics*. 2003;23:1073–1091.
4. Fletcher JG, Johnson CD, MacCarty RL, et al. CT colonography: potential pitfalls and problem-solving techniques. *Am J Roentgenol*. 1999;172:1271–1278.
5. Galdino GM, Yee J. Appearance of a carpet lesion on CT colonography: a potential pitfall. *Am J Roentgenol*. 2003; 180:1332–1334.
6. Taylor SA, Halligan S, Bartram CI. CT colonography: methods, pathology, and pitfalls. *Clin Radiol*. 2003;58:179–190.
7. Silva AC, Vens EA, Hara AK, et al. Evaluation of benign and malignant rectal lesions with CT colonography and endoscopic correlation. *Radiographics*. 2006;26:1085–1099.
8. Regge D, Gallo TM, Nieddu G, et al. Ileocecal valve imaging on computed tomographic colonography. *Abdom Imaging*. 2004;30:20–25.
9. El-Amin LC, Levine MS, Rubesin SE, et al. Ileocecal valve: spectrum of normal findings at double-contrast barium enema examination. *Radiology*. 2003;227:52–58.
10. Hoeffel C, Crema MD, Belkacem A, et al. Multi-detector

row CT: spectrum of diseases involving the ileocecal area. *Radiographics*. 2006;26:1373–1390.
11. Koff JM, Choi JR, Hwang I. Inverted appendiceal orifice masquerading as a cecal polyp on virtual colonoscopy. *Gastrointest Endosc*. 2005;62:308.
12. Prout TM, Taylor AJ, Pickhardt PJ. Inverted appendiceal stumps simulating large pedunculated polyps on screening CT colonography. *Am J Roentgenol*. 2006;186:535–538.
13. Posner R, Salomon A. Dilemma of an inverted cecal diverticulum simulating a pedunculated polyp: CT appearance. *Abdom Imaging*. 1995;20:440–441.
14. Moore CJ, Corl FM, Fishman EK. CT of cecal volvulus: unraveling the image. *Am J Roentgenol*. 2001;177:95–98.
15. Bobroff LM, Messinger NH, Subbarao K, et al. The cecal bascule. *Am J Roentgenol Radium Ther Nucl Med*. 1972;115:249–252.
16. Stringer D. Pediatric small bowel. In: Freeny PC, Stevenson GW, eds. *Margulis and Burhenne's Alimentary Tract Radiology*, 5th ed. St. Louis: Mosby; 1994:1878–1931.
17. Fulcher AS, Turner MA. Abdominal manifestations of situs anomalies in adults. *Radiographics*. 2002;22:1439–1456.
18. Zissin R, Rathaus V, Oscadchy A, et al. Intestinal malrotation as an incidental finding on CT in adults. *Abdom Imaging*. 1999;24:550–555.
19. Sosna J, Blachar A, Amitai M, et al. Colonic perforation at CT colonography: assessment of risk in a multicenter large cohort. *Radiology*. 2006;239:457–463.
20. Chang AE. Colorectal cancer. Greenfield LJ, Mulholland MW, Zelenock GB, etal. eds. *Surgery: Scientific Principles and Practice*, 2nd ed. Philadelphia: Lippincott-Raven; 1997:1128–1146.
21. Burling D, Halligan S, Slater A, et al. Potentially serious adverse events at CT colonography in symptomatic patients: National Survey of the United Kingdom. *Radiology*. 2006;239:464–471.
22. Laks S, Macari M, Bini EJ. Positional change in colon polyps at CT colonography. *Radiology*. 2004;231:761–766.
23. Stevenson GW. Normal anatomy and techniques of examination of the colon: barium, CT, and MRI. In: Freeny PC, Stevenson GW, eds. *Margulis and Burhenne's Alimentary Tract Radiology*, 5th ed. St. Louis: Mosby; 1994:692–694.
24. Wolfer JA, Beaton LE, Anson BJ. Volvulus of the cecum: anatomical factors in its etiology. *Surg Gynecol Obstet*. 1942; 74:882.
25. Rogers RL, Harford FJ. Mobile cecum syndrome. *Dis Colon Rectum*. 1984;27:399–402.
26. Chen JC, Dachman AH. Cecal mobility: a potential pitfall of CT colonography. *Am J Roentgenol*. 2006;186:1086–1089.
27. Yee J, Kumar NN, Hung RK, et al. Comparison of supine and prone scanning separately and in combination at CT colonography. *Radiology*. 2003;226:653–661.
28. Savitt DL, Hawkins HH, Roberts JR. The radioopacity of ingested medications. *Ann Intern Med*. 1987;16:331–339.
29. Eisenberg RL. Single filling defects in the colon. Eisenberg RL, ed. *Gastrointestinal Radiology, a Pattern Approach*, 4th ed. Philadelphia: Lippincott Williams & Wilkins; 2002:667–698.
30. Madoff RD, Fleshman JW. American Gastroenterological Association technical review on the diagnosis and treatment of hemorrhoids. *Gastroenterology*. 2004;126:1463–1473.
31. Heiken JP, Zuckerman GR, Balfe DM. The hypertrophied anal papilla: recognition on air-contrast barium enema examinations. *Radiology*. 1984;151:315–318.
32. Schutte AG, Tolentino MG. A second study of anal papillae. *Dis Colon Rectum*. 1971;14:435–450.
33. Castro EB, Stearns MW. Lipoma of the large intestine: a review of 45 cases. *Dis Colon Rectum*. 1972;15:441–444.
34. Heiken JP, Forde KA, Gold RP. Computed tomography as a definitive method for diagnosing gastrointestinal lipomas. *Radiology*. 1982;142:409–414.
35. Abou-Nukta F, Gutweiler J, Khaw J, et al. Giant lipoma causing a colo-colonic intussusception. *Am Surg*. 2006;72:83–84.
36. Buetow PC, Buck JL, Carr NJ, et al. Intussuscepted colonic lipomas: loss of fat attenuation on CT with pathologic correlation in 10 cases. *Abdom Imaging*. 1996;21:153–156.
37. Miettinen M, Majidi M, Lasota J. Pathology and diagnostic criteria of gastrointestinal stromal tumors (GISTs): a review. *Eur J Cancer*. 2002;38:S39–S51.
38. Stewart ET, Dodds WJ. Neoplastic colonic lesions. In: Freeny PC, Stevenson GW, eds. *Margulis and Burhenne's Alimentary Tract Radiology*, 5th ed. St. Louis: Mosby; 1994: 762–800.
39. Meyers WC, Kelvin FM, Jones RS. Diagnosis and surgical treatment of colonic endometriosis. *Arch Surg*. 1979; 114:169–175.
40. Macrae FA, Young GP. Neoplastic and nonneoplastic polyps of the colon and rectum. Yamada T, Alpers DH, Laine L, etal. eds. *Textbook of Gastroenterology*, 3rd ed, Vol. 2. Philadelphia: Lippincott Williams & Wilkins; 1999: 1965–1994.
41. Yee J, Hung RK, Akerkar GA, et al. The usefulness of glucagon hydrochloride for colonic distention in CT colonography. *Am J Roentgenol*. 1999;173:1–4.
42. Ota Y, Matsui T, Ono H, et al. Value of virtual computed tomographic colonography for Crohn's colitis: comparison with endoscopy and barium enema. *Abdom Imaging*. 2003;28:778–783.
43. Biancone L, Fiori R, Tosti C, et al. Virtual colonoscopy compared with conventional colonoscopy for structuring postoperative recurrence in Crohn's disease. *Inflamm Bowel Dis*. 2003;9:343–350.
44. Coady-Fariborzian L, Angel LP, Procaccino JA. Perforated colon secondary to virtual colonoscopy: report of a case. *Dis Colon Rectum*. 2004;47:1247–1249.
45. Triester SL, Hara AK, Young-Fadok TM, et al. Colonic perforation after computed tomographic colonography in a patient with fibrostenosing Crohn's disease. *Am J Gastroenterol*. 2006;101:189–192.
46. Rubesin SE, Saul SH, Laufer I, et al. Carpet lesions of the colon. *Radiographics*. 1985;5:537–552.
47. Glick SN, Teplick SK, Balfe DM, et al. Large colonic neoplasms missed by endoscopy. *Am J Roentgenol*. 1989; 152:513–517.
48. Morson BC. Pathology of diverticular disease of the colon. *Clin Gastroenterol*. 1975;4:37–52.
49. Balthazar EJ. Diverticular disease of the colon. In: Gore RM, Levine MS, eds. *Textbook of Gastrointestinal Radiology*, 2nd ed. Philadelphia: WB Saunders; 2000.
50. Gollub MJ, Jhaveri S, Schwartz E, et al. CT colonography features of sigmoid diverticular disease. *Clin Imaging*. 2005; 29:200–206.
51. Lefere P, Gryspeerdt S, Baekelandt M, et al. Diverticular disease in CT colonography. *Eur Radiol*. 2003; 13(Suppl 4):L62–L74.
52. Glick SN. Inverted colonic diverticulum: air contrast barium enema findings in six cases. *Am J Roentgenol*. 1991;156:961–964.
53. Fenlon HM, Clarke PD, Ferruci JT. Virtual colonoscopy: imaging features with colonoscopic correlation. *Am J Roentgenol*. 1998;170:1303–1309.

CHAPTER 7 ACCURACY

Judy Yee

Multiple studies have been performed to evaluate the sensitivity and specificity of computed tomographic colonography (CTC) for the detection of polyps and cancer in various types of patient cohorts. Most published studies have been carried out at a single center in symptomatic or high-risk patients (see Table 7.1). There are also several large multicenter trials that have been published.

Over the last 10 years, significant advances in image acquisition and image display capabilities have occurred and these still continue to evolve. In evaluating the results of performance studies it is important to note that specific study parameters may affect performance results. Variations in these parameters are likely the cause for some of the conflicting results in the published literature.

PATIENT RISK

CTC studies may include average-risk patients, high-risk patients, or both types of patients. Most of the published studies evaluating the performance of CTC have been performed in patients who are at increased risk for developing colorectal cancer. These are patients who may have a personal or family history of colorectal cancer or adenomatous polyp. They may have symptoms or signs of colorectal cancer such as iron-deficiency anemia, positive fecal occult blood test or hematochezia.

The use of CTC as a screening tool for colorectal carcinoma is optimally validated by testing performance in average-risk patients who have a low prevalence of disease (see Figure 7.1). Several studies have been published evaluating the performance of CTC in a screening type patient population.[1–3] The American College of Radiology Imaging Network (ACRIN) National CT Colonography Trial is the largest study evaluating the performance of CTC in a screening population to date.[4]

PATIENT PREPARATION

The results from most published studies examining the accuracy of CTC for polyp detection are based on patients who have undergone bowel cleansing using a wet preparation method with the ingestion of polyethylene glycol. Polyethylene glycol lavage solution is often the preferred agent by gastroenterologists and study patients typically must undergo both the CT examination and colonoscopy on the same day, often within several hours of each other. A large amount of residual fluid in the colon may cause decreased sensitivity for polyp detection on CTC. Saline cathartics such as sodium phosphate (phosphosoda) and magnesium citrate are osmotic agents that often leave the colon relatively dry. However, these "dry preparations" may leave more adherent solid stool, which can lead to an increased number of false positives.

The colon is distended by retrograde insufflation using either room air or carbon dioxide. Most published studies have included a protocol using air insufflation of the colon for CTC. However, more current published studies include the use of electronic insufflation of the colon with carbon dioxide as a method that provides optimal colonic distention more consistently. Earlier studies of CTC performance included the injection of glucagon as an antispasmodic agent. However, glucagon is no longer used routinely for CTC because it has not been found to be effective in improving colonic distention or lesion detection.[5–7] This also avoids additional cost and is less invasive to the patient. Hyoscine butylbromide (Buscopan) has been found to be a more effective spasmolytic agent and is often used in Europe to improve colonic distention for CTC.[8,9]

COMPUTED TOMOGRAPHY PROTOCOL

Earlier CTC performance studies employed single detector helical CT technology. Single detector computed tomography (SDCT) scan protocols required collimations of 3 mm or larger. Thicker collimation such as 5 mm or larger may make it more difficult to detect lesions, particularly smaller polyps. There are now multiple published studies

TABLE 7.1 Polyp Detection: Single-Center Studies

			≥10 mm				6–9 mm			
Study	**Scan Parameters**	**No. of Patients and Type**	**No. of Polyps**	**Per-Polyp Sensitivity**	**Per-Patient Sensitivity**	**Per-Patient Specificity**	**No. of Polyps**	**Per-Polyp Sensitivity**	**Per-Patient Sensitivity**	**Per-Patient Specificity**
Hara et al., 1997	SD/5/120/140	70 high risk	15	70%	75%	91%	21	63% (≥5 mm)	66% (≥5 mm)	63% (≥5 mm)
Dachman et al., 1998	SD/5/120/100	44 high risk	6	83% (>8 mm)	–	100%	3	33%	–	–
Rex et al., 1999	SD/5/120/200	46 asymptomatic	14	25–60%	75–83%	89%	14	43%	43%	–
Fenlon et al., 1999	SD/5/110/110	100 high risk	22	91%	96%	96%	36	82%	94%	92%
Pescatore et al., 2000	SD/5/110/200	50 high risk	11	–	37–62%	74%	8	–	71% (<10 mm)	75% (<10 mm)
Fletcher et al., 2000	SD/5/120/70	180 high risk	121	75%	85%	93%	142	47%	88% (≥5 mm)	72% (≥5 mm)
Morrin et al., 2000	SD+MD/2.5–5/ 120/120–200	81 high risk	20	90%	87%	100%	20	65%	73%	96%
Spinzi et al., 2001	SD/5/120/ 230–260	96 high risk	13	62%	–	100%	32	56% (<10 mm)	–	–
Hara et al., 2001	SD+MD/5/ 120/50–70	283 high risk	19	80–89%	78–100%	90–93%	–	–	–	–
Yee et al., 2001	SD/3/120/ 120–150	300 (204 high risk)	82	90%	100%	72% (overall)	141	80%	93%	–
Gluecker et al., 2002	MD/5/120/90	50 high risk	11	82%	–	90% (overall)	15	33%	–	–
Macari et al., 2002	MD/1/120/50	105 high risk	14	93%	–	98% (overall)	27	70%	–	–
McFarland et al., 2002	SD/5/120/200	70 high risk	40	68%	88%	60% (overall)	45	36%	71%	–
Iannaccone et al., 2003	MD/2.5/120/50	158 (127 high risk)	13	100%	–	97% (overall)	24	83%	–	–
Pineau et al., 2003	SD/5/120/200	205 (157 high risk)	27	78%	90%	95%	48	75%	84% (≥6 mm)	83% (≥6 mm)
Johnson et al., 2003	SD+MD/5/120/ 70–80	703 high risk, asymptomatic	59	32,34,73%	35,38,72%	97,98,98%	94	29,35,57%	41,46,69%	88,93,95%
Van Gelder et al., 2004	MD/2.5/120/ 100	249 high risk	48	75–77%	84%	92%	36	64–75%	–	69–71% (≥6 mm)
Macari et al., 2004	MD/1/120/50	68 asymptomatic	3	100%	100%	99%	17	53%	–	–
Iannaccone et al., 2005	MD/2.5/ 140/10	88 (76 high risk)	11	100%	100%	99%	26	86% (≥6 mm)	84% (≥6 mm)	82% (≥6 mm)
Yasumoto et al., 2006	MD/1.25/120/ 120	50 mixed	29	98%	–	–	70	87%	–	–

SD, single detector; MD, multidetector/collimation (mm)/kVp/mAs.

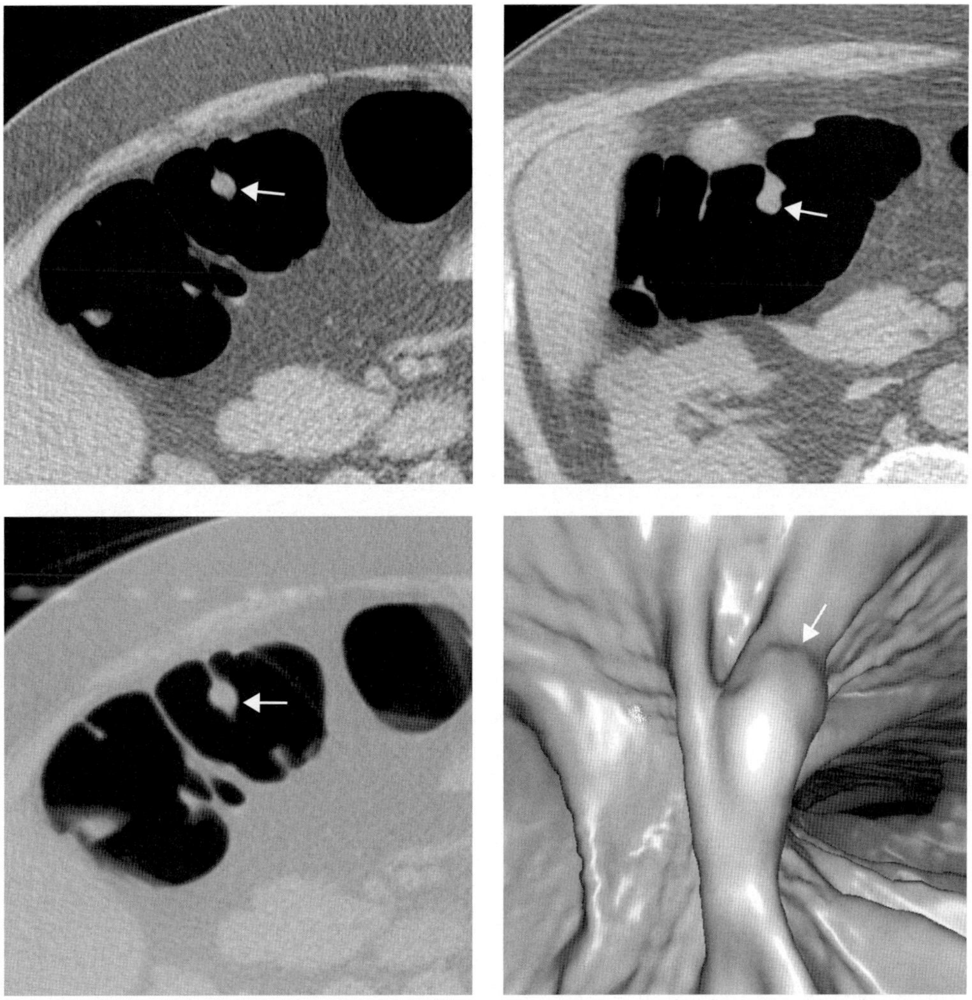

A B C D

FIGURE 7.1 Large Polyp in an Asymptomatic Screening Patient. A large polyp is visualized on the axial images in abdominal window in both supine **(A)** and prone **(B)** images. The appearance of the lesion is more prominent using a colon window **(C)**. The lesion was also identified on the 3D endoluminal view **(D)**.

evaluating the sensitivity and specificity of CTC using multidetector row CT. Multidetector computed tomography (MDCT) allows for thinner collimation of 1.25 mm or smaller. This may lead to improved spatial resolution and increased sensitivity, particularly for smaller polyps and flat lesions. Additionally, narrower collimation may allow easier differentiation between a true polyp versus stool so that there are fewer false positives, leading to increased specificity. However, the use of thinner collimation includes drawbacks such as higher effective radiation dose to the patient, noisier images, and larger data sets for evaluation and storage.

Almost all published CTC performance studies employ dual position scanning typically in the supine and prone positions. Standard CTC protocol includes the use of dual position scanning because this allows shifting of residual fluid and stool to reveal the underlying colon wall for examination and it can increase segmental distention leading to improved lesion detection.[10–12]

IMAGE DISPLAY

Options for image display include two-dimensional (2D) views, including axial images and multiplanar reformations, as well as various three-dimensional (3D) views, including the traditional endoluminal fly-through and the subvolume cube view. The performance of alternative displays has been studied less extensively and includes the dissection view, unfolded cube display, map projections, and planar virtual pathology view. Currently, most published CTC performance studies have included readers that employ 2D views primarily with the use of 3D views for problem solving. This has been found to be time efficient although a wide range of results has been reported. The 2D axial images may be easily and rapidly correlated with sagittal or coronal multiplanar reformats to identify true lesions. 2D views allow easy orientation from the extraluminal point of view and the inherent ability to evaluate lesion density. The 3D endoluminal views can provide rapid differentiation of a polyp from a fold and is the preferred interpretation technique by some readers because it may be easier to learn and identify polyps. Primary 3D interpretation has been found in several published studies to be an accurate visualization technique for lesion detection.[3,13]

READER TRAINING

The level of training and experience of readers for CTC performance trials has been variable. This has been partly due to the lack of clear guidelines until the American College of Radiology Practice Guidelines for the Performance of CTC in Adults was published in 2005.[14] These guidelines recommend that a supervising or interpreting physician should have reviewed at least 50 CTC cases either by taking a course with interactive training, double-readings performed by a trained physician, or correlation of CTC cases with colonoscopy.

It has become increasingly apparent that the level of training and experience of the reader is one of the most important factors influencing the diagnostic performance of CTC.[15] Studies with good or excellent performance results are often carried out at single centers using experienced readers. The inclusion of inexperienced readers is considered to be one of the contributing factors to the poor performance of CTC.[16–18] Some of the more recently published performance studies and large multicenter trials that are currently under way ensure reader training by proficiency testing or documenting adequate reader case experience.[4] One to three readers or consensus readings has been typically included in most published CTC performance trials.

DETECTION OF POLYPS: 1997 TO 2000

An initial evaluation of the sensitivity and specificity of CTC for polyp detection was performed by Hara et al.[19] CTC was performed in the supine position using 5-mm collimation, pitch 1.3, 120 kVp, and 140 mA followed by colonoscopy in 70 high-risk patients. Images were independently interpreted by two observers who evaluated the axial images or the 3D endoluminal views using proprietary software. Only adenomatous polyps were considered for analysis. The per-patient sensitivity for adenomas measuring 10 mm and larger was 75% (9/12) with a specificity of 91% for both observers. The sensitivity and specificity for patients with adenomas 5 cm and larger averaged 66% and 63% respectively. Patients with adenomas <5 mm were detected with a sensitivity and specificity of 45% and 80% respectively. Interpretation of axial images only yielded lower sensitivity and specificity for 10 mm or larger adenomas (58% and 74%, respectively) compared with use of the 3D endoluminal views. It was concluded in this early study that CTC was a promising test for the detection of polyps 5 mm and larger.

In a prospective study of 44 high-risk patients undergoing CTC followed by colonoscopy, Dachman et al. used axial images for primary interpretation and use of the 3D endoluminal views for problem solving only.[20] Dual position scanning was performed using SDCT with 5-mm collimation, pitch 1.5, 120 kVp, and 100 mA. The sensitivity and specificity for detection of polyps >8 mm were 83% (5/6) and 100% for two observers. There were only three polyps measuring 5 to 8 mm and both observers had a sensitivity of 33%. The average interpretation time was 28 minutes. The 3D endoluminal view was employed by the readers in 52% of patients and did not significantly impact on interpretation times. The authors concluded that CTC may be performed using axial images to initially search for polyps of significant size and that the endoluminal views should be used only when needed to distinguish folds from polyps.

Rex et al. published a study of their early experience with CTC cases that had been performed in 1995 to 1996.[1] CTC was performed in 46 asymptomatic patients using dual-slice technique with 5-mm collimation, pitch 1.5, 120 kVp, and 300 mA. Interpretation was performed by two readers in batches using proprietary software. They found that 3D endoluminal views were superior to axial imaging for polyp detection but still did poorly. CTC detected only 1 of 4 (25%) adenomas 2 cm or larger, 6 of 10 (60%) adenomas 1 to 1.9 cm, 6 of 14 (43%) adenomas 6 to 9 mm, and 7 of 65 (11%) 5 mm or smaller. The sensitivity for the detection of patients with adenomas 1 to 1.9 cm was 83% and the specificity for patients with adenomas 1 cm or larger was 89%. Three large, flat adenomas of the right colon were missed. Critical factors for accurate interpretation of CTC were meticulous bowel cleansing and adequate distention. On the basis of these results, the authors concluded that CTC was not yet ready to be used as a screening test.

Fenlon et al. evaluated 100 high-risk patients using CTC and colonoscopy.[21] CT scanning was performed using 5-mm collimation with 2-mm reconstructions, pitch 1.25, 110 kVp, and 110 mA. Interpretation was performed by two reviewers who used axial images and 3D endoluminal views. The CT studies were reviewed jointly and a consensus reading was obtained. The per-polyp sensitivity of CTC was 91% (20/22) for polyps 10 mm or larger, 82% (33/40) for polyps 6 to 9 mm, and 55% (29/53) for polyps 1 to 5 mm. Per-patient sensitivity and specificity as well as positive predictive value (PPV) and negative predictive value (NPV) were all 96% for polyps 10 mm or larger. For polyps between 6 and 9 mm per patient sensitivity, specificity, PPV, and NPV were 94%, 92%, 92%, and 94% respectively. All three carcinomas were identified by CTC. The average time required was <20 minutes for CT scanning, 30 minutes for image manipulation, and 10 minutes for interpretation. The authors concluded that CTC and colonoscopy had similar efficacy for identifying 6 mm or larger polyps in patients at high risk for colorectal neoplasia. Fenlon et al. also found significantly lower sensitivity for hyperplastic polyps compared to similar size adenomatous polyps. This was thought to be possibly related to the tendency for effacement of hyperplastic polyps with colonic distention.

CTC and colonoscopy were performed in 50 high-risk patients in a study by Pescatore et al.[22] Patients were scanned using 5-mm collimation, pitch 1.5, 110 kVp, and 200 mA. Two teams independently interpreted the CTC data sets using two dimensional and surface-rendered 3D endoluminal views. The sensitivity of CTC for the detection of patients with polyps of any size was 75% and 71%, and specificity was 62% and 69% for teams 1 and 2 respectively. The per-patient sensitivity for polyps 10 mm or larger was 38% and 64% with a specificity of 74% and 74% for teams 1 and 2 respectively. A learning curve effect was noted with improved accuracy comparing the results of the first 24 cases with the last 26 patients. The poor results were explained in this study as related to frequent suboptimal preparation quality, lower resolution of the surface rendering technique used, and lack of reader expertise.

Fletcher et al. recruited 180 patients with known polyps or risk factors for colorectal cancer and performed CTC using 5-mm collimation, pitch 1.3, 120 kVp, and 70 mA and a 3 mm reconstruction interval.[10] Three or four 20-second breathholds were required to scan the entire colon with 3-cm overlap between gaps. Colonoscopy was performed on the same day in all patients. There was also random assignment of 89 patients who received oral iodinated contrast with the bowel-cleansing regimen the day before the CT. Using proprietary software, one reader interpreted the supine images alone and another reader evaluated both supine and prone data sets. Per-polyp sensitivity for lesions 10 mm or larger and for polyps between 5 and 9 mm were 75.2% (91/121) and 47.2% (67/142) respectively. Per-patient sensitivity and specificity for 10 mm or larger polyps were 85.4% and 93% respectively. The use of the combination of supine and prone images significantly improved identification of patients with polyps 5 mm or larger. Administration of oral iodinated contrast in this study did not improve polyp detection.

Morrin et al. evaluated 81 high-risk patients who underwent CTC and colonoscopy or surgery.[23] A subset of 48 patients received intravenous contrast. CTC was performed using single and multidetector scanners. SDCT was performed on most patients and the protocol consisted of 3-mm collimation, pitch 2, 120 kVp, 120 mA, and 1.5-mm reconstructions. MDCT protocol consisted of 2.5- to 5-mm slice thickness, 11.25- to 15-mm/second table speed, 120 kVp, and 200 mA in high-speed mode. Per-polyp sensitivity for 10- to 19-mm polyps, 5- to 9-mm polyps, and <5-mm polyps was 90% (18/20), 65% (13/20), and 33% (9/27) respectively. Per-patient sensitivity for the 10- to 19-mm polyps and 5- to 9-mm polyps was 87% and 73% with a specificity of 100% and 96% respectively. The use of intravenous contrast was found to improve the detection of medium-sized polyps (75% vs. 58%).

DETECTION OF POLYPS: 2001 TO PRESENT

In a study of 96 high-risk or symptomatic patients, Spinzi et al. compared the performance of CTC to colonoscopy.[24] CTC was performed using 5-mm collimation, pitch 2, 120 kVp, 230 to 260 mA, and 2.5-mm reconstructions. One reader evaluated the 2D images and 3D surface rendered endoluminal view. The per-polyp sensitivity for 10 mm or larger lesions was 62% (8/13) with a specificity of 100%. There was also low per-polyp sensitivity of 56% (18/32) for polyps <10 mm. CTC detected seven of eight carcinomas for a sensitivity of 88%. The sensitivity for polyp detection was significantly lower (32%) for the first 25 cases compared to the last 20 patients (92%).

Hara et al. compared single detector versus multidetector CTC for lesion detection in 237 high-risk patients.[25] Single-detector CTC was performed on 77 patients with 5-mm collimation, pitch 1.3, 120 kVp, 70 mA, and 3-mm reconstructions. Three to four CT volumes were obtained with 3-cm overlap. The remaining patients underwent MDCT scanning with 5-mm collimation, pitch 0.75, 50 mA, 120 kVp, and 3-mm reconstructions. Two of three radiologists interpreted each of the studies using primary 2D interpretation with 3D volume rendered views for problem solving. No significant differences in performance were identified for SDCT versus MDCT. Per-polyp sensitivity for lesions >10 mm was 89% (8/9) for SDCT versus 80% (8/10) for MDCT. Per-patient sensitivity and specificity were 100% (5/5) and 90% (65/72) for SDCT versus 78% (7/9) and 93% (140/151) for MDCT. CTC using MDCT showed significantly improved colonic distention with fewer respiratory artifacts.

Yee et al. evaluated the performance of CTC for polyp and cancer detection in a study of 300 patients.[26] Ninety-six patients were asymptomatic and referred for screening. Scanning was performed using SDCT with 3-mm collimation, pitch 1.5 to 2, 120 kVp, 120 to 150 mA, and 1.5-mm reconstructions. A consensus reading was obtained from two readers who evaluated both 2D and 3D surface rendered images. The per-polyp sensitivity was 90% (74/82) for detecting polyps 10 mm or larger, 80% (113/141) for identifying polyps between 5 and 9.9 mm and 59% (178/301) for finding polyps <5 mm. The sensitivity was 100% (49/49) for identifying patients with polyps measuring 10 mm or larger, 93% (50/54) for detecting patients with polyps measuring between 5 and 9.9 mm, and 82% (65/79) for finding patients with polyps <5 mm. The PPV and NPV for clinically significant polyps measuring ≥10 mm was 80.8% and 97.2%, respectively. Overall specificity was 72%, although this included a large number of diminutive polyps. All eight carcinomas were detected on CTC. Performance results for polyp and cancer detection showed no significant difference comparing asymptomatic and symptomatic patients.

In a study of 50 high-risk patients, Gluecker et al. performed MDCT colonography and colonoscopy on the same day.[27] The CT protocol consisted of 5-mm collimation, pitch 3, 120 kVp, and 90 mA. One experienced reader used a primary 2D interpretation method with surface rendered 3D endoluminal views for problem solving. The per-polyp sensitivity was 82% (9/11) for lesions ≥10 mm, 33% (5/15) for lesions 6 to 9 mm, and 4% (1/41) for ≤5 mm lesions. The overall per-patient specificity was 90% (19/21). Median interpretation time was 13 minutes with evaluation of the supine and prone 2D data sets requiring an average of 10 minutes. It was concluded that

MDCT colonography has good sensitivity and specificity for detecting colonic lesions 10 mm or larger.

Thin-section low-dose MDCT colonography was performed on 105 high-risk patients in a study by Macari et al.[28] Images were acquired using 4 × 1 mm detector collimation, pitch 6 to 7, 120 kVp, effective mAs of 50, and 1.25 mm reconstructions. One radiologist evaluated the images using primary 2D interpretation. The median CT interpretation time was 12 minutes. Sensitivity was 93% (13/14) for 10 mm and larger lesions, 70% (19/27) for 6 to 9 mm lesions, and 12% (11/91) for polyps 5 mm or smaller. Overall specificity was found to be 98%. The PPV for detecting 10 mm or larger polyps was 93% and the NPV was 85%. The effective dose for MDCT colonography was 5 mSv for men and 7.8 mSv for women.

Multiobserver diagnostic performance was evaluated by McFarland et al. in a study of 70 patients with known or suspected colorectal polyps who underwent CTC using SDCT with 5-mm collimation, 120 kVp, 200 mA, and a 2-mm reconstruction interval.[29] Four trained radiologists independently evaluated the cases using primary 2D interpretation and volume rendered 3D endoluminal views for problem solving. The per-polyp sensitivity for polyps measuring 10 mm or larger, 6 to 9 mm, and 5 mm or smaller ranged between 60% and 78%, 20% and 44%, and 6% and 38% respectively. Pooled results of sensitivity for polyps measuring 10 mm or larger and 6 to 9 mm were 68% (with 75% agreement among four readers) and 36% respectively. There was more individual variability among readers for 6 to 9 mm polyps than for lesions 10 mm or larger. A trend for readers with higher sensitivity to also have more false-positive findings was noted. Pooled results of sensitivity per-patient for polyps measuring 10 mm or larger, 6 to 9 mm, and 5 mm or smaller were 88% (with 94% agreement), 71%, and 48% respectively. Individual specificity for the four readers ranged between 36% and 73%. The average interpretation time was 20 minutes. The two readers with relatively longer reader times had the highest per-polyp sensitivity and the two readers with lower sensitivity had shorter reader times.

Iannaccone et al. used low-dose CTC with a beam collimation of 4 × 2.5 mm, pitch 0.875, 140 kVp, and 10 mAs (effective) to evaluate 158 patients followed by colonoscopy.[30] Thirty-one patients were referred for colorectal cancer screening. Two radiologists used primary 2D interpretation with 3D for problem solving. All 22 cancers were identified on CTC. The per-polyp sensitivity for detecting polyps 10 mm or larger, 6 to 9 mm, and 5 mm or smaller were 100% (13/13), 83% (20/24), and 51% (19/37) respectively. Overall per-patient sensitivity for CTC was 96% with a specificity of 97%, a PPV of 94% and a NPV of 98%. The simulated effective doses for CTC were 1.8 mSv in men and 2.4 mSv in women. Excellent sensitivity and specificity were achieved using a low-dose CTC protocol, which allowed a significant decrease in radiation dose to patients.

Single-detector CTC was used to evaluate 205 subjects followed by colonoscopy using segmental unblinding in a study by Pineau et al.[31] Seventy-six patients were asymptomatic and referred for screening or surveillance. Although this study was published in 2003, older technique was employed with 5-mm collimation, pitch 2, 120 kVp, 200 mAs, and 1-mm reconstructions. Limited prone position scanning was performed which included the pelvis only. These factors may have contributed to the poor per-polyp sensitivity results. A single radiologist performed primary 2D interpretation using proprietary software. The per-polyp sensitivity for identifying lesions 10 mm or larger, 6 to 9 mm, and 1 to 5 mm were 78% (21/27), 75% (36/48), and 29% (37/126) respectively. The sensitivity, specificity, PPV, and NPV of CTC for the detection of patients with lesion 10 mm or larger were 90%, 95%, 64%, and 99% respectively. When the cut-off was decreased to 6 mm or larger the sensitivity, specificity, PPV, and NPV of CTC were 84%, 83%, 59%, and 95% respectively.

Johnson et al. performed a large single-center study evaluating CTC in 703 asymptomatic individuals who were at higher than average risk for colorectal cancer.[32] SDCT was used for 16% of the patients with 5-mm collimation, pitch 1.3, 120 kVp, 70 mAs, and 3-mm reconstructions. MDCT was used for most patients (83%) with 5-mm collimation, 120 kVp, and 80 mAs. Two of three experienced readers were randomly assigned to interpret each case using a primary 2D method on proprietary software. Reviewers were asked to ignore diminutive lesions <5 mm. The prevalence of 10 mm or larger lesions was low at 5% reflecting a screening population. CTC had poor sensitivity of 34%, 32%, 73%, and 63% for 59 polyps measuring 10 mm or larger for readers 1, 2, 3, and double-reading. There was a sensitivity of 35%, 29%, 57%, and 54% for the 94 polyps 5 to 9 mm in size for readers 1, 2, 3, and double-reading. Per-patient sensitivities for each of the size categories were similar to per-polyp sensitivities. Specificity of CTC ranged between 95% and 98% and 86% to 95% for 10 mm or larger polyps and 5 to 9 mm polyps respectively. Interobserver variability was noted to be high in this study.

A prospective study investigating the ability of CTC to detect large polyps in 249 patients at increased risk for colon cancer was performed by van Gelder et al.[33] The MDCT protocol used included 4 × 2.5 mm collimation, pitch 1.25, 120 kVp, and ≤100 mAs. Two observers interpreted each case independently. The per-polyp sensitivity for identifying polyps 10 mm or larger and 6 to 9 mm were 75% to 77% (36–37/48) and 64% to 75% (23–27/36) respectively for the two readers. Nine of the missed polyps were noted to be flat lesions. The per-patient sensitivity and specificity for large polyps were 84% and 92% with a PPV of 59% to 60% and a NPV of 98%. It was concluded that CTC and colonoscopy have a similar ability to identify subjects with large polyps in patients with increased risk for colon cancer.

Sixty-eight asymptomatic men at average risk for colorectal cancer were evaluated by MDCT colonography and colonoscopy in a study by Macari et al.[2] CT parameters included 4 × 1 mm collimation, pitch 6 to 7, 120 kVp, 50 effective mAs and 1.25-mm reconstructions. One radiologist performed primary interpretation of the axial images and used the multiplanar reformats and volume rendered 3D endoluminal views for problem solving. Mean interpretation time was 9 minutes. The per-polyp sensitivity for the identification of lesions 10 mm or larger, 6 to 9 mm, and 1 to 5 mm were 100% (3/3), 53% (9/17), and 12% (9/78) respectively. Overall per-patient specificity was 90% and the specificity for large polyps at least 10 mm in size was 99%. It was concluded that CTC is an effective test for the detection of polyps 10 mm or larger in average risk patients.

Low-dose MDCT colonography followed by two sequential colonoscopies on different days were performed in 88 patients in a study by Iannaccone et al.[34] Twelve patients were referred for colorectal cancer screening and the remaining patients were symptomatic or at increased risk for colorectal cancer. A low-dose CT protocol was used consisting of 4 × 2.5 mm collimation, 140 kVp, and 10 effective mAs. Three readers independently interpreted each case using a primary 2D technique with 3D for problem solving. The per-polyp sensitivities for the detection of polyps 6 mm or larger for CTC and initial colonoscopy were 86% (32/37) and 84% (31/37), respectively. The per-polyp sensitivities for the detection of polyps 10 mm or larger for CTC and initial colonoscopy were 100% (11/11) and 91% (10/11) respectively. For patients with polyps 6 mm or larger sensitivity, specificity, PPV, and NPV of CTC and initial colonoscopy were 84% and 90%, 82% and 100%, 70% and 100%, and 91% and 95% respectively. Low-dose CTC compared favorably with colonoscopy for the detection of polyps 6 mm or larger.

Primary 3D interpretation (one-way vs. two-way) was evaluated for polyp detection on MDCT Colonography in 50 patients in a study by Yasumoto et al.[13] Average-risk patients as well as individuals at increased risk for colorectal cancer were included. Only supine scanning was performed to reduce radiation dose. The CT parameters used included 8 × 1.25 mm collimation, pitch 13.75, 120 kVp, 120 mA, and 1.25-mm reconstructions. Three experienced radiologists independently reviewed each case using surface-rendered 3D endoluminal navigation as the primary interpretation method with 2D views used to confirm findings. During each of two interpretation sessions, 25 cases were reviewed using a one-way method and 25 cases were read using a two-way method. The average per-polyp sensitivity using standard two-way 3D interpretation for lesions measuring 10 mm or larger, 6 to 9 mm, and 5 mm or smaller were 98%, 87%, and 85% respectively. The average per-polyp sensitivity using only one-way 3D interpretation for lesions measuring 10 mm or larger, 6 to 9 mm, and 5 mm or smaller were 91%, 79%, and 70% respectively. The average interpretation time with two-way was 39 minutes which was significantly longer than for one way (25 minutes).

MULTICENTER STUDIES

Multicenter trials performed in the United States have reported conflicting results (see Table 7.2). Similar to the discrepant results found in single-center studies, differences in trial parameters likely accounted for these variable results. This includes differences in CT protocol, the use of fecal and fluid tagging, image display and interpretation method, and reader training and experience.

Pickhardt et al. evaluated 1,233 asymptomatic patients at three sites using MDCT colonography followed by colonoscopy with segmental unblinding in a study supported by Advances in Medical Practice funds from the Department of Defense.[3] The CT protocol consisted of 1.25- to 2.5-mm collimation, 120 kVp, 100mAs with a 1-mm reconstruction interval. This study was the first to be carried out in a large average-risk screening patient cohort. Fecal and fluid tagging was included and patients ingested 500 mL of 2.1% barium and 120 mL of diatrizoate meglumine and diatrizoate sodium (Gastrografin) before CTC. One of six trained radiologists (each trained with a minimum of 25 cases) reviewed the cases using primary 3D interpretation with 2D reserved for problem solving. Performance was evaluated for adenomatous polyps. The per-polyp sensitivity for polyps measuring 10 mm or larger, 8 mm or larger, and 6 mm or larger were 92% (47/51), 93% (88/95), and 86% (180/210) respectively. The per-patient sensitivity for polyps measuring 10 mm or larger, 8 mm or larger, and 6 mm or larger were 94% (45/48), 94% (77/82), and 89% (149/168) respectively. Specificity for patients with polyps measuring 10 mm or larger, 8 mm or larger, and 6 mm or larger were 96%, 92%, and 80% respectively. The test-positive rates for patients with polyps measuring 10 mm or larger, 8 mm or larger, and 6 mm or larger were 7.5%, 13.5%, and 29.7% respectively. This study also reported the sensitivity of colonoscopy using the CT findings as the reference standard as determined by segmental unblinding. CTC outperformed colonoscopy for 8 mm or larger adenomas. The sensitivity of colonoscopy for polyps measuring 10 mm or larger, 8 mm or larger, and 6 mm or larger were 88%, 92%, and 92% respectively.

Cotton et al. evaluated CTC followed by colonoscopy with segmental unblinding in 600 high-risk patients at nine centers that was carried out from 2000 to 2001.[16] This study was funded by the Office of Naval Research of the United States Department of Defense. CT protocol included 2.5- to 5-mm collimation with 1- to 1.5-mm reconstructions. Other CT parameters were not specified. Primary 2D interpretation was used and focal 3D snapshot reconstructions were reviewed when needed. Radiologists were required to have read only 10 CTC studies before participation in the trial. Full 3D navigations were examined later without referral back to the initial 2D reviews. Per-polyp sensitivity for detecting lesions sized 10 mm or larger, 6 to 9 mm, and 1 to 5 mm were 52% (28/54), 23% (27/119), and 8% (50/654), respectively. Per-patient sensitivity for identifying lesions measuring 10 mm or larger, 6 to 9 mm, and 1 to 5 mm were 55% (23/42), 30% (23/76), and 14% (37/274), respectively. Although there was suboptimal sensitivity, specificity was excellent for all size categories. Specificity for patients with polyps 10 mm or larger, 6 to 9 mm, and 1 to 5 mm were 96%, 93%, and 91%, respectively. PPV and NPV for patients with polyps 10 mm or larger were 50% and 97% respectively. CTC missed two of eight cancers. The accuracy of CTC varied considerably between centers and did not improve as the study progressed. Only one center had substantial prior experience with CTC and had the best results with a sensitivity of 82%.

TABLE 7.2 Polyp Detection: Multicenter Studies

			≥10 mm				6–9 mm			
Study	**Scan Parameters**	**No. of Patients and Type**	**No. of Polyps**	**Per-Polyp Sensitivity**	**Per-Patient Sensitivity**	**Per-Patient Specificity**	**No. of Polyps**	**Per-Polyp Sensitivity**	**Per-Patient Sensitivity**	**Per-Patient Specificity**
Pickhardt et al., 2003	MD/1.25–2.5/ 120/100	1,233 asymp-tomatic	51	92%	94%	96%	210	86% (≥6 mm)	89% (≥6 mm)	80% (≥6 mm)
Cotton et al., 2004	MD/2.5–5/–/–	600 high risk	54	52%	55%	96%	119	23%	30%	93%
Rockey et al., 2005	MD/2.5/–/–	614 high risk	76	53%	59%	96%	158	47%	51%	89%

SD, single detector; MD, multidetector/collimation (mm)/kVp/mAs.

In a multicenter study funded by the National Cancer Institute (NCI), Rockey et al. evaluated 614 high-risk patients at 14 centers who underwent air contrast barium enema (ACBE) and then after seven to 14 days all subjects underwent same-day CTC and colonoscopy.[35] MDCT protocol included 2.5-mm collimation with 1-mm reconstruction intervals. Other CT parameters were not specified. Primary 2D interpretation with 3D for problem solving was used by readers. Approximately half the number of readers had experience with 50 or more CTC cases and the other half had to complete a training module although no testing was performed. Performance results of CTC were similar to those reported by Cotton et al. for large polyps.[16] Per-polyp sensitivity of CTC for detecting lesions sized 10 mm or larger and 6 to 9 mm were 53% (40/76) and 47% (74/158), respectively. Per-patient sensitivity of CTC for identifying lesions measuring 10 mm or larger and 6 to 9 mm were 59% (37/63) and 51% (59/116). ACBE had lower performance levels for polyp detection compared to CTC. Per-polyp sensitivity of ACBE for detecting lesions sized 10 mm or larger and 6 to 9 mm were 45% (34/76) and 30% (48/158), respectively. Per-patient sensitivity of ACBE for identifying lesions measuring 10 mm or larger and 6 to 9 mm were 48% (30/63) and 35% (40/116). CTC and ACBE had high specificity for detection of patients with polyps 10 mm or larger reported at 96% and 90% respectively. CTC missed two of nine cancers and ACBE missed eight of nine cancers. There was large variability in the number of patients recruited at the various sites, with the maximum number of patients examined at any one site reported at 165 and the minimum at 2. The median number of patients enrolled per site was 22.5.

The Special Interest Group for Gastrointestinal and Abdominal Radiology (SIGGAR), a subspecialty group of the United Kingdom Royal College of Radiologists, is conducting a multicenter trial comparing CTC, barium enema, and optical colonoscopy in 4,500 symptomatic patients age 55 or older.[36] The study is funded by the NHS Health Technology Assessment (HTA) program. The SIGGAR 1 study consists of two parallel randomized trials (CTC vs. barium enema, CTC vs. colonoscopy) held in at least 10 centers. The goal of the study is the detection or exclusion of significant colorectal neoplasia (cancer and/or polyps >10 mm). The incidence and significance of extracolonic findings will also be determined. Psychological and physical morbidity will be evaluated and a cost analysis will be performed. The trial started in February 2004 and results are expected to be published in mid-2009.

ACRIN 6664: NATIONAL COMPUTED TOMOGRAPHIC COLONOGRAPHY TRIAL

The American College of Radiology Imaging Network (ACRIN 6664) National CT Colonography Trial funded by the NCI is a multicenter study that evaluates the performance of CTC in 2,607 asymptomatic screening patients.[4] The study was activated in February 2005 and recruitment was completed in November 2006. Fifteen institutions are included. The goal of the study is to validate the widespread use of CTC in a screening population for the detection of colorectal neoplasia. Primary aims include evaluation of per-patient sensitivity of CTC for the detection of patients with 10 mm or larger polyps and 5- to 10-mm polyps. Secondary aims include evaluation of interobserver variability, the benefit of primary 3D interpretation and independent second read, colonic cleansing protocols, patient acceptance, and extracolonic findings. Broader themes include generation of a CTC database for development of computer-aided detection and evaluating the cost-effectiveness of CTC.

Patients who were prescheduled for a screening colonoscopy aged 50 or older and who had not had a prior colonoscopy within the last 5 years were recruited for the study. Exclusion criteria were inflammatory bowel disease, familial adenomatous polyposis, pregnancy, lower gastrointestinal symptoms such as melena or hematochezia, anemia (hemoglobin <10 gm/dL), positive fecal occult blood test, and patients with comorbid conditions that would increase the risk of colonoscopy.

In addition to bowel cleansing, fecal and fluid tagging was achieved with 40 mL of high-density barium sulfate and 60 mL of water-soluble contrast. Mechanical insufflation of the colon was performed with carbon dioxide on all patients. One milligram of glucagon was administered subcutaneously unless contraindicated. Participants underwent MDCT colonography followed by colonoscopy on the same day. Scanning was performed on 16 row MDCT or higher with a maximum slice thickness of 1 to 2 mm and a reconstruction interval of 1 to 1.25 mm, 120 kVp and variable mA depending upon the display field of view (DFOV).

All readers were to have interpreted at least 500 CTC cases or had to attend a CTC interpretation course. Readers were also required to take a competency examination in CTC interpretation and had to achieve at least 90% accuracy. Each case was interpreted twice, once locally and once off-site, with the reader randomized to either primary 2D interpretation with 3D problem solving or primary 3D interpretation with 2D problem solving. All lesions 5 mm or larger and identified locally were sent for central review. An independent radiologist performed lesion matching. A positive match was one where a lesion found on the CT was identified on colonoscopy located in the same or adjacent colon segment and if the lesion was within 50% of the reported size on colonoscopy.

Results of ACRIN 6664 are anticipated to further promote more widespread acceptance and use of CTC for both diagnostic and screening purposes. The sensitivity and specificity of CTC on a per-polyp and a per-patient basis will likely fall somewhere between the excellent results of the trial by Pickhardt et al. and the suboptimal results of Cotton et al. and Rockey et al. However, additional large multicenter trials are already under way both in the United States and Europe, which will continue to provide evidence of CTC performance that can only improve with technological advances and increasing reader experience.

META-ANALYSES OF CTC PERFORMANCE

Several meta-analyses of CTC performance have been published. Sosna et al. compiled the results of 14 studies with a total of 1,324 patients and 1,411 polyps.[37] All studies included 5-mm collimation except for two and all patient cohorts were high risk except for 2. The pooled per-polyp sensitivity for lesions measuring 10 mm or larger, 6 to 9 mm, and 5 mm or smaller were 81%, 62%, and 43%. The pooled per-patient sensitivity for lesions measuring 10 mm or larger, 6 to 9 mm, and 5 mm or smaller were 88%, 84%, and 65%. The sensitivity for polyp detection increased with increasing polyp size. The pooled overall specificity for detecting polyps 10 mm or larger was 95%. It was concluded that the sensitivity and specificity of CTC are high for polyps 10 mm or larger.

Halligan et al. searched the MEDLINE database for CTC reports published between 1994 and 2003.[38] Twenty-four studies met established criteria and were included for evaluation. Meta-analysis of 2,610 patients showed average per-patient sensitivity and specificity for 10 mm or larger polyp to be 93% and 97% respectively. This decreased to 86% and 96% respectively for medium sized polyps. There was a 96% sensitivity for the detection of cancers with 144 of 150 tumors identified. This meta-analysis concluded that CTC had sufficient sensitivity and specificity for the detection of large and medium polyps and high sensitivity for the detection of symptomatic cancers.

Mulhall et al. searched PubMed, MEDLINE, and EMBASE databases and the Cochrane Controlled Trials Register for CT colonography studies published between 1975 and 2005.[39] Thirty-three studies were identified that included data on 6,393 patients. Heterogeneous sensitivity was found for CTC, which improved with increasing polyp size. The pooled sensitivity for lesions measuring 10 mm or larger, 6 to 9 mm, and 5 mm or smaller were 85%, 70%, and 48%. The pooled specificity for lesions measuring 10 mm or larger, 6 to 9 mm, and 5 mm or smaller were 97%, 93%, and 92%. It was concluded that although CTC has high specificity, there is a wide range of sensitivities not fully accounted for by patient or scanner characteristics.

DETECTION AND STAGING OF COLORECTAL CARCINOMA

In an early study by Royster et al., CTC was performed in 20 patients who initially had findings on colonoscopy suggestive of colorectal carcinoma (see Table 7.3).[40] Supine and prone scanning was performed using 5-mm collimation, 110 kVp, 110 mA and images were analyzed on commercially available software. 2D and complete 3D volume rendered images were evaluated by two radiologists with a consensus reading obtained. Masses were defined as intraluminal projections measuring 2 cm or larger and polyps were defined as lesions projecting into the colonic lumen <2 cm. All 20 masses and 14/15 polyps were detected using axial images. Endoluminal views demonstrated 19/20 masses and 13/15 polyps. Per-polyp sensitivity for lesions measuring 11 to 20 mm and for those between 6 and 10 mm were 100% (2/2) and 90% (9/10) respectively.

Laghi et al. evaluated 165 high-risk patients using SDCT with 3-mm collimation, pitch 2, 130 kVp, 120 mAs, and 2-mm reconstructions or MDCT with 1-mm collimation, 8 mm/second table speed, 120 kVp, 80 mAs, and 1-mm reconstructions.[41] Intravenous contrast was administered to 67 patients (130 mL 2.5 to 3.5 mL/sec, 60-second delay). Interpretation was performed by two observers who used both 2D and 3D endoluminal views and a consensus reading was obtained. There was 100% (30/30) sensitivity for cancers, 92% (11/12) sensitivity for ≥10 mm polyps, 82% (14/17) sensitivity for 6- to 9-mm polyps, and 50% (4/8) sensitivity for ≤5 mm polyps. Overall per-patients sensitivity and specificity were 93% and 97% respectively. It was concluded that CTC has a diagnostic sensitivity similar to that of conventional colonoscopy.

In a study of 80 patients with symptoms of colorectal disease, Munikrishnan et al. performed MDCT colonography followed by colonoscopy.[42] MDCT technique included 1-mm collimation, variable table speed, 120 kVp, and 120 to 200 mA. All patients received 100 to 130 mL of intravenous contrast. CTC had a sensitivity of 97% (28/29) for cancers, 100% (12/12) for polyps 10 mm or larger,

TABLE 7.3 Detection of Colorectal Carcinoma

Study	Scan Parameters	No. of Patients and Type	No. of Cancers	Sensitivity	Specificity
Royster et al., 1997	SD/5/110/110	20 high risk	20	100%	–
Laghi et al., 2002	SD+MD/1,3/120,130/ 80–120 + IV contrast (67 patients)	165 high risk	30	100%	97% (overall)
Munikrishnan et al., 2003	MD/1/120/120–200 + IV contrast	80 high risk	29	97%	98%
Chung et al., 2005	MD/0.75/120/120–160 + IV contrast	51 high risk	21	100%	–

SD, single detector; MD, multidetector/collimation (mm)/kVp/mAs.

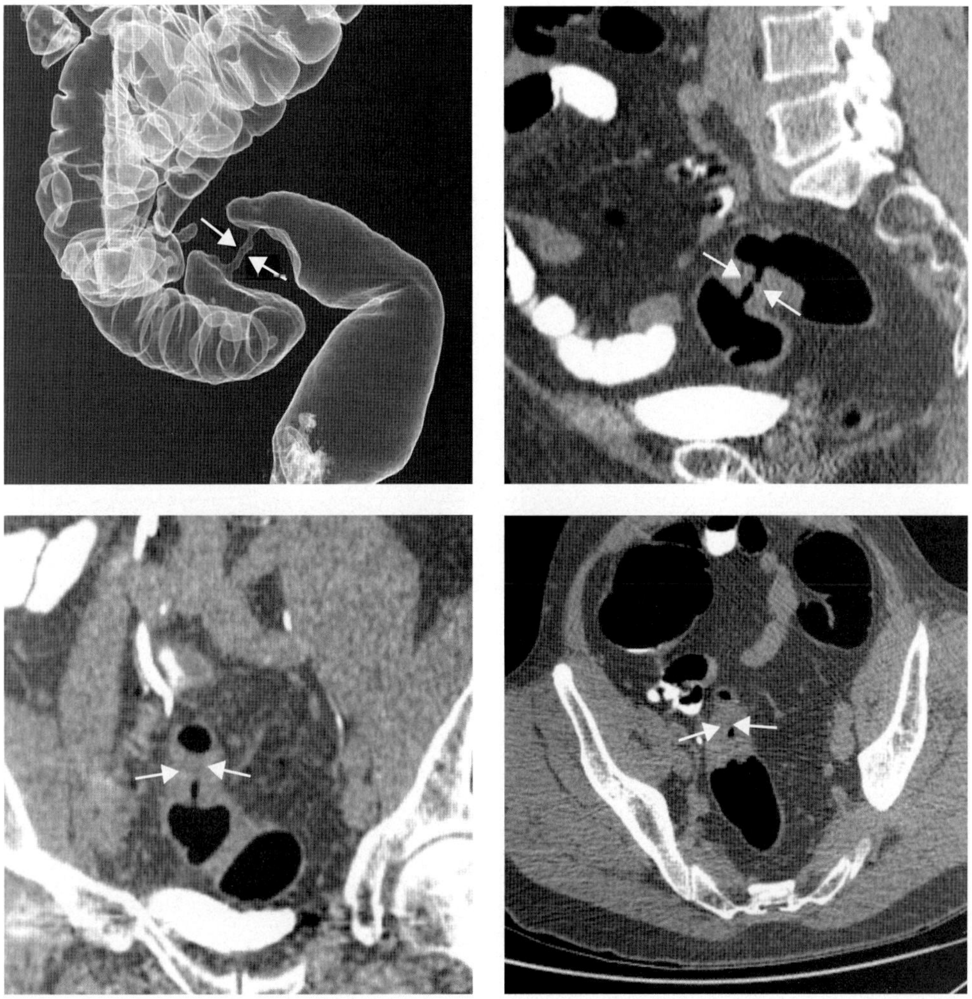

A B C D

FIGURE 7.2 Annular Sigmoid Carcinoma. An annular carcinoma in the sigmoid was the cause of a failed colonoscopy in this patient as seen on the BE overview **(A)**, sagittal reformat **(B)**, coronal reformat **(C)** and axial **(D)** views.

83% (5/6) for 6- to 9-mm polyps, and 53% (8/15) for 5 mm or smaller polyps. The specificity, PPV, and NPV for detecting patients with cancer were 98%, 96%, and 98% respectively. Overall specificity for polyp detection was 96% with a PPV of 88% and an NPV of 90%. It was concluded that CTC had the same efficacy as colonoscopy for the detection of colorectal cancers and 6 mm or larger polyps.

Chung et al. evaluated 51 patients who were thought to have colorectal cancer.[43] All patients underwent colonoscopy first followed by 16-row MDCT scanning using 0.75-mm collimation, pitch 1 to 1.3, 120 kVp, and 120 to 160 mAs. Eleven patients had incomplete colonoscopy due to distally occluding lesions (see Figure 7.2). Twenty patients had surgery and 21 cancers were identified. Unenhanced prone scanning was performed followed by contrast-enhanced supine CT with the administration of 140 mL of intravenous contrast at 3 mL/second and a scan delay of 60 seconds. The sensitivity of CTC for cancer detection was 100% (21/21). The diagnostic accuracies of CTC for TNM staging were 95% (20/21), 85% (17/20), and 100% (1/1) for tumor, node, and metastasis respectively. Per-polyp sensitivity for the detection of lesions 10 mm or larger, 6 to 9 mm and 5 mm or smaller were 100% (6/6), 94% (15/16), and 84% (16/19) respectively.

Sun et al. investigated the use of CTC for preoperative staging of 64 patients with known colorectal cancer from August 1998 to December 2002.[44] Only supine CT scanning was performed using 10-mm collimation, pitch 1 to 2, and 200 mA. All patients received intravenous contrast (1.5 mL/kg) at a rate of 3 mL/sec with a 60-second scan delay. A consensus reading was obtained from two radiologists blinded to the surgery and pathology findings. CTC demonstrated the tumor in all patients. The sensitivity and specificity were 95% and 41% for detection of local invasion and 75% and 91% for detection of metastasis (see Figure 7.3). Overall, CT correctly staged 64% of patients. CT staging accuracy for Dukes A, B, C, D tumors were 33%, 78%, 67%, and 88%.

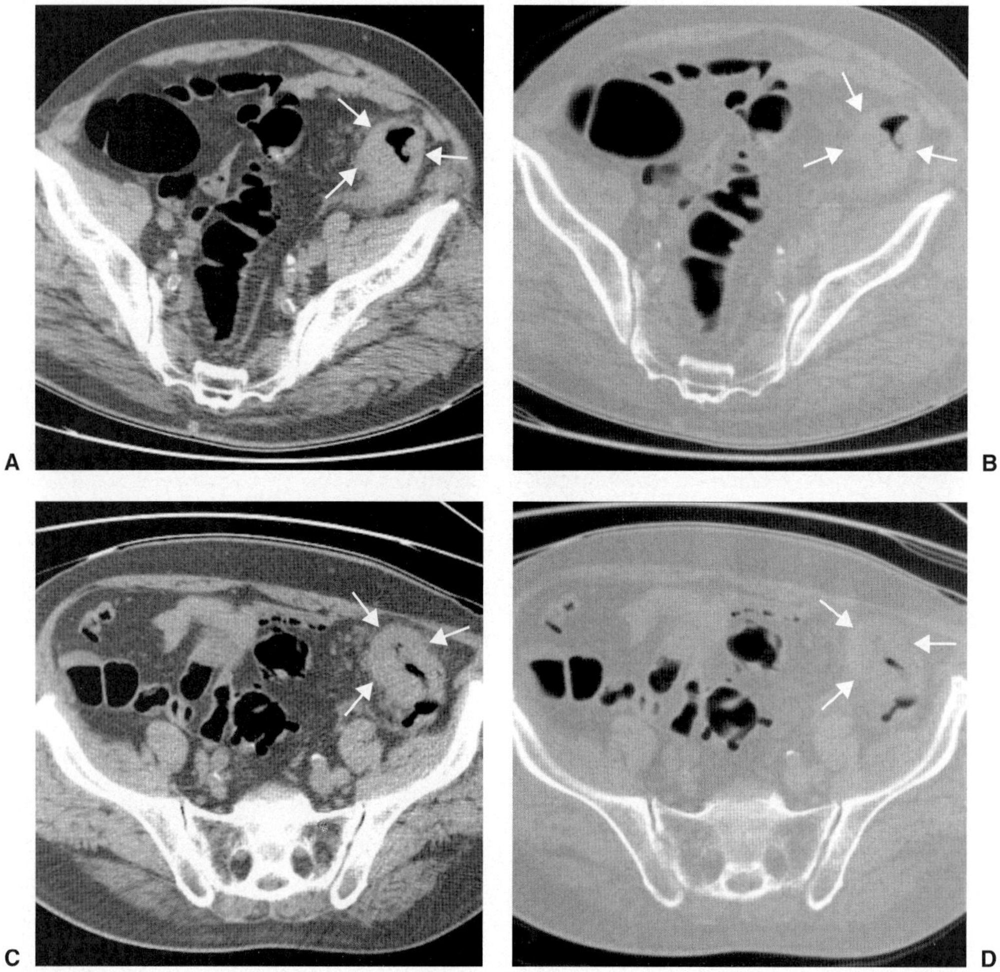

FIGURE 7.3 Local Extension of Sigmoid Cancer. A large annular carcinoma is shown on 2D axial supine images in both abdominal **(A)** and colon **(B)** windows. The same lesion is shown in abdominal **(C)** and colon **(D)** window images obtained from the prone series. Note extensive stranding in the pericolonic fat on the abdominal windows clearly indicating local extension of tumor through the colon wall.

Mainenti et al. performed a study evaluating 52 patients with known colorectal cancer using contrast-enhanced MDCT colonography.[45] The CT protocol consisted of 2.5-mm collimation, pitch 1.25, 120 kVp, and 200 mAs. The CT was performed 70 seconds after the administration of 120 mL of intravenous contrast at a rate of 3 mL/second. Two radiologists independently reviewed the depth of tumor invasion into the colon wall (T), regional lymph node involvement (N), and extra-colonic metastasis (M). CTC staging accuracy for T, N, M were 93%, 71%, and 93%, respectively.

CONCLUSION

In the presentation of 20 single-center studies evaluating CTC performance, it is clear that there is a wide range of results for per-polyp and per-patient sensitivities for polyp detection. This is also true for the three multicenter trials and even for the three meta-analyses presented. Specific parameters of the studies must be considered that can account for the level of performance reported such as the type of patients included in the study, patient preparation, CT protocol, the specific image display and version of the display used for interpretation, and reader training and experience. The results indicate that CTC has high specificity for the detection of large polyps. CTC also has high sensitivity and specificity for the detection of colorectal cancer.

REFERENCES

1. Rex DK, Vining D, Kopecky KK. An initial experience with screening for colon polyps using spiral CT with and without CT colography (virtual colonoscopy). *Gastrointest Endosc*. 1999;50:309–313.

2. Macari M, Bini EJ, Jacobs SL, et al. Colorectal polyps and cancers in asymptomatic average-risk patients: evaluation with CT colonography. *Radiology*. 2004;230:629–636.
3. Pickhardt PJ, Choi R, Hwang I, et al. Computed tomographic virtual colonoscopy to screen for colorectal neoplasia in asymptomatic adults. *N Engl J Med*. 2003;349:2191–2200.
4. http://www.acrin.org/6664_protocol.html. Accessed January 5, 2007.
5. Yee J, Hung RK, Akerkar GA, et al. The usefulness of glucagon hydrochloride for colonic distention in CT Colonography. *AJR Am J Roentgenol*. 1999;173:1–4.
6. Yee J, Hung RK, Steinauer-Gebauer AM, et al. Colonic distention and prospective evaluation of colorectal polyp detection with and without glucagon during CT Colonography [Abstract]. *Radiology*. 1999;213(Suppl):256.
7. Morrin MM, Farrell RJ, Keogan MT, et al. CT colonography: colonic distention improved by dual positioning but not intravenous glucagon. *Eur Radiol*. 2002;12:525–530.
8. Taylor SA, Halligan S, Goh V, et al. Optimizing colonic distention for multi-detector row CT colonography: effect of hyoscine butylbromide and rectal balloon catheter. *Radiology*. 2003;229:99–108.
9. Rogalla P, Lembcke A, Ruckert JC, et al. Spasmolysis at CT colonography: butyl scopolamine versus glucagon. *Radiology*. 2005;236:184–188.
10. Fletcher JG, Johnson CD, Welch TJ, et al. Optimization of CT colonography technique: prospective trial in 180 patients. *Radiology*. 2000;216:704–711.
11. Chen SC, Lu DS, Hecht JR, et al. CT colonography: value of scanning in both the supine and prone positions. *AJR Am J Roentgenol*. 1999;172:595–599.
12. Yee J, Kumar NN, Hung RK, et al. Comparison of supine, prone and both supine and prone scans in CT colonography. *Radiology*. 2003;226:653–661.
13. Yasumoto T, Murakami T, Yamamoto H, et al. Assessment of two 3D MDCT colonography protocols for observation of colorectal polyps. *AJR Am J Roentgenol*. 2006;186:85–89.
14. American College of Radiology. ACR practice guideline for the performance of Computed Tomography (CT) colonography in adults. In *practice Guidelines and Technical Standards 2005*. Reston, VA: American College of Radiology; 2005;295–299.
15. Soto JA, Barish MA, Yee J. Reader training in CT Colonography: how much is enough? *Radiology*. 2005;237:26–27.
16. Cotton PB, Durkalski VL, Benoit PC, et al. Computed tomographic colonography (virtual colonoscopy)—a multicenter comparison with standard colonoscopy for detection of colorectal neoplasia. *JAMA*. 2004;291:1713–1719.
17. Ferruci J, Barish M, Choi R, et al. Working Group on Virtual Colonoscopy. Virtual colonoscopy [Letter]. *JAMA*. 2004; 292:431–432.
18. Halligan S, Taylor S, Burling D. Virtual colonoscopy [Letter]. *JAMA*. 2004;292:432.
19. Hara AK, Johnson CD, Reed JE, et al. Detection of colorectal polyps with CT colography: initial assessment of sensitivity and specificity. *Radiology*. 1997;205:59–65.
20. Dachman AH, Kuniyoshi JK, Boyle CM, et al. CT colonography with three-dimensional problem solving for detection of colonic polyps. *AJR Am J Roentgenol*. 1998;171:989–995.
21. Fenlon HM, Nunes DP, Schroy PC, et al. A comparison of virtual and conventional colonoscopy for the detection of colorectal Polyps. *N Engl J Med*. 1999;341:1496–1503.
22. Pescatore P, Glucker T, Delarive J, et al. Diagnostic accuracy and interobserver agreement of CT colonography (virtual colonoscopy). *Gut*. 2000;47:126–130.
23. Morrin MM, Farrell RJ, Kruskal JB, et al. Utility of intravenously administered contrast material at CT colonography. *Radiology*. 2000;217:765–771.
24. Spinzi G, Belloni G, Martegani A, et al. Computed tomographic colonography and conventional colonoscopy for colon diseases: a prospective, blinded study. *Am J Gastroenterol*. 2001;96:394–400.
25. Hara AK, Johnson CD, MacCarty RL, et al. CT colonography: single-versus multi-detector row imaging. *Radiology*. 2001; 219:461–465.
26. Yee J, Akerkar GA, Hung RK, et al. Colorectal neoplasia: performance characteristics of CT colonography for detection in 300 patients. *Radiology*. 2001;219:685–692.
27. Gluecker T, Dorta G, Keller W, et al. Performance of multidetector computed tomography colonography compared with conventional colonoscopy. *Gut*. 2002;51:207–211.
28. Macari M, Bini EJ, Xue X, et al. Prospective comparison of thin-section low-dose multislice CT colonography to conventional colonoscopy in detecting colorectal polyps and cancers. *Radiology*. 2002;224:383–392.
29. McFarland EG, Pilgram TK, Brink JA, et al. CT colonography: multiobserver diagnostic performance. *Radiology*. 2002; 225:380–390.
30. Iannaccone R, Laghi A, Catalano C, et al. Detection of colorectal lesions: lower-dose multi-detector row helical CT colonography compared with conventional colonoscopy. *Radiology*. 2003;229:775–781.
31. Pineau BC, Paskett ED, Chen GJ, et al. Virtual colonoscopy using oral contrast compared with colonoscopy for the detection of patients with colorectal polyps. *Gastroenterology*. 2003;125:304–310.
32. Johnson CD, Harmsen WS, Wilson LA, et al. Prospective blinded evaluation of computed tomographic colonography for screen detection of colorectal polyps. *Gastroenterology*. 2003;125:311–319.
33. Van Gelder RE, Nio CY, Florie J, et al. Computed tomographic colonography compared with colonoscopy in patients at increased risk for colorectal cancer. *Gastroenterology*. 2004;127:41–48.
34. Iannaccone R, Catalano C, Mangiapane F, et al. Colorectal polyps: detection with low-dose multi-detector row helical CT colonography versus two sequential colonoscopies. *Radiology*. 2005;237:927–937.
35. Rockey DC, Paulson E, Niedzwiecki D, et al. Analysis of air contrast barium enema, computed tomographic colonography, and colonoscopy: prospective comparison. *Lancet*. 2005;365:305–311.
36. http://www.htacolonography.co.uk/. Accessed January 22, 2007.
37. Sosna J, Morrin MM, Kruskal JB, et al. CT colonography of colorectal polyps: a meta-analysis. *AJR Am J Roentgenol*. 2003;181:1593–1598.
38. Halligan S, Altman DG, Taylor SA, et al. CT colonography in the detection of colorectal polyps and cancer: systematic review, meta-analysis, and proposed minimum data set for study level reporting. *Radiology*. 2005;237:893–904.
39. Mulhall BP, Veerappan GR, Jackson JL. Meta-analysis: computed tomographic colonography. *Ann Intern Med*. 2005;142:635–650.
40. Royster AP, Fenlon HM, Clarke PD, et al. CT colonoscopy of colorectal neoplasms: two dimensional and three dimensional virtual reality techniques with colonoscopic correlation. *AJR Am J Roentgenol*. 1997;169:1237–1242.

41. Laghi A, Iannaccone R, Carbone I, et al. Detection of colorectal lesions with virtual computed tomographic colonography. *Am J Surg*. 2002;183:124–131.
42. Munikrishnan V, Gillams AR, Lees WR, et al. Prospective study comparing Multislice CT colonography in the detection of colorectal cancer and polyps. *Dis Colon Rectum*. 2003; 46:1384–1390.
43. Chung DJ, Huh KC, Choi WJ, et al. CT colonography using 16-MDCT in the evaluation of colorectal cancer. *AJR Am J Roentgenol*. 2005;184:98–103.
44. Sun CH, Li ZP, Meng , et al. Assessment of spiral CT pneumocolon in preoperative colorectal carcinoma. *World J Gastroenterol*. 2005;11:3866–3870.
45. Mainenti PP, Cirillo LC, Camera L, et al. Accuracy of single phase contrast enhanced multidetector CT colonography in the preoperative staging of colorectal cancer. *Eur Radiol*. 2006;60:453–459.

CHAPTER 8

EXTRACOLONIC FINDINGS

Gregory M. Galdino and Judy Yee

Computed tomographic colonography (CTC) is a major advance in colon cancer diagnosis and screening, and will likely join mammography as a first-line imaging modality in the prevention of cancer. Cancer screening has the potential benefits of early discovery of curable lesions and early treatment of the diseases being screened for. However, it may also have the unexpected result of leading to the discovery of incidental findings. This may result in further diagnostic evaluation or intervention with the possibility for increased patient morbidity and health care costs.

ADVANTAGES

The ability of CTC to identify extracolonic lesions is often viewed as advantageous particularly by patients who are increasingly becoming advocates for their own health care (see Table 8.1). Unlike all of the other colon cancer screening tests, CTC (and magnetic resonance colonography) has the ability to directly detect lesions outside of the colon that may be completely incidental or may account for the patients presenting symptoms for CTC.

Abdominal aortic aneurysms (AAA) are often identified as completely incidental findings on CTC and those that are large enough (≥5 cm) will require surgical or endovascular repair (see Figure 8.1). In a study of 243 patients undergoing elective repair of abdominal aortic aneurysm, 62% of cases were discovered incidentally.[1] The impact on future risk to the patient is significant. The mortality rate associated with AAA is much lower for elective surgery (5%) than for surgery after aneurysm rupture (85% to 95%).[2] Aneurysms that are identified incidentally on CTC and are not large enough for elective surgery are followed with serial imaging to assess stability. The recommendation of the United States Preventive Services Task Force is to perform one-time screening for AAA by ultrasonography in men between the ages of 65 and 75 years who have ever smoked.[3] Screening programs for AAA using ultrasonography have demonstrated that almost 5% of men at age 65 have an asymptomatic AAA,[4] and that screening has effectively reduced the incidence of ruptured aneurysms by 49%.[5]

Extracolonic malignancies such as renal cell carcinoma (RCC) or ovarian carcinoma that are discovered incidentally on CTC may be found at an earlier stage when they are more likely to be curable (see Figure 8.2). Tsui et al. studied the prognostic significance of incidentally discovered RCC retrospectively in 633 consecutive patients. The authors found that patients with incidentally detected RCC had significantly lower grade and stage than tumors producing symptoms, leading to better patient survival and decreased recurrence. The 5-year survival rate was 85% for incidentally discovered RCC compared to 63% for symptomatic tumors.[6]

Although some extracolonic carcinomas that are discovered may not be operable or curable, they may be found when the patient is asymptomatic and still able to plan knowledgeably for their future before the onset of significant symptoms. Early discovery of disease with timely intervention could prevent the high cost of health care due to prolonged hospitalization

TABLE 8.1 Advantages and Disadvantages of the Discovery of Extracolonic Findings

Advantages	Disadvantages
Detection of diseases at an earlier stage when curable	Additional diagnostic workup or treatment of disease ultimately proved to be benign leading to increased:
Avoid expenses associated with prolonged hospitalization and procedures due to later presentation of diseases	*Patient morbidity/mortality* *Radiation exposure* *Health care expenses*
Patient has time to knowledgeably plan for the future	Undue patient inconvenience and anxiety associated with findings
Requires trained radiologist for CTC interpretation	

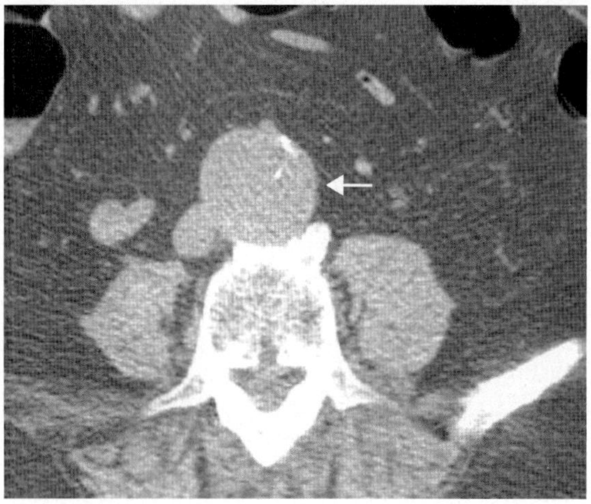

FIGURE 8.1 Abdominal aortic aneurysm is a finding of major clinical importance. This large infrarenal abdominal aortic aneurysm which approximates 5 cm in largest diameter will likely require surgical or endovascular repair.

or extensive diagnostic and surgical procedures from later presentation of disease. Similarly if metastases are identified at the time of diagnosis of colon carcinoma on CTC, this can help direct patient management without additional diagnostic evaluation or intervention.

DISADVANTAGES

The investigation and treatment of incidental lesions that are ultimately found to be benign may be associated with increased health care costs, increased patient morbidity or mortality, and unnecessary radiation exposure to patients. Additionally, patients often experience anxiety and inconvenience associated with the discovery and workup of incidental findings. These disadvantages must be offset by the gains that may arise from the early detection of clinically important or malignant incidental lesions on CTC. Cost-effectiveness as estimated by the number of life years saved due to incidental lesions is yet unknown. The negative effect on patient well-being has been difficult to assess for CTC.[7] However, in a parallel study by Lerman et al. there was significantly increased anxiety in women who underwent additional evaluation of suspicious mammographic findings for breast lesions that were later found to be benign.[8] With continuing increases in image utilization in health care, the discovery of clinically unimportant findings will rise, and outcome studies will need to further explore cost effectiveness and direct benefits to patients.

COMPUTED TOMOGRAPHY COLONOGRAPHY TECHNIQUE

The CTC technique uses thin sections ($\leq$5 mm, preferably $\leq$3 mm) and small reconstruction intervals ($\leq$2 mm) allowing for the detection of colorectal polyps as well as well as extracolonic lesions.[9] Axial images are primarily used to examine for extracolonic findings. Multiplanar reformats are often helpful for further evaluation of questionable lesions identified on the axial views. CTC allows visualization of the lung bases as well as structures in the abdomen and pelvis. A soft tissue window (width 400, level 40) should be used for evaluation of the solid organs and most structures in the abdomen and pelvis. Lung windows (width 1,500, level −700) should be

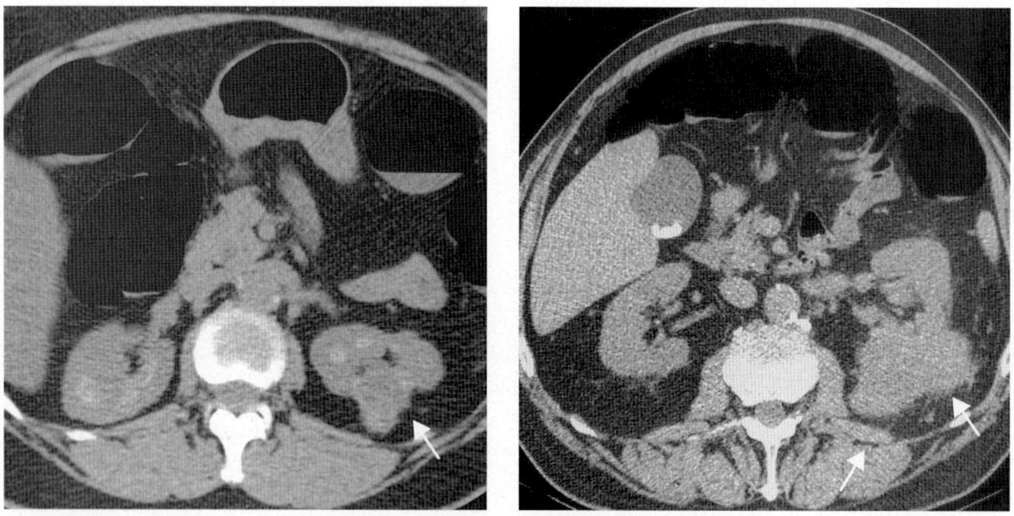

A B

FIGURE 8.2 Solid malignant mass in the left kidney discovered incidentally in a patient who had no symptoms of renal cell carcinoma **(A)**. A different patient with a larger left renal cell carcinoma found on CTC **(B)**. Gallstones are also noted in this patient.

used to examine the lung bases. Bone windows (width 2,000, level 300) should be used to examine the skeletal system.

Standard CTC technique requires supine and prone scanning which increases radiation dose. Many multidetector computed tomography (MDCT) colonography protocols employ low tube currents (≤100 mAs) to decrease radiation dose. However, even with these lower dose protocols, detection of extracolonic pathology is feasible. Iannaccone et al. evaluated ultra low-dose CTC and was able to successfully detect colorectal polyps and cancers using 10 mAs resulting in a 40% to 70% decrease in radiation dose compared with prior studies.[10] Although low mAs may not compromise the ability to detect colorectal polyps and cancers because of the inherently high contrast between the gas-filled lumen and the soft tissue density of the colonic wall, increased image noise will decrease the ability to evaluate for extracolonic lesions, particularly of the solid organs. More studies are needed to define the ability to detect extracolonic findings on CTC with decreasing radiation dose.

CLASSIFICATION OF EXTRACOLONIC FINDINGS

Extracolonic findings may be classified according to their clinical importance (see Table 8.2). Site-specific differences in the classification of lesions are possible. The size and/or location of a lesion may impact on its classification.

Findings of major importance are defined as those requiring prompt or immediate additional evaluation, including further diagnostic imaging, surgery, or medical attention. Examples of these include AAA defined as an infrarenal aorta measuring >3 cm,[11] solid masses in abdominal organs, indeterminate pulmonary nodules, adenopathy, suspected bony metastases (see Figures 8.3 to 8.5). Pneumothorax, pneumonia, and pneumoperitoneum are of major importance and should be immediately communicated to the referring physician. Evidence of acute infection or inflammation such as pancreatitis, diverticulitis, and appendicitis are major findings that require immediate medical attention.

Findings of moderate importance are defined as those that are likely benign but may require additional evaluation or treatment in the future, such as cholelithiasis and nephrolithiasis (unless obstructing then major), enlarged ovary or uterus, splenomegaly (unless massive then major), cardiomegaly, and pleural effusion (see Figures 8.6 to 8.10). Uncomplicated ventral, inguinal, or other hernias are of moderate importance unless large and may be classified as of major importance if surgical or medical treatment may be necessary.

Findings of minor importance are benign and do not warrant any additional evaluation. These findings include simple renal and hepatic cysts (<20 Hounsfield units), liver steatosis, calcified granulomata in the lungs and abdomen, lipomas, vertebral hemangioma, and vascular calcifications (see Figures 8.11 to 8.15). Uncomplicated small hiatal hernias are of minor importance.

TABLE 8.2 Classification of Extracolonic Findings[a]

Classification	Definition	Examples
Major	Requires prompt or immediate additional evaluation (imaging, surgery, medical attention)	Abdominal aortic aneurysm >3 cm Solid organ mass Pulmonary nodule Lymphadenopathy Suspected bony metastases Pneumothorax Pneumoperitoneum Pneumonia Acute infection
Moderate	Likely benign, may require additional evaluation in the future	Cholelithiasis Nephrolithiasis Enlarged ovary or uterus Splenomegaly Cardiomegaly Pleural effusion
Minor	Benign, no additional diagnostic evaluation	Simple hepatic and renal cysts Liver steatosis Calcified granulomata Lipoma Vertebral hemangioma Vascular calcification

[a]Alternative classification is to divide lesions as those that require additional workup or those that do not. C-RADS uses five categories to document extracolonic findings.[12]

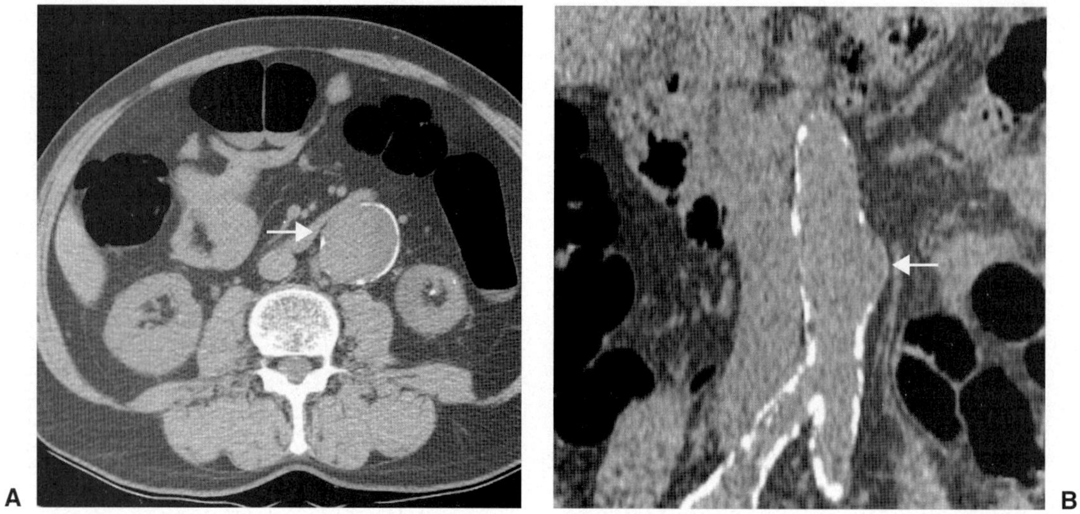

FIGURE 8.3 Abdominal aortic aneurysm seen on axial **(A)** and coronal reformatted **(B)** views which was first discovered on CTC. Left nephrolithiasis is also identified.

An alternative scheme for classifying extracolonic findings simply divides lesions into those that are clinically important and require further workup or intervention and clinically unimportant lesions that require no further workup and with no change in management of the patient.

A consensus proposal for a CTC reporting and data system (C-RADS) developed by the Working Group on Virtual Colonoscopy includes a classification system for extracolonic findings that consists of five categories.[12] This system is useful for documentation and reporting of extracolonic findings. Category E0 is used for a nondiagnostic study where there is significant degradation of image quality due to technical factors. Category E1 is for an essentially normal study and includes anatomic variants. Category E2 is used for minor findings that do not warrant further evaluation. Category E3 includes findings that are likely unimportant, but may require further workup according to site-specific practice. Category E4 represents findings of major importance that will require prompt evaluation.

INCIDENCE OF EXTRACOLONIC FINDINGS

In comparing the studies that have been performed evaluating extracolonic findings on CTC it is important to

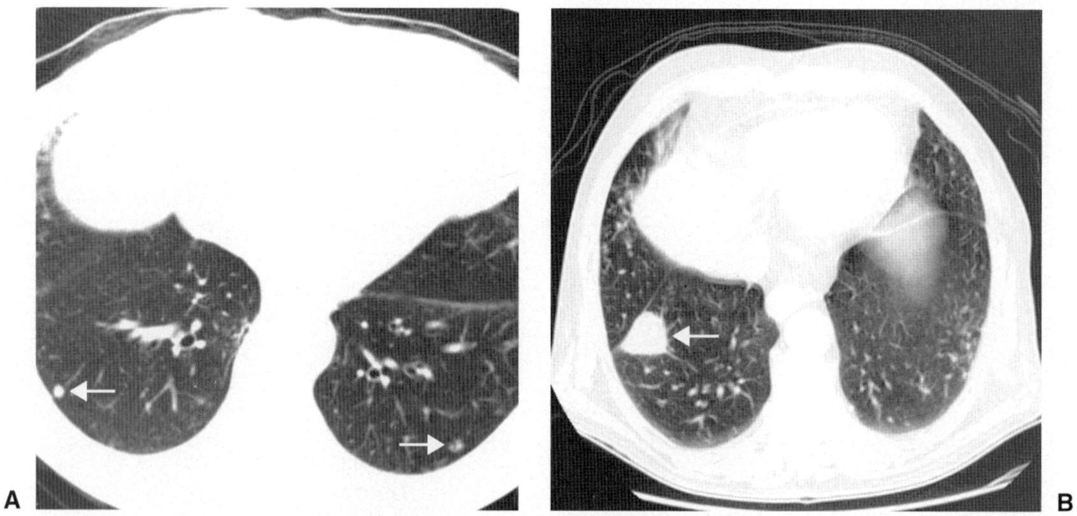

FIGURE 8.4 Small lung nodules first discovered at CTC, one in the right lower lobe and one in the left lower lobe **(A)**. These are indeterminate and follow-up CT scan is needed. A large right lower lung mass due to bronchogenic carcinoma found in a different patient with a long smoking history **(B)**.

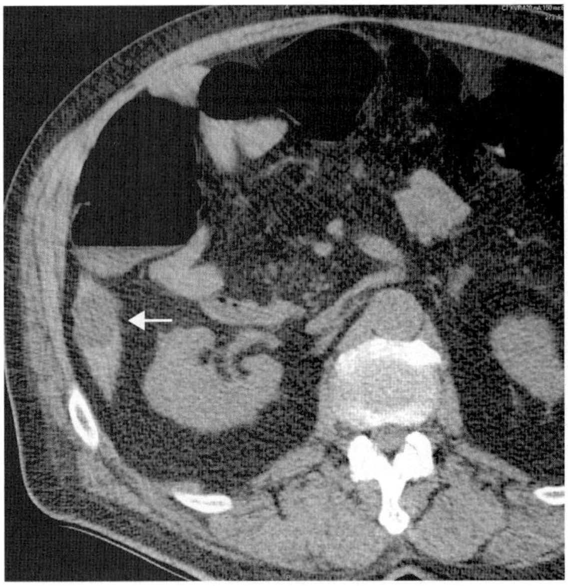

FIGURE 8.5 Hepatocellular carcinoma first identified on CTC appearing as a lobulated mass that deforms the contour of the liver.

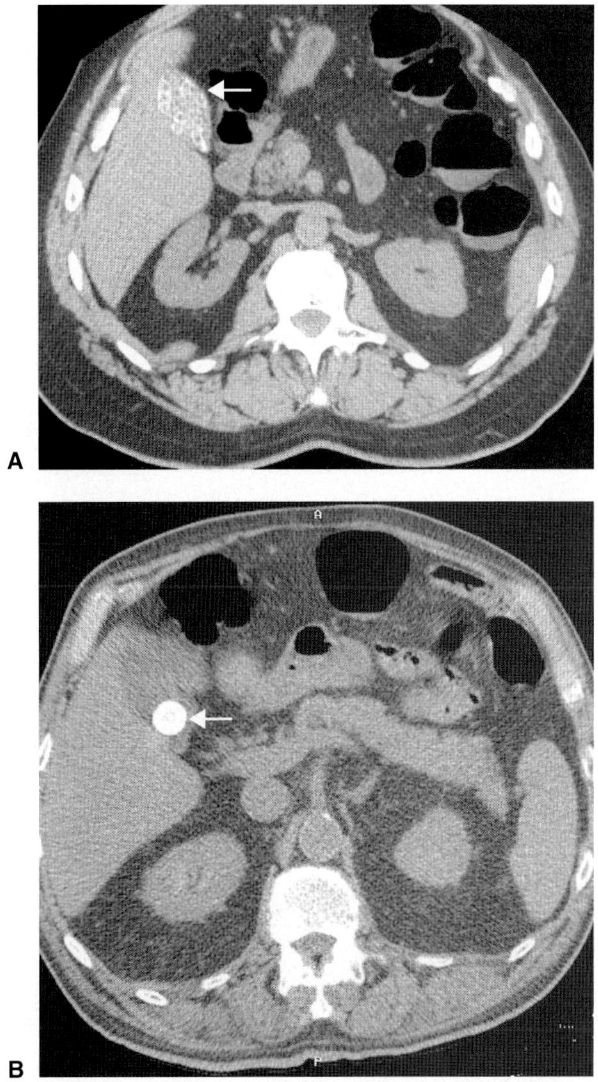

FIGURE 8.6 Axial image from a patient undergoing CTC revealed multiple small calcific gallstones filling the gallbladder **(A)**. Another patient with a solitary large calcific gallstone discovered incidentally **(B)**.

consider how the extracolonic findings were defined and classified, the patient population being evaluated, radiation dose used, and how cost assessment, if applicable, was determined (see Table 8.3). Extracolonic findings that were previously known are typically not included for data analysis. The use of intravenous contrast can also influence the ability to identify and characterize extracolonic findings.

Hara et al. published the first study on extracolonic findings and evaluated 264 patients (mean age 64 years) at high risk for colorectal carcinoma who underwent CTC.[13] Two radiologists independently interpreted the computed tomography (CT) scan studies for evidence of extracolonic findings. The CT scan protocol consisted of 5-mm collimation, 3-mm reconstruction, 70 mA, and pitch 1.3. Findings were classified as having high, moderate, or low clinical importance. Maximum interval for follow-up was 22 months. Extracolonic findings known to be preexisting were not included in the cost analysis because these did not require further diagnostic workup. A total of 151 lesions were found in 109 (41%) of the 264 patients. Thirty patients (30/264, 11%) had a highly important extracolonic finding. There were 34 (34/151, 23%) highly important lesions, 49 (49/151, 32%) moderately important lesions, and 68 (68/151, 45%) lesions of low importance. The most common highly important finding was an indeterminate renal mass, followed by a lung nodule, and then abdominal aortic aneurysm. Eighteen of the 30 patients (60%) (or 18/264, 7% of all patients) underwent further diagnostic evaluation of a highly important finding. The remaining 12 of 30 patients had findings of a previously diagnosed condition. Six patients (6/264, 2.3%) underwent surgery, including two patients with a malignant lesion. Three malignancies were missed by CTC and found subsequently on additional contrast CT imaging within a year of the study. The total cost for additional diagnostic workup of all findings was $7,324, or a mean of $28 per CTC performed. Twenty-three percent of this total was spent on further evaluation of malignant or surgical disease; 44% was for indeterminate lesions, and 33% was for benign findings.

Edwards et al. evaluated extracolonic findings in 100 patients at high risk for colorectal carcinoma who underwent CTC.[14] The mean age of patients included in this study was 65 years. CTC was performed using 5-mm collimation, 1- to 2-mm reconstructions, pitch 1.5, and 70 mAs. Axial images were reviewed for extracolonic findings by one radiologist. Fifteen patients (15%) had extracolonic abnormalities, including one probable renal cell cancer (patient expired of other causes before complete evaluation), one AAA, two liver lesions and three

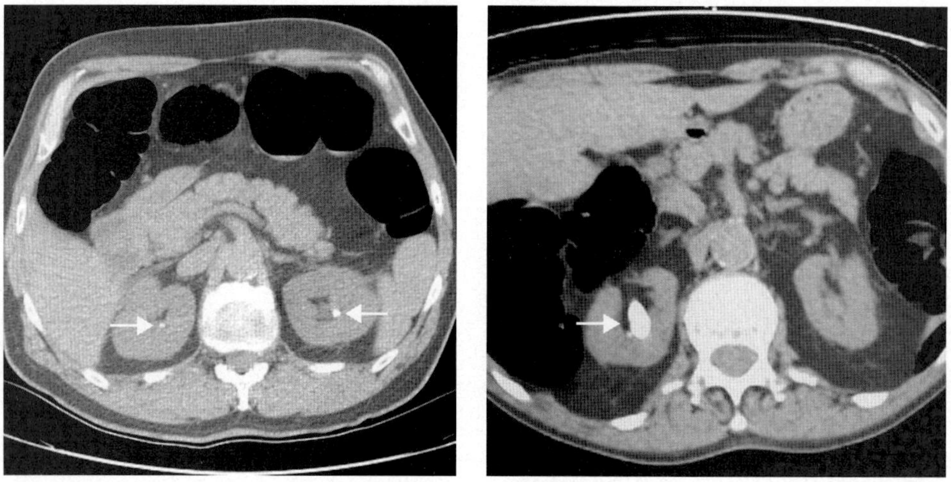

A B

FIGURE 8.7 Axial images from two patients with incidentally discovered renal calculi of various sizes. Small bilateral renal stones are identified in the first patient **(A)** and a much larger right-sided renal calculus is seen in the second patient **(B)**.

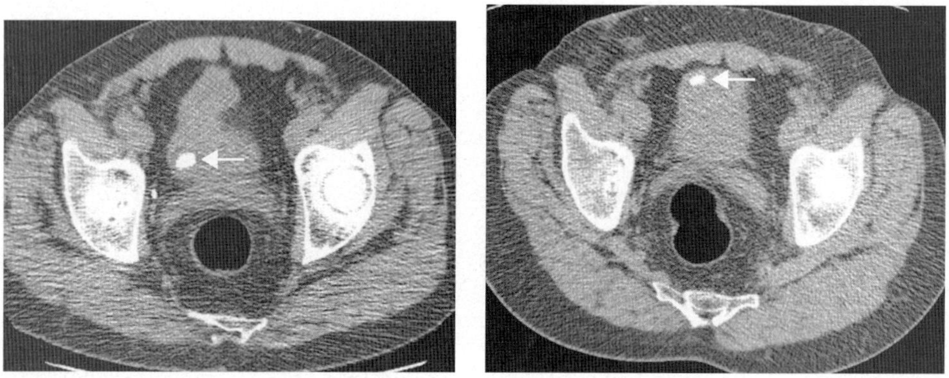

A B

FIGURE 8.8 Large mobile bladder stone found on CTC in an asymptomatic patient seen on supine **(A)** and prone **(B)** axial images.

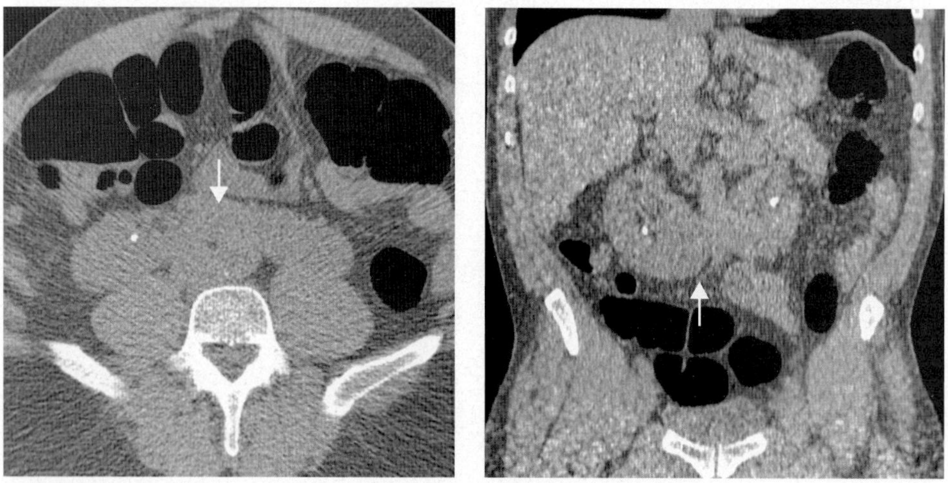

A B

FIGURE 8.9 Horseshoe kidney which was previously unknown found on CTC shown on axial **(A)** and coronal multiplanar reformat **(B)** views. Small right renal calculus is also present.

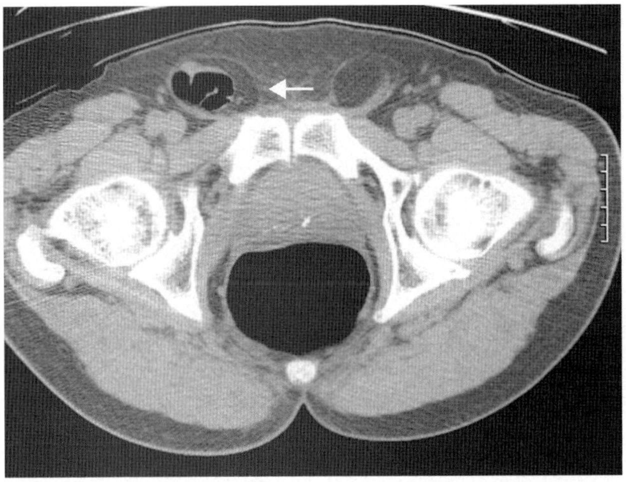

FIGURE 8.10 Right inguinal hernia containing small bowel seen on axial view. There were no findings to indicate bowel obstruction and the hernia was easily reduced on physical examination.

ovarian cysts. Four patients had findings that had been diagnosed previously. Eleven percent of patients underwent further medical review. Two patients (2%) with large ovarian cysts had surgical intervention, both of which were found to be benign. No cost analysis was performed. The prevalence of total extracolonic findings was significantly lower than that reported in most other studies.

Gluecker et al. studied extracolonic findings in 681 asymptomatic screening type patients with a median age of 64.[15] CTC protocol consisted of 5-mm collimation, 2.5- to 3-mm reconstructions, pitch 1.3, and 40 to 70 mA. One of three radiologists interpreted the CTC. Extracolonic findings were divided into high, medium, and low clinical importance. Mean time interval for follow-up was approximately 31 months. There were 858 extracolonic findings in 469/681 (69%) patients of which 10% (71/681) were of high clinical importance, 27% (183/681) of moderate clinical importance, and 50% (341/681) of low clinical importance. Ninety-four follow-up procedures were performed for highly important lesions and 1.3% of the patients required subsequent medical or surgical intervention. Extracolonic findings were detected most commonly in the kidneys, ovaries, lung, and aorta. The resulting cost of additional workup was $34.33 per CTC performed. The average cost in this study was slightly higher than in Hara et al., likely due to the higher overall prevalence found of extracolonic findings (69% vs. 41%).

Pickhardt et al. also studied an asymptomatic screening population and reported the extracolonic findings in 1,233 patients.[16] The mean age was 58 years. MDCT was performed using 1.25- to 2.5-mm collimation, 1-mm reconstruction interval, and 100 mAs. Lesions were classified as high, moderate, or low clinical significance. Of note, a much lower percentage (4.5%, 56/1,233) of patients were identified with a highly significant finding. The incidence of extracolonic malignancy was 0.4% (5/1,233), which included one case each of RCC, ovarian carcinoma and lymphoma as well as two cases of bronchogenic carcinoma. Approximately 8% of patients were documented to have nephrolithiasis and approximately 6% of patients had cholelithiasis. In contrast to Gluecker et al., results of this study showed that the frequency of extracolonic findings of major importance in a screening population was less than half that identified in other studies carried out in high-risk and symptomatic patients. This may also be related to the younger mean age of the patients included in this study (58 years vs. 62 to 66 years).

Ginnerup Pedersen et al. performed a study of extracolonic findings detected on MDCT colonography in 75 asymptomatic patients undergoing surveillance for prior adenomatous polyps or cancer.[17] The median age of patients was 61 years. Patients were scanned

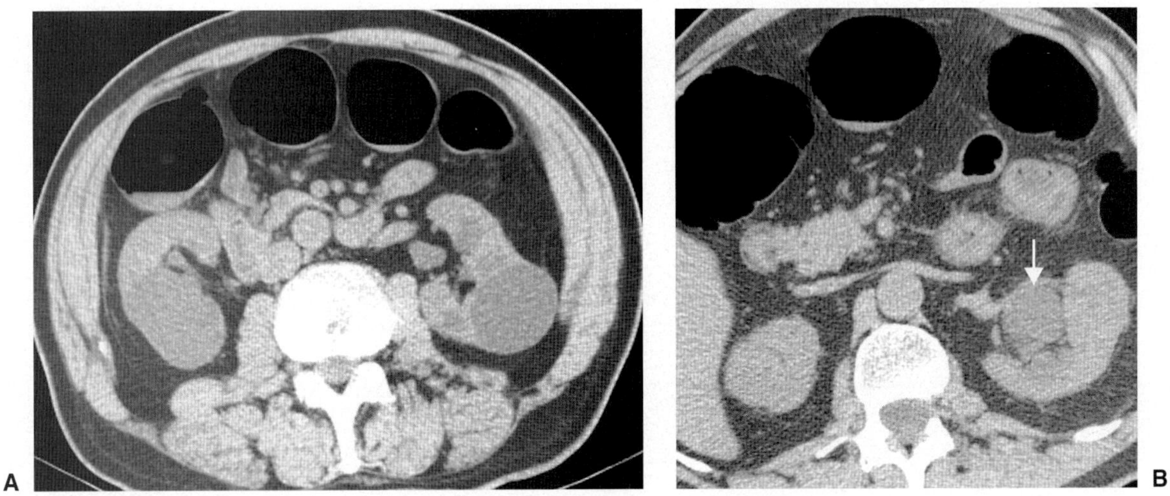

FIGURE 8.11 Renal cysts are often discovered on CTC. Axial image shows several large bilateral simple renal cysts which all measured less than 20 Hounsfield Units **(A)**. A parapelvic cyst is demonstrated in a different patient **(B)**.

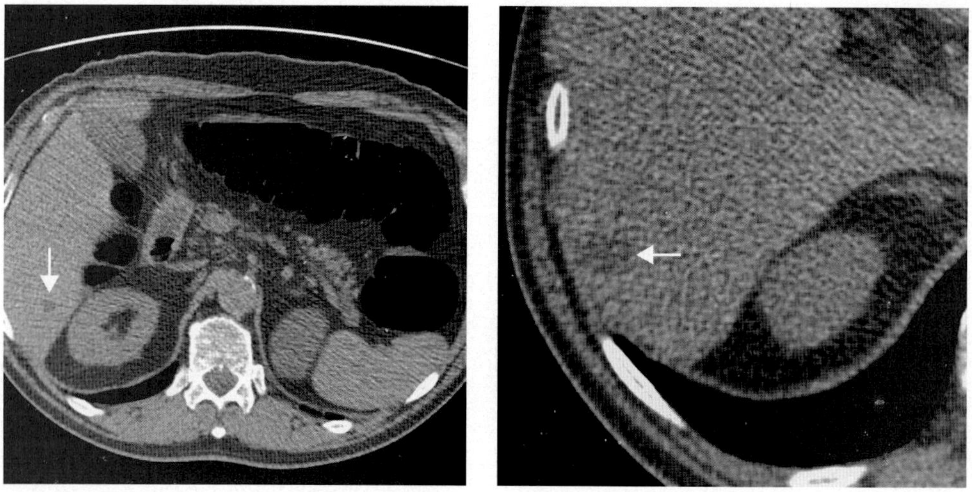

FIGURE 8.12 Axial images show benign liver cysts of varying sizes located in the right lobe found incidentally on CTC in two different patients **(A, B)**.

using 2.5-mm collimation, pitch 1.25, and 70 mAs. Two radiologists independently interpreted the CTC examinations. Follow-up was performed at 6 months following the CTC. Preexisting lesions were excluded. There were 68 extracolonic findings detected in 49/75 patients (65%). Additional workup was suggested in 12% (9/75) of patients. Two patients (3%) underwent surgery because of what was found during workup or as a complication of the workup.

Hellström et al. analyzed the frequency and clinical importance of extracolonic findings in 111 symptomatic patients referred for colonoscopy.[18] The median age of patients was 66 years. All patients underwent CTC using 5-mm slice thickness, pitch 1.25, and 125 mAs. The images were jointly reviewed by a radiologist and a trained resident. Findings were classified as major, moderate, or minor clinical importance. Cost analysis was not performed. The follow-up time was approximately 3 years and chart review for preexisting findings was performed. Most (85%) patients were found to have an extracolonic finding. A major finding was identified in 23% (26/111) of patients with the most common being lymphadenopathy, abdominal aortic aneurysm, and solid hepatic or renal mass. A finding of moderate importance was found in 52% (58/111) of patients and the most common were cholelithiasis, indeterminate renal mass, and benign appearing adrenal mass. Forty-one percent (46/111) had no extracolonic findings or findings or low importance. In 13% of patients (14/111), the finding was a previously unknown major finding. The authors attributed the high incidence of extracolonic findings overall to the high risk or symptomatic population studied. Eleven percent (12/111) of patients had documented malignant disease at the time of CTC and accounted for 43% of the major findings. Extracolonic findings of major importance occurred with much higher frequency in 9/12 (75%) patients with malignancy versus 17/99 (17%) patients with no malignancy.

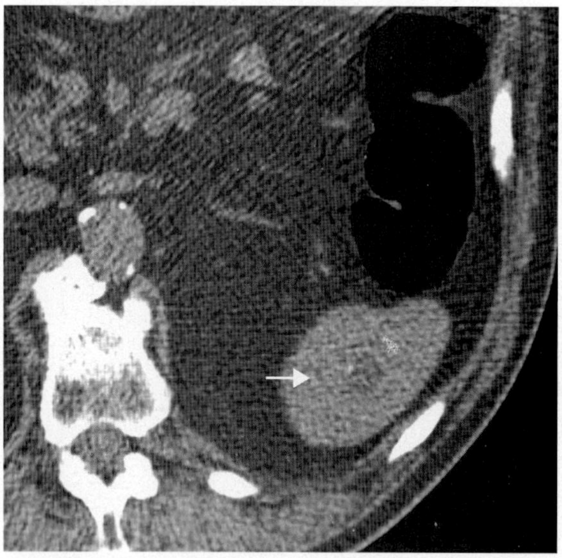

FIGURE 8.13 A splenic epithelioid cyst discovered incidentally at CTC is shown on axial view. Note the small associated calcification. This is a benign lesion that does not require any additional follow-up.

Rajapaksa et al. looked at extracolonic findings in 250 symptomatic patients undergoing CTC who were referred for colonoscopy.[19] The patient cohort was predominantly male with a mean age of 62.5 years. Low-dose CTC was performed using 1-mm collimation, 1.25-mm reconstructions, pitch 6 to 7, effective 50 mAs. There was a single-blinded reader who divided findings into having high, moderate, or low clinical significance. The median follow-up time was 509 days (almost 17 months). A total of 136 extracolonic findings were identified in 83/250 (33%) patients. Of the 136 findings, 17 (12.5%) were considered to be highly significant, 53 (39%) were of moderate significance, and 66 (49%) were of low significance.

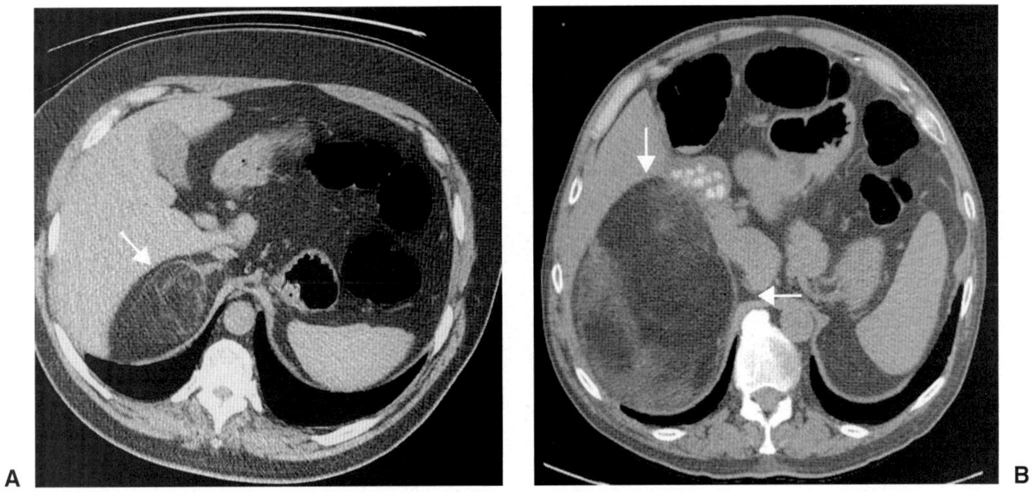

FIGURE 8.14 Axial image shows the fatty density of a right adrenal myelolipoma, a rare benign neoplasm, which was identified incidentally on CTC and classified as a finding of minor importance **(A)**. A much larger right adrenal myelolipoma found on CTC in a different patient presenting with right upper quadrant pain **(B)**. This is a finding of major importance in a symptomatic patient due to the large size of the benign lesion. Gallstones are incidentally noted.

Common findings of major importance included lung nodules, adenopathy, adrenal, and liver lesions as well as bony metastases. Eighty-two percent (14/17) of the highly significant lesions were new findings. Additional diagnostic testing was performed in 4.4% (11/250) of patients. This study also found that patients with extracolonic findings were significantly older than patients without any findings (64.2 vs. 61.6 years).

Chin et al. reported the prevalence and clinical significance of extracolonic findings identified within a community-based CTC screening program in Australia.[20] The mean age of the patients was 59 years. Low-dose CTC was performed using 3- or 5-mm collimation, 1- to 2-mm reconstruction intervals, pitch 1.5 or 2, 70 or 96 mA to evaluate 432 asymptomatic, average-risk individuals. Two of three experienced observers concurrently read the axial images. In contrast to other studies, the authors classified extracolonic findings as either clinically relevant or not clinically relevant. Clinically relevant lesions were those that required further medical or surgical attention, further blood tests or imaging. The interval of follow-up was 2 years after the completion of each study. A total of 146 extracolonic findings were identified in 118 patients (27%). Thirty-two (32/432, 7.4%) patients had clinically relevant extracolonic findings. It was found that 9/432 (2.1%) patients might benefit from the detection of the clinically relevant findings outside of the colon. The cost for making a definitive diagnosis of the clinically relevant extracolonic lesions was $24.37 per CTC or an additional 14% to the cost of each CTC.

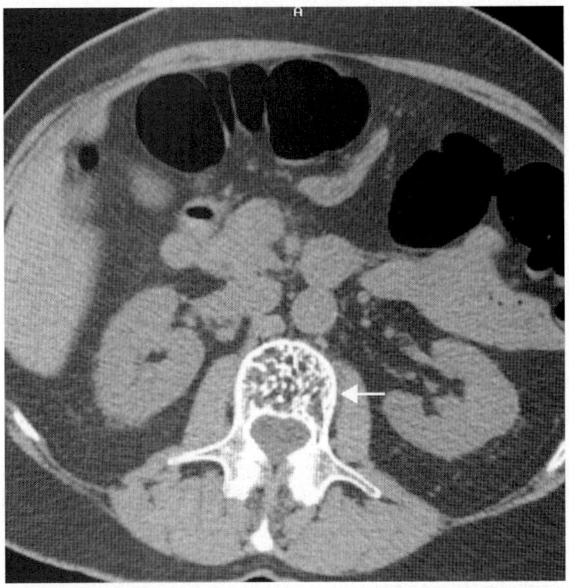

FIGURE 8.15 Vertebral hemangioma seen in the lumbar spine on axial view which is a finding of minor clinical importance and requires no further workup.

Yee et al. investigated the prevalence of clinically relevant incidentally discovered extracolonic findings on CTC and associated costs incurred by further diagnostic investigation in a male population.[21] The study evaluated 500 male patients with a mean age of 62.5 years. Thirty-nine percent of patients were asymptomatic and 61% of patients were symptomatic or high risk for colon cancer. CTC was performed using 3-mm collimation, 1.5-mm reconstruction interval, pitch 1.5 to 2.0, and 150 mA. Findings were divided into only two categories, those that were considered clinically significant, defined as any abnormality requiring further diagnostic evaluation or follow-up, and those that were clinically insignificant. The mean follow-up time was 3.6 years.[20] Sixty-three percent (315/500) of patients had a total of 596 extracolonic findings. Fourteen percent (45/315) of these patients

TABLE 8.3 Comparison of Studies Examining Extracolonic Findings at Computed Tomographic Colonography

Study	No. of Patients and Type	mA(s)	% Patients With ECF	% Patients With Major ECF	Cost/CTC Performed	% Patients With Health Care Altered	% Patients Requiring Surgery
Hara et al., 2000	264 HR/symptomatic	70	41%	11%	$28	7%	2.3%
Edwards et al., 2001	100 HR/symptomatic	70	15%	11%	–	7%	2%
Gluecker et al., 2003	681 asymptomatic	40–70	69%	10%	$34.33	10%	1.3%
Pickhardt et al., 2003	1,233 asymptomatic	100	–	4.5%	–	–	–
Ginnerup Pedersen et al., 2003	75 HR/symptomatic	70	65%	12%	–	12%	3%
Hellstrom et al., 2004	111 HR/symptomatic	125	85%	23%	–	13%	–
Rajapaksa et al., 2004	250 HR/symptomatic	50	33%	12.5%	–	4%	<1%
Chin et al., 2005	432 asymptomatic	79–96	27%	7.4%	$24.37	2%	–
Yee et al., 2005	500 mixed	150	63%	9%	$28	5%	1%

HR, high risk.

and 9% (45/500) of all patients had clinically significant findings, with no statistical difference noted between the symptomatic and asymptomatic groups. Fifty (50/596, 8.4%) of the extracolonic findings were thought to be clinically significant. Seventy-two percent (36/50) of these findings were new. Of the 36 new clinically significant findings in 35 patients, 34% (12/35) were found to have benign lesions on further evaluation, 37% (13/35) had the finding confirmed as clinically significant, and 28% (10/35) had no follow-up imaging after CTC. Therefore 71% (25/35) of these patients had their health care altered, and 52% of these patients confirmed to have the new finding as clinically significant (12/25) had further surveillance imaging or surgery. In all, 5% (25/500) of patients had their health care altered. Only 2% of (12/500) patients underwent further diagnostic evaluation for benign disease without any complications. Three percent (15/500) of patients had missed extracolonic findings. The total cost for additional diagnostic imaging was $14,058. Of this total, 35% ($4,872) was spent on further evaluation of clinically significant findings, and 65% ($9,186) was spent on clinically insignificant findings. This averaged $28.12 per CTC performed.

META-ANALYSIS

Xiong et al. identified primary studies of extracolonic findings on CTC using electronic databases, reference lists, and manual searches of pertinent journals and conference proceedings.[22] Seventeen studies involving 3,488 patients were identified, of which 13 were full papers and the remaining were abstracts. A total of 2,015 incidental lesions were identified in 3,488 patients (58%). Approximately 14% (188/1,362) of patients had additional workup and 0.8% required immediate treatment (17/2,237). Extracolonic cancers were found in 2.7% (81/3,005) of patients and 0.9% (24/2,549) of patients had early stage (N0 M0) malignancies. This study concluded that although only a small population was determined to be clinically important, the prevalence of serious extracolonic lesions was higher than in other screening programs.

INTRAVENOUS CONTRAST

Screening CTC does not typically include the administration of intravenous contrast. Although some incidental lesions may be identified on a noncontrast CT scan, the characterization of specific lesions such as differentiating cystic versus solid hepatic and renal masses often requires intravenous contrast. Vascular lesions that do not deform the contour of an organ may not be identified without the use of intravenous contrast. Hara et al. studied 163 patients who received intravenous contrast for CTC using a standard tube current of 180 mAs.[23] The precontrast scans had significantly more highly important findings compared with postcontrast scans (24% vs. 17%). Fewer follow-up studies were ordered using contrast-enhanced CTC. It was noted that the prevalence of highly important extracolonic findings was significantly larger than in series evaluating noncontrast CTC.

Spreng et al. compared the clinical importance of extracolonic lesions in 102 symptomatic patients using contrast-enhanced CTC ($n = 72$) versus nonenhanced CTC ($n = 30$).[24] CT scan parameters included 2-mm collimation, 2-mm reconstructions, pitch 1.375, and 200 mAs. Incidental lesions were classified into two groups—those requiring further workup or having an impact and those that did not. Eighty-nine percent (91/102) of patients had at least one extracolonic finding. There were 303 extracolonic findings identified of which 215 (71%) were found on contrast-enhanced CTC and 88 (29%) were found on nonenhanced CTC. Additional workup or change in treatment was suggested for 25% (26/102) of patients. Of these, 22 patients (22/26) underwent contrast-enhanced

CTC. A higher percentage of extracolonic findings leading to further workup or a change in therapy was found using contrast-enhanced CTC compared to nonenhanced CTC (31% vs. 13%, respectively).

COST CONSIDERATIONS

There has been limited evaluation of the cost of follow-up care for incidental extracolonic findings detected on CTC. Four of the studies reviewed include cost analyses and have found that there is a cost of an additional $24 to $34 per CTC study.[13,15,20,21] It was concluded from these studies that the cost of workup of significant extracolonic lesions is low given the potential benefit. Typically these calculations are based on the relevant Medicare reimbursement costs for follow-up studies. However, although the costs evaluated include additional diagnostic workup, the cost of interventional procedures such as surgery, endoscopy, and hospital stays are not included leading to falsely low total costs. Xiong et al. assessed the clinical resources and costs associated with the evaluation and treatment of extracolonic lesions in the United Kingdom.[25] They evaluated 225 symptomatic patients and found that 116 (52%) had one or more extracolonic findings. Twenty-four patients (24/225, 11%) had further workup or treatment of the previously unknown extracolonic lesion. It was found that most costs incurred were for surgical procedures. The resources that were used due to the workup of extracolonic lesions almost doubled the cost of diagnostic CTC. Other than financial cost, there is the inconvenience and distress experienced by the patient who is found to have an unexpected extracolonic lesion and requires workup. There is also the risk of a complication from the workup itself, which incurs more cost as well as patient anxiety.

SUMMARY

CTC allows assessment of the abdomen and pelvis for extracolonic lesions, adding the potential benefit of early disease detection and early intervention. Potential negative consequences include additional costs for further diagnostic workup of benign disease as well as detrimental effects on the psychological well-being of patients and the possibility of increased patient morbidity.

The incidence of extracolonic findings on CTC is high, occurring in 15% to 85% (average 50%) of patients. The incidence of findings of major clinical importance varies depending on the particular patient cohort studied. Patients at high risk for colon cancer or who are symptomatic have been found to have 11% to 23% incidence of highly important findings whereas asymptomatic screening patients have a much lower incidence (4.5% to 7.4%). Although most patients suspected of having a finding of major importance will end up having a benign lesion (up to 80%), approximately 1% to 3% of patients will have surgery for the previously unsuspected extracolonic finding.

A limited number of studies have been performed that indicate the additional cost per study is not significant; however, additional larger controlled studies will need to be performed that include procedural costs incurred. Low-dose radiation protocol increases image noise and may limit the ability to detect extracolonic findings on CTC. The minimum acceptable radiation dose that maintains the diagnostic quality of images for the detection of extracolonic findings must be established.

REFERENCES

1. Chervu A, Clagett GP, Valentine RJ, et al. Role of physical examination in the detection of abdominal aortic aneurysms. *Surgery*. 1995;117:454–457.
2. Nevitt MP, Ballard DJ, Hallett JW. Prognosis of abdominal aortic aneurysms: a population-based study. *N Engl J Med*. 1989;321:1009–1014.
3. United States Preventive Services Task Force. Screening for abdominal aortic aneurysm: recommendation statement. *Ann Intern Med*. 2005;142:198–202.
4. Kyriakides C, Byrne J, Green S, et al. Screening of abdominal aortic aneurysm: a pragmatic approach. *Ann R Coll Surg Engl*. 2000;82:59–63.
5. Wilmink T, Quick C, Hubbard C, et al. The influence of screening on the incidence of ruptured abdominal aortic aneurysms. *J Vasc Surg*. 1999;30:203–208.
6. Tsui K, Shvarts O, Smith R, et al. Renal cell carcinoma: prognostic significance of incidentally detected tumors. *J Urol*. 2000;163:426–430.
7. Westbrook JI, Braithwaite J, McIntosh JH. The outcomes for patients with incidental lesions: serendipitous or iatrogenic? *Am J Roentgenol*. 1998;171:1193–1196.
8. Lerman C, Trock B, Rimer BK, et al. Psychological side effects of breast cancer screening. *Health Psychol*. 1991;10: 259–267.
9. Sosna J, Kruskal JB, Bar-Ziv J, et al. Extracolonic findings at CT colonography. *Abdom Imaging*. 2005;30:709–713.
10. Iannaccone R, Laghi A, Catalano C, et al. Feasibility of ultra-low-dose multislice CT colonography for the detection of colorectal lesions: preliminary experience. *Eur Radiol*. 2003; 13:1297–1302.
11. Johnston KW, Rutherford RB, Tilson MD, et al. Suggested standards for reporting on arterial aneurysms. Subcommittee on Reporting Standards for Arterial Aneurysms, Ad Hoc Committee on Reporting Standards, Society for Vascular Surgery and North American Chapter, International Society for Cardiovascular Surgery. *J Vasc Surg*. 1991;13:452–458.
12. Zalis M, Barish M, Choi R, et al. CT colonography reporting and data system (C-RADS): a consensus statement. *Radiology*. 2005;236:3–9.
13. Hara AK, Johnson CD, MacCarty RL, et al. Incidental extracolonic findings at CT colonography. *Radiology*. 2000;215: 353–357.
14. Edwards JT, Wood CJ, Mendelson RM, et al. Extracolonic findings at virtual colonoscopy: implications for screening programs. *Am J Gastroenterol*. 2001;96:3009–3012.
15. Gluecker TM, Johnson CD, Wilson LA, et al. Extracolonic findings at CT Colonography: evaluation of prevalence ad cost in a screening population. *Gastroenterology*. 2003; 124:911–916.
16. Pickhardt PJ, Choi R, Hwang I, et al. Computed tomographic virtual colonoscopy to screen for colorectal neoplasia in asymptomatic adults. *N Engl J Med*. 2003;349:2191–2200.
17. Ginnerup Pedersen B, Rosenkilde M, Christiansen TE, et al. Extracolonic findings at computed tomography colonography are a challenge. *Gut*. 2003;52:1744–1747.

18. Hellstrom M, Svensson MH, Lasson A. Extracolonic and incidental findings on CT colonography (virtual colonoscopy). *AJR Am J Roentgenol*. 2004;182:631–638.
19. Rajapaksa RC, Macari M, Bini E. Prevalence and impact of extracolonic findings in patients undergoing CT colonography. *J Clin Gastroenterol*. 2004;38:767–771.
20. Chin M, Mendelson R, Edwards J, et al. Computed tomographic colonography: prevalence, nature, and clinical significance of extracolonic findings in a community screening program. *Am J Gastroenterol*. 2005;100:2771–2776.
21. Yee J, Kumar N, Godara S, et al. Extracolonic abnormalities discovered incidentally at CT Colonography in a male population. *Radiology*. 2005;236:519–526.
22. Xiong T, Richardson M, Woodroffe R, et al. Incidental lesions found on CT colonography: their nature and frequency. *Br J Radiol*. 2005;78:22–29.
23. Hara AK. Extracolonic findings at CT Colonography. *Semin Ultrasound CT MRI*. 2005;26:24–27.
24. Spreng A, Netzer P, Mattich J, et al. Importance of extracolonic findings at IV contrast medium-enhanced CT colonography versus those at non-enhanced CT colonography. *Eur Radiol*. 2005;15:2088–2095.
25. Xiong T, McEvoy K, Morton DG, et al. Resources and costs associated with incidental extracolonic findings from CT colonography: a study in a symptomatic population. *Br J Radiol*. 2006;79:948–961.

CHAPTER 9 REPORTING

Judy Yee

Effective communication of the results of imaging studies is an important part of radiology. Results of imaging studies should be communicated in a timely manner so that appropriate modifications in patient management may be made when necessary. The American College of Radiology (ACR) has published practice guidelines for the communication of diagnostic imaging findings.[1] Suggested components of the report include demographic information such as location of where the study was performed, patient identification, referring physician versus self-referred, and name and date of the study. Relevant clinical information should be included as available. The body of the report should include a description of the procedure and materials, complications encountered, and findings of the study. Potential limitations and clinical issues should be addressed in the report. Comparison with prior relevant studies should be made and also reported.

The documentation of the findings made on computed tomographic colonography (CTC) in a report must be accurate and complete. CTC reports share an overall similar format to other radiology reports. The ACR Practice Guideline for the performance of CTC in adults states that reporting should be in accordance with the ACR Practice Guideline for Communication of Diagnostic Imaging Findings.[1,2] There are also certain elements of the report specific to CTC that are discussed in the subsequent text (see Figures 9.1 to 9.6). Template reports that contain the needed elements of CTC documentation are useful and an efficient method of reporting findings.

IDENTIFIERS

Basic demographic information included in the radiology report is patient name and another identifier. Patient gender, birth date, or age may be stated. The name and address of the site where the CTC is performed are included. The name and date of the examination are stated. The ACR Practice Guideline for Communication of Diagnostic Imaging Findings also encourages inclusion of the date of dictation and the date and time of transcription of the report.[1]

METHOD OF REFERRAL

The name of the physician or health care provider who refers the patient for CTC is recorded. The inclusion of contact information such as the phone number of the physician or health care provider makes it easier and more efficient for the communication of significant findings. If the patient is self-referred then that should be stated. Some states do not allow patient self-referral for CTC. The ACR Practice Guideline for Communication of Diagnostic Imaging Findings states that diagnostic imagers should recognize that performing imaging studies on self-referred patients establishes a doctor–patient relation that includes responsibility for communicating the study results directly to the patient and arranging for appropriate follow-up.[1]

PATIENT HISTORY

Clinicians should be encouraged to provide relevant clinical information. If the patient is symptomatic then the specific symptoms for which the CTC is being obtained should be included such as abdominal pain, diarrhea, constipation, weight loss, possible bowel obstruction, hematochezia, bright red blood per rectum, positive fecal occult blood test, and/or iron deficiency anemia. Pertinent patient history such as personal or family history of prior polyps or colorectal carcinoma should be included. Patients with one first-degree relative (mother, father, brother, sister, or child) with colorectal neoplasia before the age of 60 or who have multiple relatives who develop colorectal neoplasia at any age are considered to be at increased risk.[2] Individuals who are asymptomatic but with a history of prior benign or malignant colorectal neoplasm undergo CTC as a surveillance examination and this should be noted. If the patient undergoing CTC for screening is asymptomatic and at average risk for colorectal carcinoma, then this is stated.

Patients undergoing CTC because of a failed or incomplete colonoscopy should have this documented with the portion of the colon successfully evaluated by

CT Colonography Report

University Hospital

123 Main St.
Anytown, USA 00000

Patient Name:	Jane Doe		
Patient Age:	65	Referring MD:	JudyYee,MD
Patient Gender:	F	Scan Date:	12/10/2007
Date of Birth:	04/06/1942	Patient ID:	LP7

Procedure: Screening CT Colonography

Following bowel cleansing (magnesium citrate and bisacodyl) and air distention of the colon, CT colonography was performed in supine and prone positions using a detector configuration of 16 X 0.625, pitch 1.375, 100 mA, and 120 kVP. There were no complications and the patient tolerated the procedure well. The examination resulted in positive findings which are described below.

Findings:

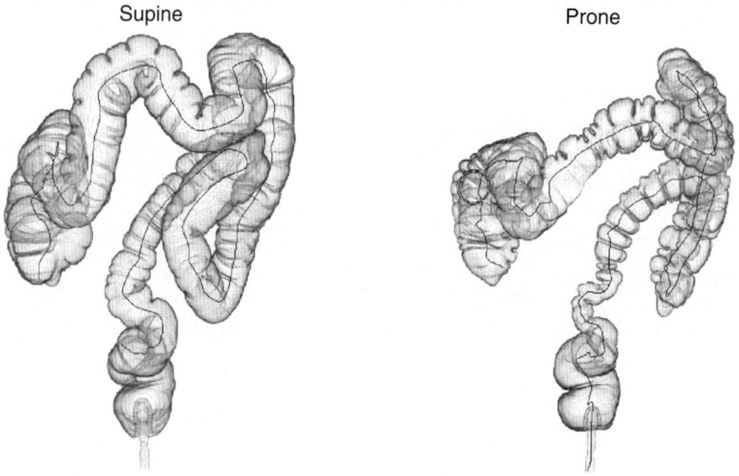

The diagram above shows supine and prone overviews of the colon in this patient, with a circle indicating the location of the finding in the ascending colon on the prone scan. There was adequate colonic distention and cleansing except for residual fluid in the ascending colon near the hepatic flexure in the prone position.

FIGURE 9.1 Tera Recon Report.

Finding

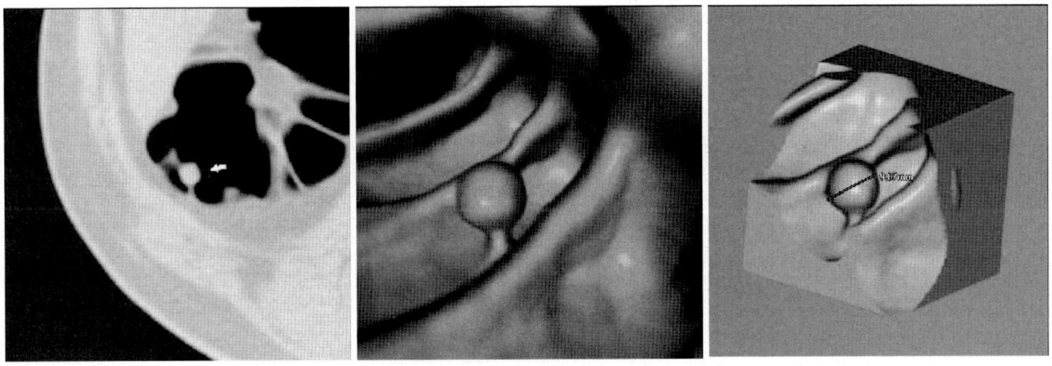

2D Axial (Prone) | 3D Endolumen (Prone) | 3D VR (Prone)

Ascending Colon

Type: Pedunculated Polyp

Size: 10 mm

Distance From Rectum: 1468 mm

Image Number: 138(Prone)

Comments: The polyp was not seen on the corresponding supine axial images secondary to residual fluid.

Recommendations

A 10 mm pedunculated polyp was seen located in the ascending colon near the hepatic flexure. The patient should be referred for optical colonoscopy and polypectomy.

Note

Segments with sub-optimal cleansing and/or distention limits the ability to detect lesions. CT Colonography has limited sensitivity for detecting diminutive (less than or equal to 5 mm) polyps and flat lesions.

FIGURE 9.1 *(Continued)*

PREVENTING COLON CANCER

Reduced animal fat in the diet, reduced alcohol intake, elimination of tobacco and possibly an increase in dietary bulk (fiber) are suggestions for prevention resulting from research into colon cancer.

In general, promotion of good health is always recommended, to include appropriate exercise and bodily fitness, a positive attitude, stress reduction and prudent food selection. Diet recommendations which may help in reducing the risk for colon cancer include:

- Avoidance of meat and animal fat
- Inclusion of fish (e.g. salmon) and occasional poultry
- Avoidance of refined grains (white rice, white bread)
- Promotion of whole grains (brown rice, whole wheat, oats) as the mainstay of the menu.
- Avoidance of refined (white) sugar.
- Promotion of vegetables that are red, orange and yellow are encouraged. (The color represents chemicals that may be beneficial.)
- Promotion of vegetables that are green and leafy, including seaweeds.
- Avoidance of fats and oils of all kinds (except olive oil and fish oil in moderation).

While many of these recommendations are solid and well-grounded in general medical research, their specific effect in preventing or curing cancer is not proven.

Sources of further information

Cancer Research Foundation of America (1-877-35-COLON)

American Cancer Society

American Digestive Health Foundation

Radiologist:

Judy Yee MD

FIGURE 9.1 *(Continued)*

University Hospital

123 Main St. Anytown, USA 00000

Patient Information

Patient ID: LP10
Patient Name: John Doe
Date of Birth: 3 Mar 1940
Gender: M

Referring Physician: Amy Smith
ExamType: VIRTUAL COLONOSCOPY
Scan Date: 5 May 2007
Report Date: 5 May 2007

INDICATIONS FOR PROCEDURE: Routine Screening Exam

TECHNIQUES: CT Colonography was performed after cathartic colonic preparation using 10 mg of magnesium citrate and bisacodyl tablets and suppository. No oral or IV contrast were used. A rectal tube was placed to insufflate the colon with carbon dioxide in order to achieve adequate distention. The patient was scanned in supine and prone positions using multi-detector helical CT scanner with 2.5 mm thick slices and 1.25 mm reconstructed slices. Images were examined using a 3D workstation.

FINDINGS: There was adequate distention and cleansing in all segments of the colon in both supine and prone positions. A 9 mm sessile polypoid lesion was detected in the distal descending colon. See images on next page.

IMPRESSIONS: 9 mm sessile polyp noted in the distal descending colon. No other colonic lesions identified.

RECOMMENDATIONS: Recommend colonoscopy for polypectomy.

Sincerely,

Judy Yee, MD
Interpreting Radiologist

Comments:

VITAL
The image of understanding

FIGURE 9.2 Vitrea Report.

Arrows demonstrate the lesion seen on both supine and prone axial images. The corresponding 3-D cube views of the polyp are shown below.

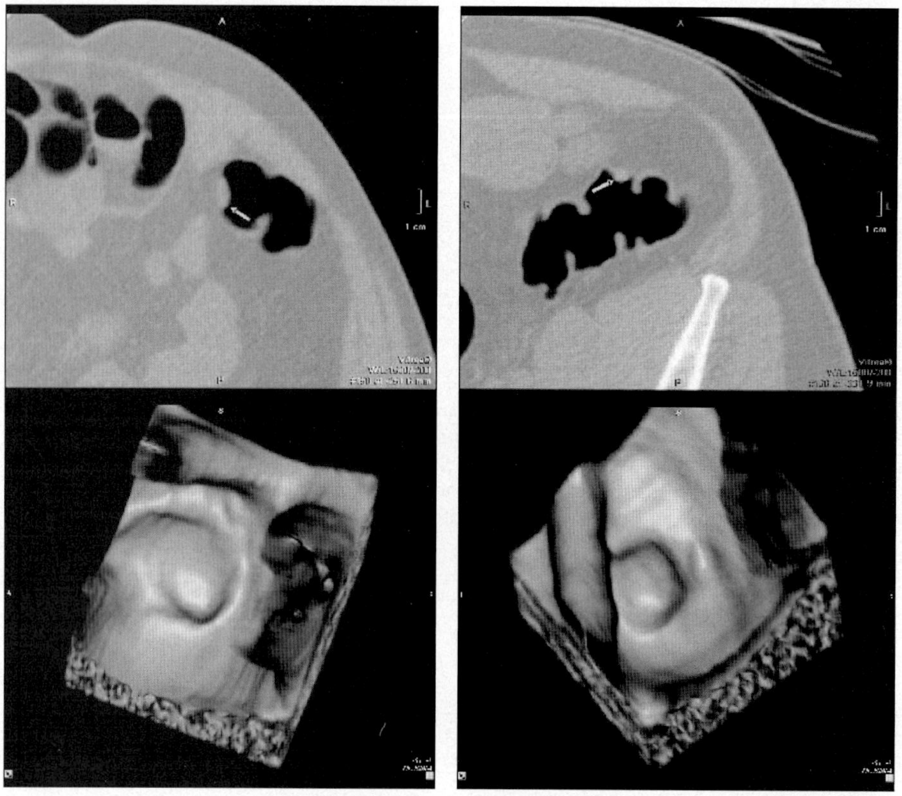

VITAL
The image of understanding

FIGURE 9.2 (*Continued*)

Virtual Colonoscopy Report

University Hospital

Patient Information

Patient Name:	Steven Doe	**Patient ID:**	LP8
Gender:	M	**D.O.B. (Age):**	1948/09/23
Accession:	000000-0000	**Study date:**	2007/05/05 10:57
Reading Date:	2007/05/05		

Procedure

Scan Orientation:	FFS (supine); FFP (prone)	**Protocol:**	VIRTUAL COLONOSCOPY
Technique:	CT KVP:120 mA:50 ms:800	**Spacing / Thickness:**	1.5 mm / 3.00mm

Reported Findings

Report 1 (merged; supine slice 211, prone slice 207)

Status:	confirmed	**Confidence:**	1 (high)
Location:	rectum	**Measurements:**	12.9 mm (prone)
Comment:	Large Pedunculated Polyp		

Technique

CT Colonography was performed following colonic cleansing with magnesium citrate and bisacodyl. The colon was electronically insufflated using carbon dioxide. There were no complications.

Findings

The colon was adequately cleansed and distended throughout. A large pedunculated polyp (12.9 mm) was identified in the rectum.

Recommendations

Colonoscopy is recommended for removal of the large pedunculated polyp.

Sincerely,

Judy Yee MD

FIGURE 9.3 Voxar Report.

Reported Findings Captures

Report 1a. Supine Axial Image with corresponding 3D cube view

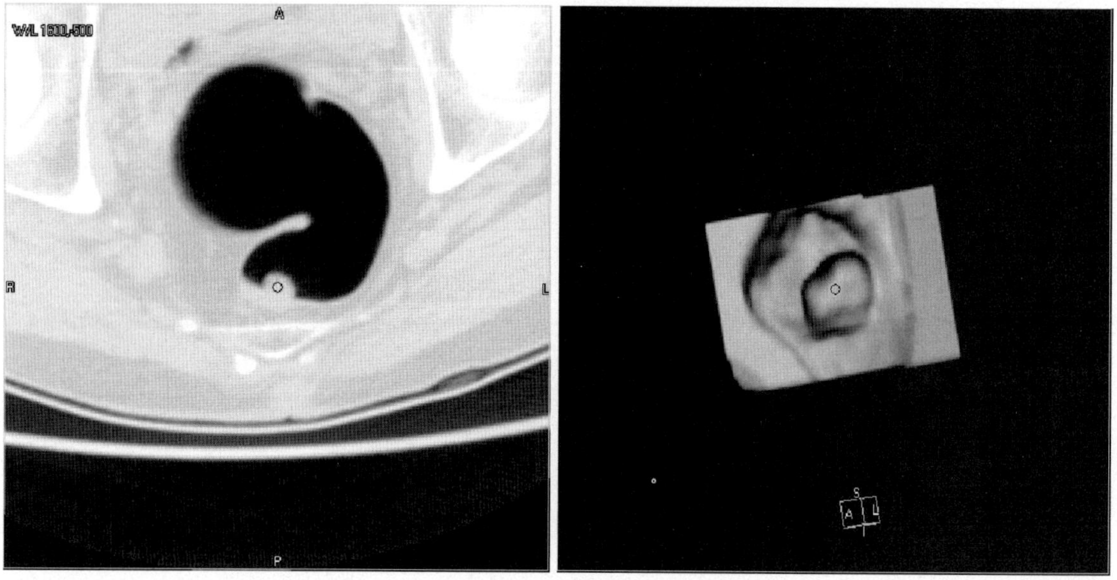

Report 1b. Prone Axial Image with corresponding 3D cube view

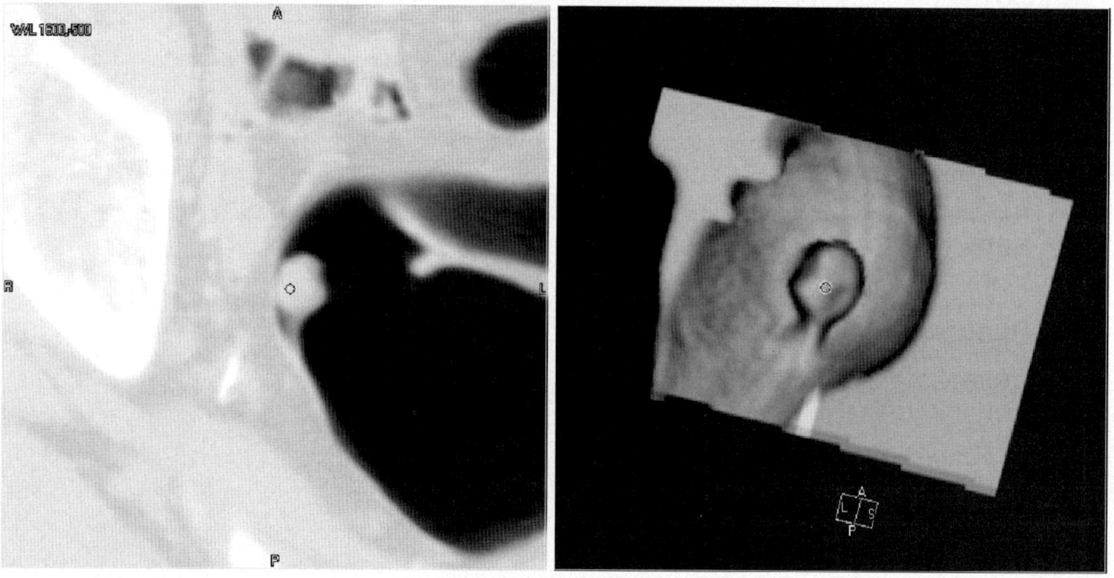

FIGURE 9.3 (*Continued*)

Diagnostic Imaging Report

Pre Exam

Family Medical history	Patient history
No family history	Negative-routine screening

Exam Preperation

CT Colonography was preformed after carthartic colon prep using 10 mg of magnesium citrate and bisacodyl tablets and suppository. No oral or IV contrast was used.A rectal tube was placed for electronic CO_2 insufflation necessary for colonic distention. The patient was scanned in the supine and prone positions using a multi-detector helical CT scanner with 2.5 mm thick slices and 1.25 mm reconstructed slices. Images were examined using a 3D workstation.

Polyp1

Location	Shape	Lesion size	Distance from Rectum
Rectum	Sessile	6.0 mm	17.0 cm

3D	Axial	Navg	Lumen

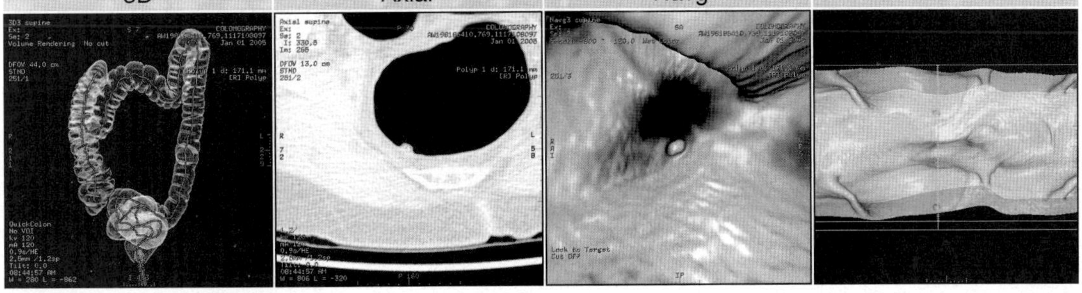

General Images

3D	3D

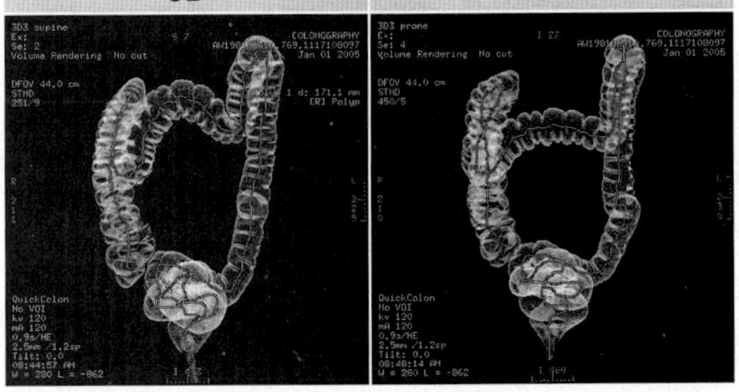

Post Exam

Conclusion

There were 1 finding when the patient was examined. There was a polyp found in the Rectal segment, a distance of 17 cm from the rectum. The polyp is 6 mm in size and can be described as sessile. Decision to undergo optical colonoscopy with polypectomy at this time should be based upon physician and patient preference and/or the presence of any other co-exisiting medical condition

FIGURE 9.4 GE Report.

PATIENT INFORMATION:

Patient:	John Doe
Patient ID:	LP9
Study Date:	1/16/2004
Referring Physician:	Yee

INTRODUCTION:

A 54 year old male presents with:

Family history of polyps
Family history of cancer

COLON FINDINGS:

(Supine) 11.8 × 0.0 mm. pedunculated (stalk perceivable) polyp identified in the cecum at 151.6 cm from anal verge.

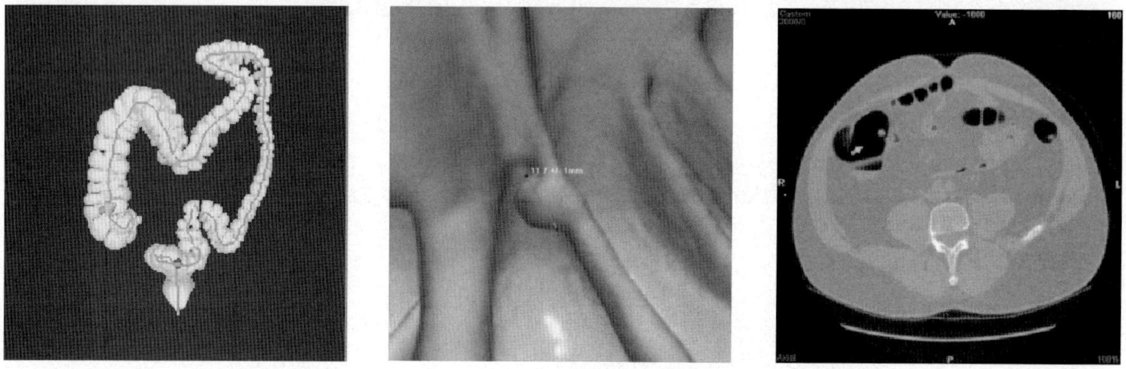

FIGURE 9.5 Viatronix Report.

(Prone) 5.0 x 0.0 mm. sessile polyp identified in the rectum at 6.3 cm from anal verge.

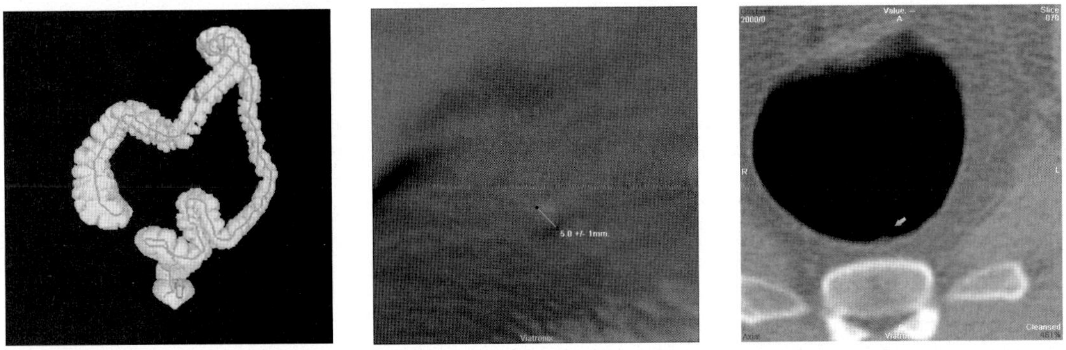

IMPRESSION

- CT colonography revealed the presence of one large polyp in the cecum and one small polyp in the rectum.

RECOMMENDATIONS:

- (Other) The patient should be scheduled for optical colonscopy and polypectomy for removal of the large lesion in the cecum.

Judy Yee, MD

FIGURE 9.5 *(Continued)*

Virtual Colonoscopy Report

Patient Info: John Smith, 70 year old male
SS# Last Four: 1234
Date of Study: 07/08/2007
Location of Study:
Radiologist: Judy Yee, M.D.
Procedure: CT Colonography was performed after cathartic colonic preparation using 10 mg of magnesium citrate and bisacodyl tablets and suppository . No oral or IV contrast were used. A rectal tube was placed for electronic CO2 insufflation necessary for colonic distention. The patient was scanned in supine and prone positions using multi-detector helical CT scanner with 2.5 mm thick slices and 1.25 mm reconstructed slices. Images were examined using a 3D workstation.

Findings:

Distention per colonic segment: 1-5 Scale (1=Excellent, 3=Adequate, 5=Poor/Collapsed)

NOTE: Poorly distended and/or collapsed segments may prevent polyp detection, especially if they occur in corresponding supine and prone segments.

Segment	Grade Supine	Grade Prone	Comments
Rectum	1	1	
Sigmoid	2	2	
Descending	1	1	
Transverse	1	1	
Ascending	1	1	
Cecum	3	2	

Residual stool/fluid per colonic segment: (1=None, 3=Moderate, 5=Excessive)

NOTE: Significant Residual Fluid/Stool indicative of poor prep may prevent polyp detection, especially if they occur in corresponding supine and prone segments.

Segment	Grade Supine	Grade Prone	Comments
Rectum	0	0	
Sigmoid	0	0	
Descending	0	0	
Transverse	1	0	
Ascending	1	1	
Cecum	2	2	

Polypoid or Mass Lesions:

Location	Size (mm)	Type of Polyp	Image Number	Comments
Ascending Colon	7.9	sessile	S119/P110	Polyp

Other Colonic Lesions: Diverticulosis present in sigmoid, descending, transverse colon segments.

Extracolonic Findings: **None**

Description	Location	Size (cm)	Image Number	Comments

FIGURE 9.6 Yee Report.

Virtual Colonoscopy Report

Images

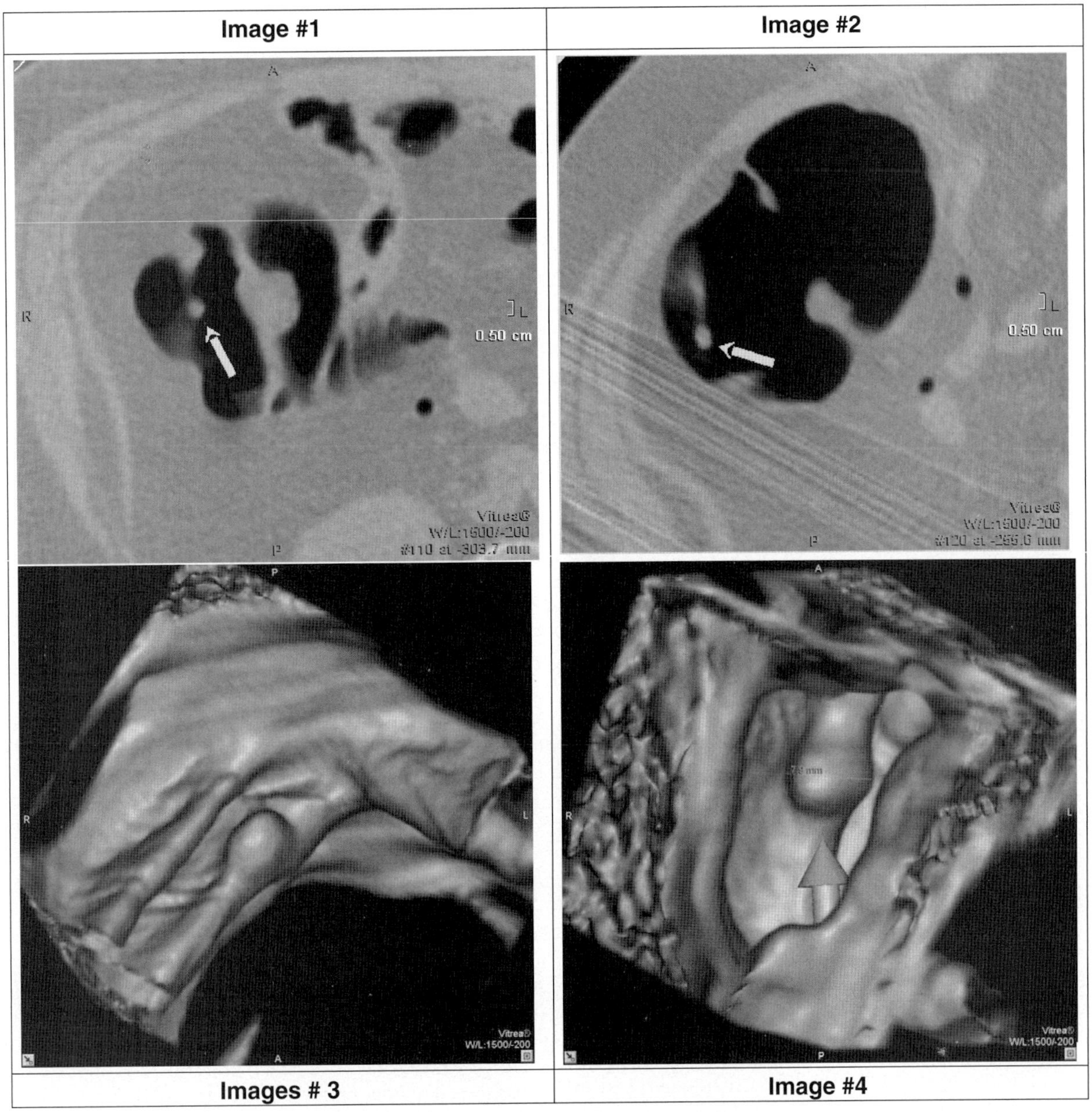

Summary / Recommendations

Summary: 7.9 mm sessile polyp found in ascending colon.
Diverticulosis present in sigmoid, descending, transverse colon segments

Recommendations: Decision to perform colonoscopy for polyp removal should be based on patient and physician preference and the presence, if any, of other medical conditions.

FIGURE 9.6 *(Continued)*

colonoscopy recorded if known. If the reason for the failed colonoscopy is identified before the CTC then this should be noted.

TECHNIQUE

A description of the procedure and materials used is a part of the report. The particular colonic cleansing regimen employed by the patient and how colonic distention was achieved (room air vs. carbon dioxide) is briefly described. Specifics of the CT scanning protocol described in the report may include the type of CT scanner used (multidetector CT scanner and the number of detector rows if preferred), collimation, and reconstruction thickness. This may be useful for future comparison of CT scan studies. Scanning of the patient is typically in two positions (typically supine and prone) and this is stated. If an antispasmodic such as glucagon is given as a part of the CTC examination then the amount and route of administration are described. If intravenous contrast is given for a diagnostic CTC then the type, volume, and route of administration should be recorded.

Any complications from the CTC examination should be recorded such as significant rectal bleeding or colonic perforation. Patient reactions to the antispasmodic and/or intravenous contrast should be documented.

FINDINGS

If there is a prior relevant comparison CT examination then previous reports and images should be reviewed and compared with the current study whenever possible.[1] The date(s) of any relevant comparison CT examinations and findings should be stated.

The report should use appropriate anatomic, pathologic, and radiologic terminology to describe findings.[1] The CTC report should include a description of the adequacy of colonic cleansing and distention. When there are suboptimally distended and/or cleansed colonic segments this should be noted in the report including whether it is in the supine, prone, or both positions. It should be noted that a colonic segment that is poorly distended and/or cleansed in both supine and prone positions is considered not adequately evaluated on CTC and is nondiagnostic for that segment. Any other potential limitations that may compromise the sensitivity or specificity of the examination should be reported. If there is a specific clinical question that the CTC is supposed to answer then this should be addressed in the report. Any limitation of the CT scan that prevents answering the clinical issue should be stated.[1]

The ACR Practice Guidelines for the Performance of CTC in Adults states that large masses should be communicated and polyps measuring 10 mm and greater should be described.[2] The reporting of medium-sized polyps measuring 6 to 9 mm is variable and depends on the reader's confidence level and the particular clinical situation. The ACR guidelines suggest that if the reader is reasonably confident of the presence of a medium-sized polyp then it should be reported. Diminutive polyps measuring 5 mm or smaller should not be reported because they are often non-neoplastic and many of these findings are not found on follow-up colonoscopy because they are false positives or due to the 25% failure rate of colonoscopy to identify such small lesions.[2]

It is also stated that characterization of extracolonic findings may be suboptimal using CTC technique and that lesions outside of the colon may be present but not detectable. The use of clinical judgment is required for reporting extracolonic findings because although these are common, most are clinically insignificant.

A detailed reporting scheme of colonic and extracolonic findings is described in the CT Colonography Reporting and Data System (C-RADS) which is a consensus proposal developed by the Working Group on Virtual Colonoscopy.[3,4] The size, morphology, location, and attenuation of colonic lesions are included in the report. Similar to the ACR Practice Guidelines for the Performance of CTC in Adults, the C-RADS suggestion is to report 6 mm or larger lesions only.[2,3] The specific view used for lesion measurement should be stated. It should be noted whether the polyp has sessile, pedunculated, or flat morphology and the segmental location of the lesion in the rectum, sigmoid, descending colon, transverse colon, ascending colon, or cecum should be stated. Soft tissue versus fat density of the lesion should be noted. Five levels are included from C0 to C4 in the classification scheme of colonic findings with specific follow-up (see Table 9.1). C2 to C4 indicate positive findings that will require a shortened interval follow-up or immediate follow-up. There are also five levels for classification of extracolonic findings from E0 to E4 (see Table 9.2). Level E4 indicates a potentially clinically significant extracolonic finding that should be communicated to the referring physician.

IMPRESSION

This section should include a conclusion or diagnosis if possible or a differential diagnosis when appropriate. A recommendation based on the findings with appropriate follow-up or additional diagnostic study should be suggested when appropriate. The ACR Practice Guidelines for the Performance of CTC in Adults states that for polyps measuring 10 mm and greater, endoscopy with polypectomy is recommended.[2] The management of medium-sized lesions is controversial. Patient factors such as age and other comorbid conditions need to be taken into account in determining a suggestion for follow-up along with the actual size of the lesion. Relatively larger lesions such as an 8- to 9-mm polyp detected with high confidence should be removed particularly if the patient is older than 70 years. A 3- to 5-year follow-up CTC might be appropriate in some patients considering individual factors.

The C-RADS scheme suggests continued routine colon cancer screening every 5 to 10 years if the CTC examination is normal or if a benign lesion is identified such as a lipoma or diverticulosis (C1). If there are only one or

TABLE 9.1 Suggested Categorization System for CT Colonography Findings and Follow-up Recommendations

C0. Inadequate study/awaiting prior comparisons
- Inadequate prep: cannot exclude lesions ≥10 mm owing to presence of fluid/feces
- Inadequate insufflation: one or more colonic segments collapsed on both views
- Awaiting prior colon studies for comparison

C1. Normal colon or benign lesion: continue routine screening[a]
- No visible abnormalities of the colon
- No polyp ≥6 mm
- Lipoma or inverted diverticulum
- Nonneoplastic findings—e.g., colonic diverticula

C2. Intermediate polyp or indeterminate finding; surveillance or colonoscopy recommended[b]
- Intermediate polyp 6–9 mm, <3 in number
- Indeterminate findings, cannot exclude polyp ≥6 mm in technically adequate examination

C3. Polyp, possibly advanced adenoma; follow-up colonoscopy recommended
- Polyp ≥10 mm
- ≥3 polyps, each 6–9 mm

C4. Colonic mass, likely malignant; surgical consultation recommended[c]
- Lesion compromises bowel lumen, demonstrates extracolonic invasion

ACR, American College of Radiology (33); prep, preparation.
[a]Every 5–10 yr.
[b]Evidence suggested surveillance can be delayed at least 3 years, subject to individual patient circumstance.
[c]Communicate to referring physician as per accepted guidelines for communication, such as ACR Practice Guideline for Communication: Diagnostic Radiology. Subject to local practice, endoscopic biopsy may be indicated.
Reprinted with permission from Zalis M, Barish M, Choi R, et al. The Working Group on Virtual Colonoscopy. CT colonography reporting and data system (C-RADS): a consensus statement. *Radiology*. 2005;236:3–9.

TABLE 9.2 Proposed Categorization System for Extracolonic Findings

E0. Limited examination. Compromised artifact; evaluation of extracolonic soft tissues is severely limited.

E1. Normal exam or anatomic variant. No extracolonic abnormalities visible.
  a. Anatomic variant: e.g., retroaortic left renal vein

E2. Clinically unimportant finding. No work-up indicated. Examples:
  a. Liver, kidney: simple cysts
  b. Gallbladder: cholelithiasis without cholecystitis
  c. Vertebra: hemangioma

E3. Likely unimportant finding, incompletely characterized. Subject to local practice and patient preference, work-up may be indicated. Examples:
  a. Kidney: minimally complex or homogeneously hyperattenuating cyst

E4. Potentially important finding. Communicate to referring physician as per accepted practice guidelines.
  a. Kidney: solid renal mass
  b. Lymphadenopathy
  c. Vasculature: aortic aneurysm
  d. Lung: non uniformly calcified parenchymal nodule ≥1 cm

A complete listing of potential extracolonic findings and descriptors is not provided here. A nonexhaustive set of examples is provided for each category.
Reprinted with permission from Zalis M, Barish M, Choi R, et al. The Working Group on Virtual Colonoscopy. CT colonography reporting and data system (C-RADS): a consensus statement. *Radiology*. 2005;236:3–9.

two medium-sized (6 to 9 mm) polyps or indeterminate findings, surveillance or colonoscopy is recommended (C2). When a large polyp (≥10 mm) or three or more medium-sized (6–9 mm) polyps are detected on CTC, colonoscopy is suggested (C3). If a colonic mass is identified which is likely malignant then endoscopic biopsy and/or surgical consultation is recommended (C4).[3]

Any complications or significant patient reactions should be stated in this section also. In emergent or nonroutine clinical situations such as pneumoperitoneum due to colonic perforation, expedited delivery of the report is suggested with documentation of the time, method of communication, and name of the person to whom the urgent finding was communicated to is suggested.[1]

DISCLAIMER STATEMENT

There are no published guidelines regarding the use of a specific disclaimer statement for CTC. However, the ACR Practice Guideline for Communication of Diagnostic Imaging Findings suggests inclusion in the report of factors that may compromise the sensitivity and specificity of the examination.[1] Segments of the colon that are not adequately evaluated because of suboptimal cleansing and/or distention (particularly if this occurs in both positions) should be reported. Some sites will also include a statement regarding the limited sensitivity of CTC for the detection of small (≤5 mm) and flat lesions.

REFERENCES

1. American College of Radiology. ACR practice guideline for communication of diagnostic imaging findings. In: *2006 Practice Guidelines and Technical Standards*. Reston, VA: American College of Radiology; 2006:3–7.
2. American College of Radiology. ACR practice guideline for the performance of computed Tomography (CT) colonography in adults. *In Practice Guidelines and Technical Standards 2005*. Reston, VA: American College of Radiology; 2005: 295–299.
3. Zalis M, Barish M, Choi R, et al. The Working Group on Virtual Colonoscopy. CT colonography reporting and data system (C-RADS): a consensus statement. *Radiology*. 2005; 236:3–9.
4. Barish MA, Soto JA, Ferruci JT. Consensus on current clinical practice of virtual colonoscopy. *AJR Am J Roentgenol*. 2005;184:786–792.

CHAPTER 10 STOOL AND FLUID TAGGING

Judy Yee

Currently patients typically undergo bowel cleansing before computed tomography colonography (CTC). However, investigators have made significant progress in identifying methods to label residual fluid and stool with positive oral contrast agents so that there is easier differentiation from the homogeneous soft tissue density of polyps. This technique has been evaluated both with and without the use of a laxative. However, if the requirement for a cathartic agent could be eliminated or if the amount of cathartic agent needed could be reduced, this would likely lead to improved patient tolerance. This can give CTC a significant advantage over colonoscopy by improving patient compliance with screening for colon cancer. Once residual fluid and stool are tagged with a positive contrast agent, electronic subtraction of the high-density material may then be performed. It has been postulated that electronic subtraction bowel cleansing may eliminate the need for scanning in both supine and prone positions because electronic removal of residual material may be performed with one acquisition. However, dual-position scanning may still be necessary in order to achieve optimal segmental distention.

Tagging of residual material in the colon may be achieved by the ingestion of iodinated contrast material and/or barium. Studies have been performed evaluating the use of iodinated contrast or barium alone as well as in combination and in some of the studies a laxative is administered. Variable results have been achieved depending upon the specific type of contrast and laxative used as well as on the volume of contrast and laxative administered and the timing of when the contrast and laxative are ingested. The employment of dietary modification and hydration before CTC can also impact on the amount of residual stool and fluid as well as the adequacy of tagging.

Optimally tagged stool has homogeneous internal high-density, which allows for easy differentiation from the soft tissue density of polyps on two-dimensional (2D) images. Optimally tagged fluid is uniformly high density allowing the detection of polyps submerged in the fluid on 2D images (see Figures 10.1 and 10.2). Homogeneous labeling of material allows for effective subtraction of the tagged material which in turn enables more efficient primary three-dimensional (3D) interpretation. An alternative method that may be employed for distinguishing tagged stool from polyp on 3D images is the use of translucency rendering, which is available using specific software.[1] Translucency rendering is a function that combines attenuation-dependent transparency with color mapping. Colors are assigned to maximize the different densities of tagged stool versus polyp. Tagged stool may be assigned a white color whereas soft tissue polyps appear as lesions with gradual density change of blue, green, and red corresponding to regions of increasing attenuation (see Figures 10.3 and 10.4). Using this color scheme, fatty lesions appear green on translucency rendering.

The use of oral contrast material as a tagging agent for CTC may also allow for the identification of polyps with villous histology. O'Connor et al. evaluated 216 patients with 338 polyps in a retrospective study and found that 46% of the 312 polyps not touching a contrast pool had adherent contrast.[2] Patients had received 500 mL of 2.1% barium for stool tagging and 120 mL of iodinated contrast material for fluid tagging as well as 90 mL of sodium phosphate and bisacodyl for colonic cleansing. Villous polyps were much more likely to have adherent contrast compared to nonvillous polyps (77% vs. 43%). In this study, villous polyps also tended to be larger on average compared to nonvillous polyps (13.9 mm vs. 7.4 mm). Pedunculated polyps were found to more likely have adherent contrast (68%) compared to sessile (45%) and flat lesions (24%).

Heterogeneous tagging of residual stool and fluid can make it difficult to distinguish polyps from unlabelled stool or fluid (see Figures 10.5 and 10.6). Electronic subtraction of heterogeneously tagged material may result in nondiagnostic images with residual unsubtracted stool confused for polyps (see Figure 10.7). Polyps may also be obscured by poorly tagged material that is not subtracted.

TAGGING WITH LAXATIVE

The labeling of residual colonic fluid with oral iodinated contrast material has been evaluated in patients who have

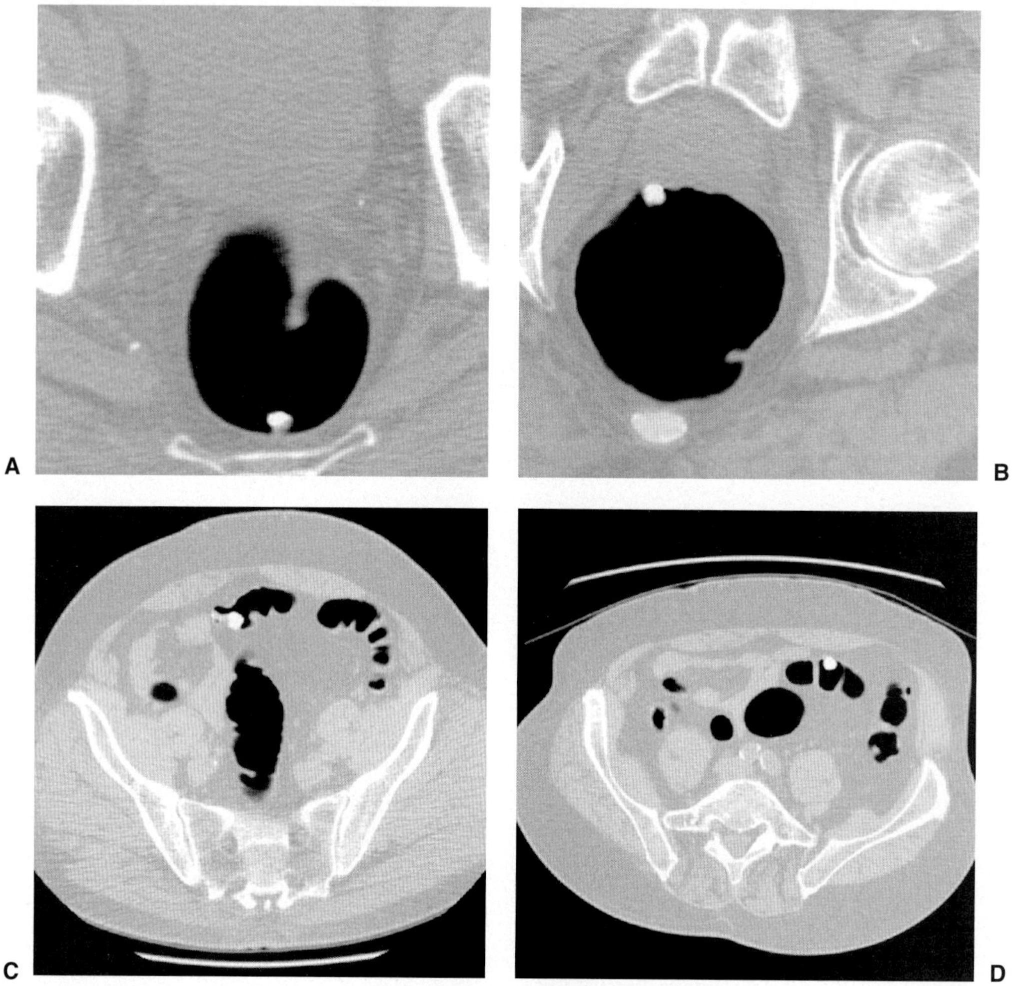

FIGURE 10.1 Tagged Stool. Axial supine **(A)** and prone **(B)** images show mobile tagged stool which is easily differentiated from a polyp. Similar findings in a different patient are shown in supine **(C)** and prone **(D)** axial images.

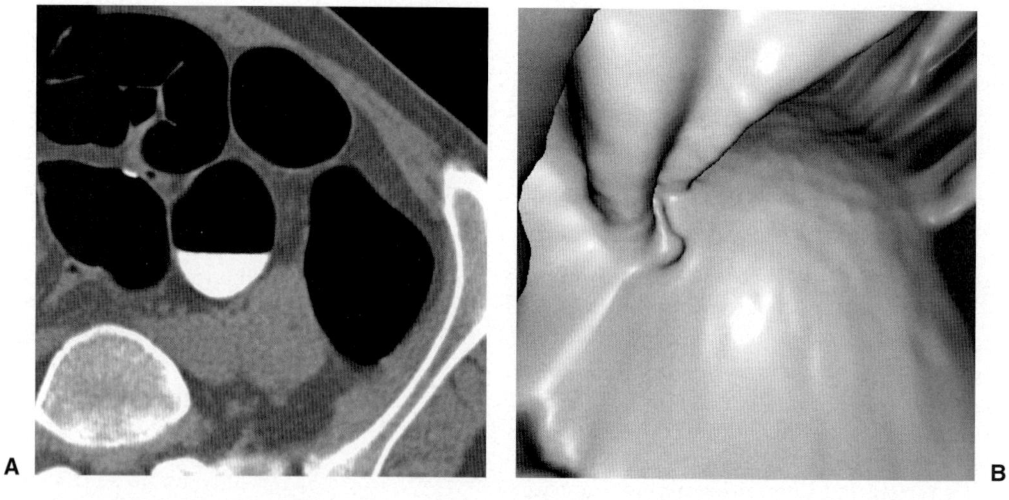

FIGURE 10.2 Tagged Fluid. Axial supine image **(A)** shows uniformly tagged fluid with no evidence of lesions. It is not possible to exclude a lesion on the unsubtracted 3D endoluminal image **(B)** which shows the top of the layering fluid.

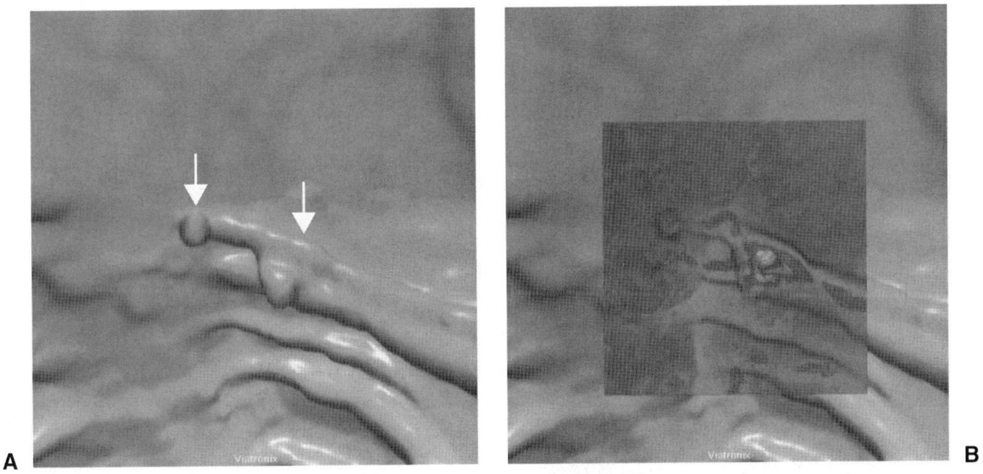

FIGURE 10.3 Polyp and Tagged Stool. 3D endoluminal view **(A)** shows two polypoid lesions on a fold. When the translucency view is employed **(B)**, the central white core in the larger lesion demonstrates it to be tagged stool. The color pattern of the smaller lesion with gradual change in the colors red, green and blue suggest a polyp. (Views A and B: See also color plate.)

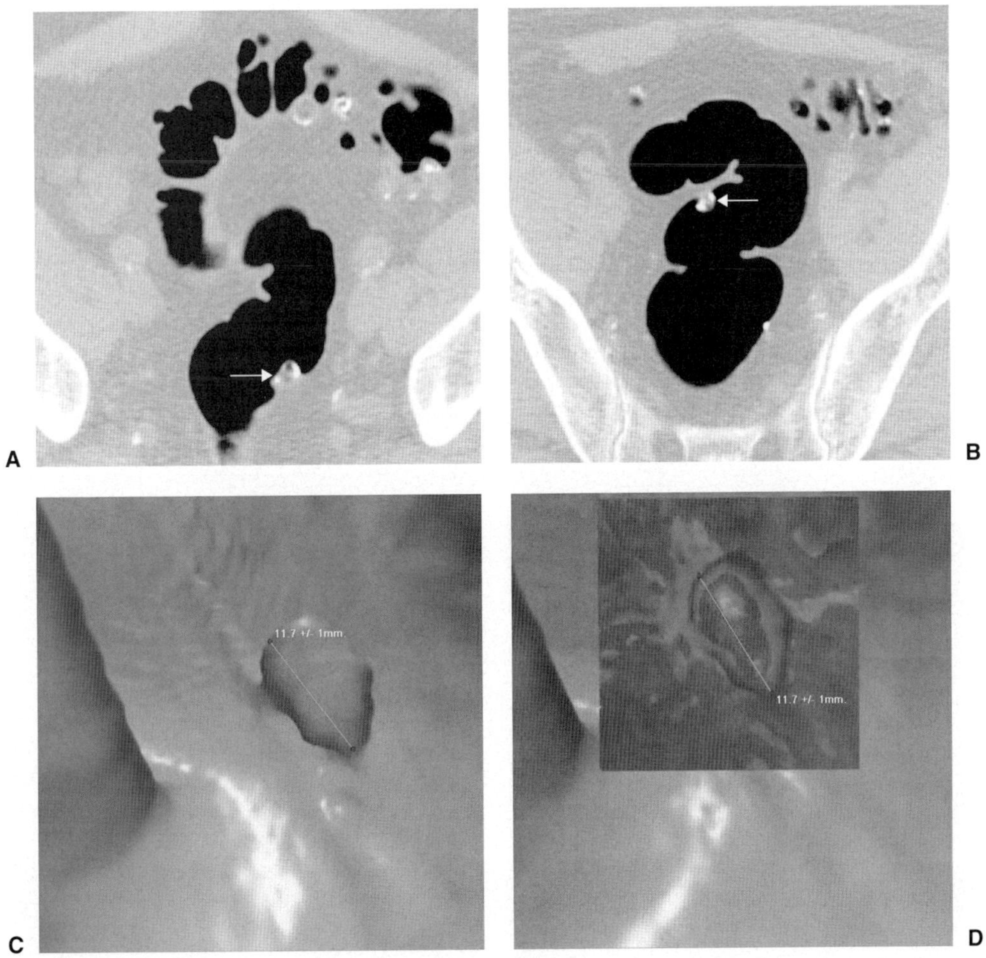

FIGURE 10.4 Heterogeneously Tagged Stool. Axial supine **(A)** and prone **(B)** images show mobile heterogeneously tagged stool. The partially tagged stool simulates a polyp on the 3D endoluminal view **(C)**. When the translucency view is applied **(D)**, the color pattern shows white centrally indicating that this lesion is tagged stool. (Views C and D: See also color plate.)

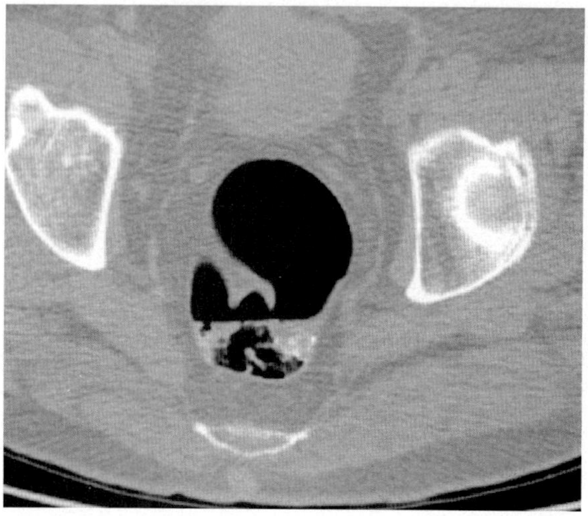

FIGURE 10.5 Poor Tagging. A large amount of untagged stool is submerged in poorly tagged fluid seen on this axial supine image. Areas of homogeneous untagged stool may not be differentiated from a polyp or mass.

also received a purgative. There are also several studies evaluating the iodinated contrast as a tagging agent without the use of a laxative and these are presented in the next section. In an earlier study by Fletcher et al., 73 patients underwent bowel cleansing with 4 L of polyethylene glycol (PEG) lavage solution and two 5-mg bisacodyl tablets.[3] Patients ingested 120 mL of iodinated contrast material the night before the computed tomography (CT) scan. Results showed that there was no increase in sensitivity or specificity for polyp detection when oral iodinated contrast material was administered. In fact there was a trend for decreased detection of medium-sized polyps (5–9 mm) with the use of oral contrast. An increase in residual fluid attenuation was found in only 48% of patients who received oral iodinated contrast according to the protocol in this study. Thomeer et al. performed a study evaluating 150 patients who received either 3 to 5 L of a home-made electrolyte solution (130 patients) or PEG before thin-slice multidetector computed tomography (MDCT) Colonography (1-mm collimation, 0.8-mm reconstruction interval, 60 effective mAs, 120 kVp).[4] Iodinated contrast material was added to the bowel preparation solution (30 mL/L) to tag residual colonic fluid and stool. Bowel cleansing and tagging occurred in the hospital up to 5 hours before the CT scan. In contrast to the results of Fletcher et al., tagging was found to be optimal with homogeneous labeling in 95% of cases and this was felt to be due to the short interval during which the patients had to ingest the iodinated contrast material before the CTC. Sensitivities were 64% to 67% for 5- to 9-mm polyps and 92% for polyps larger than 9 mm. The overall specificity was high at 94% to 95%.

Barium has been evaluated as an oral agent for stool tagging with the use of a laxative. In an initial study, Lefere et al. compared reduced colonic cleansing based on dietary fecal tagging with standard colonic cleansing.[5] Fifty patients underwent a low residue diet starting 2 days before the CT scan including a specific meal kit which was ingested the day before CTC with three separate 250-mL doses of barium (2.1% weight per volume) at each meal. In the early evening on the day before CTC, patients also underwent bowel cleansing with 16.4 g of magnesium citrate and bisacodyl tablets. A bisacodyl suppository was given the morning of the CTC examination. Fifty patients underwent standard colonic cleansing with up to 3 L of PEG the afternoon before the CTC. Results showed that patients undergoing fecal tagging had more residual stool but there was improved specificity of 88% versus 77% in the nonfecal tagging group. Overall per-patient sensitivities between the two groups were similar at 85% (nonfecal tagging) and 88% (fecal tagging). Fecal tagging

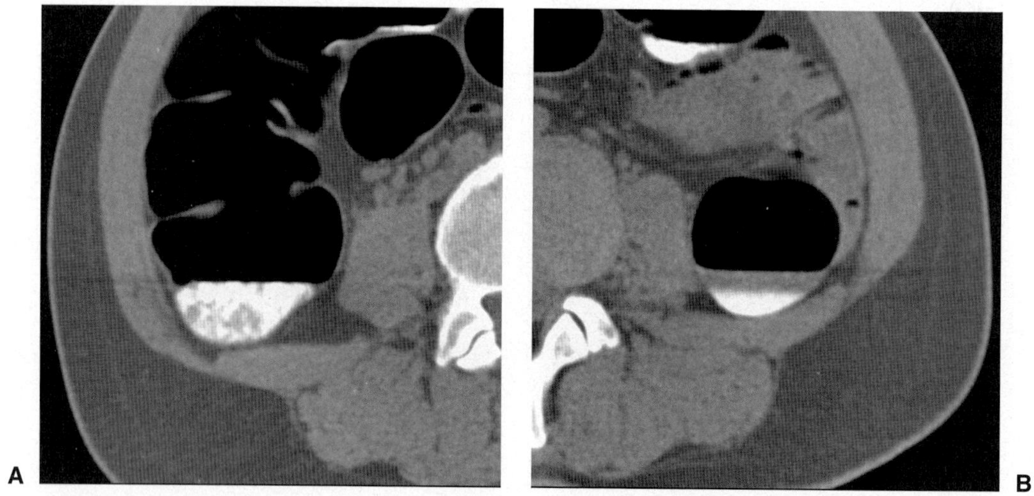

FIGURE 10.6 Variable Tagging. Axial image of the ascending colon near the cecum **(A)** shows heterogeneous stool and fluid tagging. Axial image of the descending colon **(B)** from the same patient shows a different example of heterogeneous tagging with layering of untagged fluid above tagged fluid.

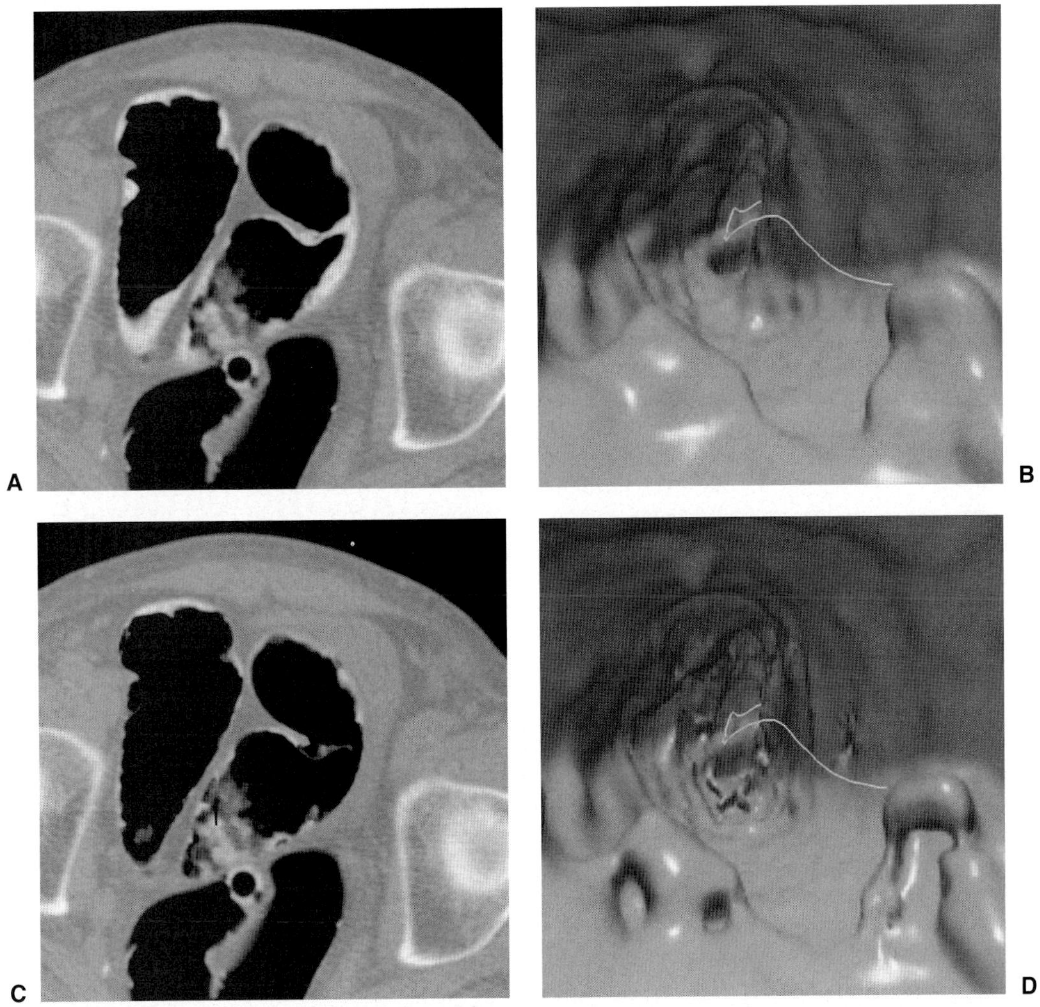

FIGURE 10.7 Adherent Poorly Tagged Stool. Axial image **(A)** shows suboptimal tagging of a large amount of residual adherent stool located in the sigmoid. The 3D endoluminal view **(B)** reveals multiple irregularities along the colonic wall that appear polypoid. Axial image after electronic cleansing **(C)** shows a large amount of unsubtracted stool with multiple artifacts seen on both the axial and the 3D endoluminal view **(D)**.

was found to significantly reduce discomfort, side effects, and sleep disturbance and produced a better final opinion of how comfortable the examination was and a trend for increased patient willingness to repeat the examination.

Gryspeerdt et al. compared three different colon cleansing techniques which were each used in 20 patients.[6] Group 1 patients received a standard PEG regimen the day of the CTC. Group 2 patients underwent reduced cleansing the day before the CTC based on a combination of diet, bisacodyl, and a decreased amount of PEG. Group 3 patients received bisacodyl, magnesium citrate, a low-residue diet, and barium for stool tagging. Results showed that the fecal tagging group had reduced fluid levels and there was improved differentiation between residual stool and polyps with the use of fecal tagging. Overall sensitivity for polyp detection was 59%, 76%, and 80% for Groups 1, 2, and 3 respectively with 100% sensitivity for polyps larger than 10 mm in all three groups. Overall specificity was 57%, 71%, and 80% for Groups 1, 2, and 3 respectively. Stool tagging with barium also reduced preparation-related discomfort compared to the other two groups. Gryspeerdt et al. also performed a study evaluating stool tagging with barium for CTC in patients following incomplete colonoscopy.[7] Twenty-four patients underwent bowel cleansing with PEG (59 g/L/20 kg body weight) the morning of the CTC examination with a delay of at least 2 hours between the administration of PEG and the CT scan. Twenty-five patients underwent stool tagging 3 to 5 weeks after incomplete colonoscopy. Patients were instructed to decrease fat intake starting 2 days before the CT scan. A low-residue diet in a meal kit was given the day before the CTC and bowel cleansing was achieved using magnesium citrate and bisacodyl. Low-density barium (2.5% weight per volume) was given in three 250-mL aliquots with meals for stool tagging. Improved colonic distention and decreased residual fluid were found in patients who underwent stool tagging. There was a higher mean score for residual stool in the fecal tagging group compared to the group of patients who received PEG (0.4 vs. 0.2). The overall sensitivity of CTC for polyp detection in endoscopically nonvisualized colon segments in the fecal tagging group was 92% compared to 50% for patients who received PEG.

Lefere et al. assessed the efficacy of stool tagging with a small volume of high-density barium combined with reduced cathartic cleansing for CTC in 200 patients and achieved promising results.[8] Patients started a low-fiber diet 2 days before the CTC and received a commercially available meal kit 1 day before the CT scan. Stool tagging was performed with a high-density 40% weight per volume barium suspension with 25 mL given at breakfast and 12.5 mL given at lunch and dinner for a total volume of 50 mL. In the early evening before the CTC, patients received 16.5 g of magnesium citrate for bowel cleansing followed by the ingestion of bisacodyl tablets. A bisacodyl suppository was administered the morning of the CT scan. Single-detector CT was performed on 115 patients using 5-mm slice thickness and 2-mm slice reconstructions. The remaining patients underwent MDCT scanning using 2.5-mm collimation, 120 kVp, and 70 mA. Two radiologists read the CTC examinations using primary 2D interpretation with 3D for problem solving. Residual stool was identified in 34% of segments with most of the stool found in the cecum and ascending colon. Stool measuring 6 mm or larger was identified in 17% of segments. Nontagged stool measuring 6 mm or larger was found in 4% of segments, most commonly in the rectum. Fecal residue in the rectum was thought to be possibly due to the use of the bisacodyl suppository. However, nontagged stool was mobile in all segments allowing differentiation from polyps. No residual fluid was found in 56% of segments or was small (covering <25% of the lumen) in 35% of segments. There was a large amount of residual fluid in 3% of segments and nontagged fluid was identified in 15% of segments. Nontagged fluid covering >50% of the lumen was present in only 0.42% of segments. There was a high sensitivity of 92% (65/71) for the detection of polyps 6 mm or larger using this tagging protocol.

Stool and fluid tagging was used in the multicenter trial by Pickhardt et al. where 1,233 patients received 500 mL of low density 2.1% barium in split doses for stool tagging and 120 mL of diatrizoate meglumine and diatrizoate sodium (Gastrografin) in split doses for fluid tagging.[9] Patients also underwent bowel cleansing with 90 mL of sodium phosphate in split doses and 10 mg of bisacodyl. MDCT colonography was performed using 1.25- to 2.5-mm collimation, 120 kVp, 100mAs with a 1-mm reconstruction interval. Primary 3D interpretation was used with the availability of translucency rendering. Excellent results were achieved with per-polyp sensitivity for polyps measuring 10 mm or larger equal to 92% (47/51) and the per-patient sensitivity for polyps measuring 10 mm or larger equal to 94% (45/48). Specificity for patients with polyps measuring 10 mm or larger was 96%.

The American College of Radiology Imaging Network (ACRIN) National CT Colonography Trial includes the use of stool and fluid tagging.[10] Patients were required to have a fully cleansed colon using one of three standardized bowel preparations according to site preference (PEG solution, magnesium citrate, sodium phosphate). All three preparations included the use of 10 mg of bisacodyl tablets. Three doses of high density 40% weight per volume barium was administered orally the day before the CTC (20 mL at 8 A.M., 10 mL at 11 A.M., 10 mL at 2 P.M.). In addition, 60 mL of iodinated contrast material (Gastrografin 37% organically bound iodine) was administered in three aliquots of 20 mL each starting the evening before the CTC. Each 20 mL of iodinated contrast material was mixed with 8 oz. of water and ingested. Adequacy of cleansing and tagging are to be assessed as part of the trial.

TAGGING WITHOUT LAXATIVE

In efforts to increase patient acceptance of CTC, investigators are looking at tagging protocols that could potentially eliminate the need for a laxative. Stool labeling was found to be feasible without cathartic use in a preliminary study by Callstrom et al.[11] Fifty-six high-risk patients were divided into five groups before CTC. Various regimens of between two to seven doses of 225 mL of 1.2% barium sulfate were given orally to the patients during 24 to 48 hours before CT. For axial image analysis, structures measuring >150 Hounsfield units (HU) were electronically labeled allowing identification of barium-labeled stool from soft tissue density polyps. It was found that the highest average stool labeling scores were in the group ingesting seven doses of barium over a 48-hour period before CT. Although electronic subtraction of tagged stool was not performed in this study, the sensitivity for polyp detection in this group was 100% and 80% both by patient and by polyp analysis.

Lefere et al. performed a pilot study evaluating laxative-free stool tagging with various concentrations of barium suspension in 15 patients.[12] Different regimens were used for five groups of three patients each consisting of different volumes and concentrations of 2.1%, 4%, and 40% weight per volume barium starting 1 to 2 days before the CTC. Patients were restricted to a maximum fluid intake of 1,250 mL. Results showed excellent labeling of 90% to 100% for almost all segments. No difference in labeling was seen between patients who ingested barium over the course of 1 versus 2 days and between patients who received 750-mL barium dose versus the 50-mL barium dose the day before CTC. The authors felt that by limiting patient hydration they were able to obtain effective stool labeling without the need for iodinated contrast material for fluid tagging. The stated preference for efficient tagging was concluded to be 50 mL of 40% weight per volume barium administered the day before CTC (25 mL at breakfast and 12.5 mL at lunch and dinner).

In another pilot study, Dachman et al. evaluated 28 patients who were randomized into uncleansed and cleansed groups.[13] Two days before the CTC, all patients avoided high-fiber foods and on the day before CT both groups received a low-residue meal kit. Both groups ingested three doses of 40% weight per volume barium at mealtimes the day before the CTC. Patients in the group receiving a laxative underwent bowel cleansing with magnesium citrate the afternoon before CT. Most of the interpretations of the uncleansed group were felt to be fairly difficult to read compared to the cleansed group where most were felt to be slightly difficult or adequate to read. Interpretation times averaged 17.5 minutes for the uncleansed group versus 17.9 minutes for the cleansed group. There were more segments with stool in the uncleansed group (160 segments) compared to the cleansed group (58 segments) and there was more stool in the uncleansed group versus the cleansed group. It was concluded that the presence of more stool in the uncleansed group made the examination subjectively harder to interpret and likely caused three polyps to be missed in this group.

Bielen et al. evaluated the feasibility of low-residue meals combined with a small volume of iodinated contrast material for stool tagging in 11 patients.[14] No laxative was administered. Three days before the CTC, patients were instructed to maintain a low-fiber diet and before each meal 5 ml of iodinated contrast material diluted in a standard glass of water was ingested. MDCT colonography was performed using 4 × 1 mm collimation, reconstructions at 1.25 mm, 120 kVp, and 60 mAs. Fecal material was found to be tagged in all patients. The degree of tagging was rated good or moderate in 92% of segments, particularly in the descending colon and sigmoid. Patient acceptance was significantly better for the CTC preparation and the examination itself compared to colonoscopy where a polyethylene lavage solution was administered for bowel cleansing.

Iannaccone et al. also used iodinated contrast as a tagging agent and compared the performance of laxative-free low-dose MDCT colonography with that of colonoscopy for the detection of polyps in 203 patients.[15] Patients started a low-fiber diet 2 days before the CTC and received a total volume of 200 mL of diatrizoate meglumine and diatrizoate sodium (Gastrografin) ingested as five 20 mL aliquots per day at meals with each diluted with a glass of water. MDCT colonography was performed using 2.5-mm collimation with 1.0-mm reconstruction interval 140 kVp, and 10 effective mAs. Primary 2D interpretation was used with 3D images for problem solving by three readers. All patients underwent same-day colonoscopy using segmental unblinding. CTC had an average sensitivity and specificity of 96% and 98% respectively for the detection of polyps 8 mm and larger and 86% and 93% respectively for detecting polyps 6 mm and larger. Most patients preferred the stool tagging method for CTC compared to cathartic bowel cleansing for colonoscopy (88%). Average interpretation time was short at 9.8 minutes. High interobserver agreement was noted for per-polyp polyp detection and with high to excellent interobserver agreement for per-patient polyp detection. It was noted that with the use of a fixed 200 mL volume of diatrizoate meglumine and diatrizoate sodium (Gastrografin), approximately 6% of patients reported a laxative effect with episodes of diarrhea.

TAGGING WITH ELECTRONIC SUBTRACTION

Subtraction CTC is a technique that was developed to decrease the need for colonic cleansing for CTC in order to remove what has been recognized as one of the major barriers to patient compliance with colorectal cancer screening. This technique may also facilitate 2D interpretation and provide suitable images for 3D endoluminal navigation. After the patient ingests barium and/or iodinated contrast material, CTC is performed. The resulting data set undergoes postprocessing using specific computer software that subtracts the residual tagged material from the colon leaving behind the colon wall, folds, and soft tissue density polyps (see Figure 10.8). Heterogeneous tagging of residual material will make electronic subtraction difficult and areas of untagged stool and/or fluid can be left behind that can simulate polyps as well as obscure lesions (see Figures 10.9 and 10.10). Interpretation of CTC studies using tagging combined with electronic subtraction requires specific training so that specific pitfalls of this technique may be avoided (see Figures 10.11 to 10.13). The most commonly encountered artifact due to electronic subtraction of fluid is a step-off around the rim of the liquid pool ("ring around the tub" appearance), which is seen on the 3D endoluminal view.

Subtraction CTC was initially evaluated in an animal model study by Sheppard et al. and found to be feasible.[16] Barium was used to tag a fecal substitute which was placed into segments of animal colon containing simulated polyps measuring between 3 and 10 mm. Using CT scanning parameters of 3-mm collimation, pitch 2, reconstruction intervals of 3 mm and a subtraction cut-off level of 150 HU, a 94% sensitivity and 80% specificity was achieved for detecting polyps larger than 3 mm. Subsequent to this study, digital subtraction bowel cleansing for CTC was performed in patients in a study by Zalis et al.[17] Five patients ingested 6 to 7 doses of 5 mL of contrast material starting at 48 hours before CT. Three patients ingested 2.1% barium sulfate and two patients were given 1:40 dilution of iodinated contrast. A final large 800 mL bolus of contrast was administered approximately 3 hours before CT to uniformly opacify cecal contents. Proprietary software was used for postprocessing of the image data sets, which used two different algorithms for subtraction. A matrix convolution method used mathematic gradient operators to identify areas in each image with high regional pixels that were then subtracted. A second method involved an extension of the roving magic squares computer graphics segmentation technique where a step-wise evaluation of neighborhood pixels was performed to detect changes in pixel value. Bone was also subtracted from the images because a threshold function was a part of the matrix algorithm. The resultant datasets in this study were found to be suitable for multiplanar and 3D endoluminal evaluation.

In a follow-up study, Zalis et al. reported that their initial experience with digital subtraction bowel cleansing was suboptimal because the postprocessed images had edge artifacts that occurred at the interface between the mucosal–air interface where there was an

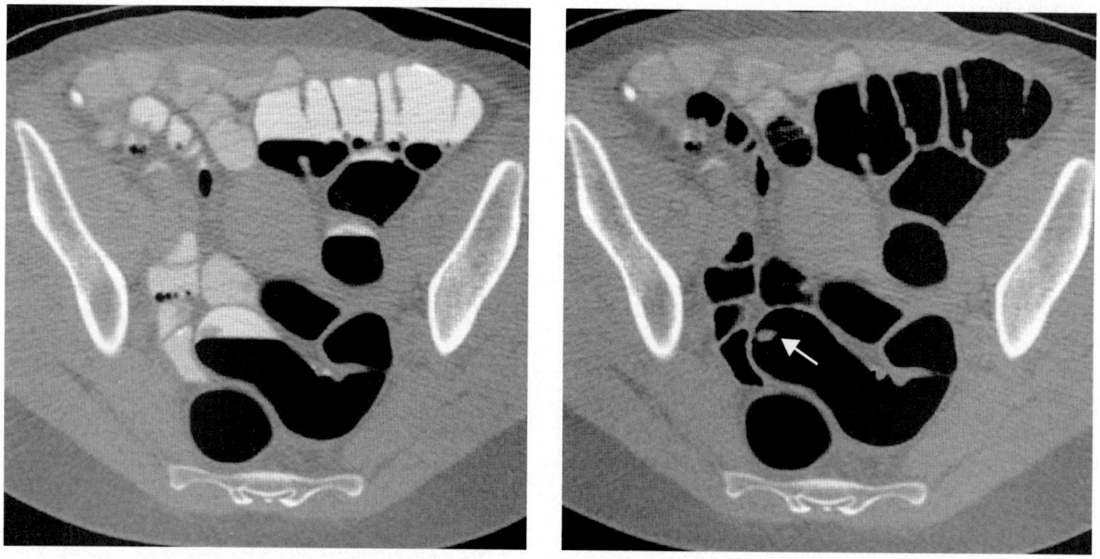

A B

FIGURE 10.8 Polyp Using Electronic Subtraction. Axial images before **(A)** and after **(B)** the application of electronic subtraction reveal a polyp in the sigmoid colon which is better seen after removal of the tagged fluid.

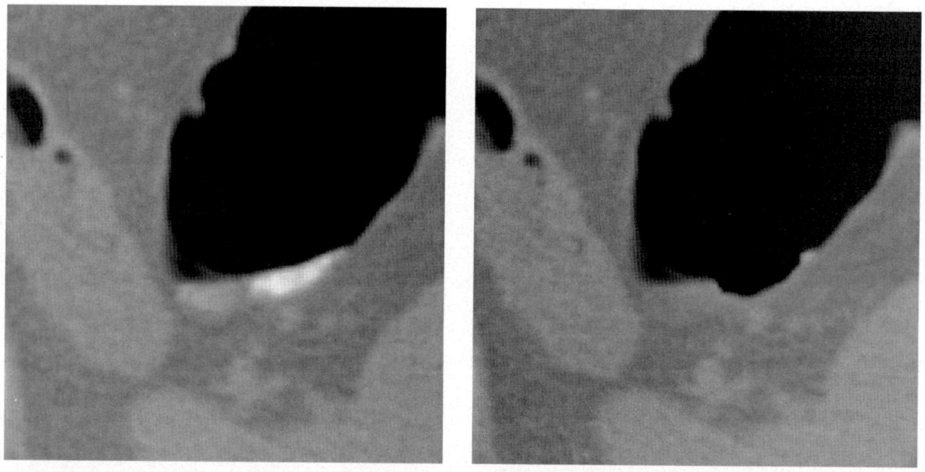

A B

FIGURE 10.9 Heterogeneous Tagging And Electronic Subtraction. Axial images before **(A)** and after **(B)** electronic subtraction show removal of only tagged portions of residual fluid and stool. Notice the artifact that is created by the remaining untagged material. The 3D endoluminal images before **(C)** and after **(D)** electronic subtraction show artifacts after partial removal of tagged material with multiple protruding lesions that can be difficult to interpret without the aid of the axial images.

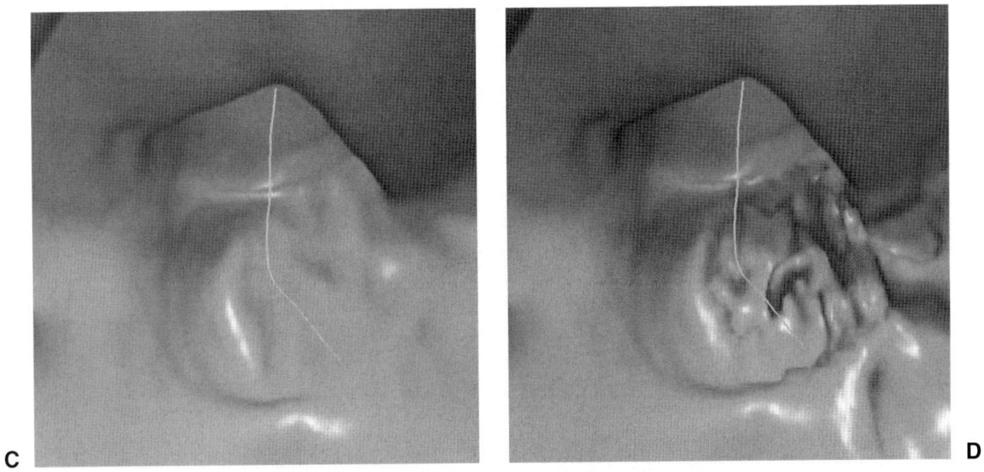

FIGURE 10.9 (*Continued*).

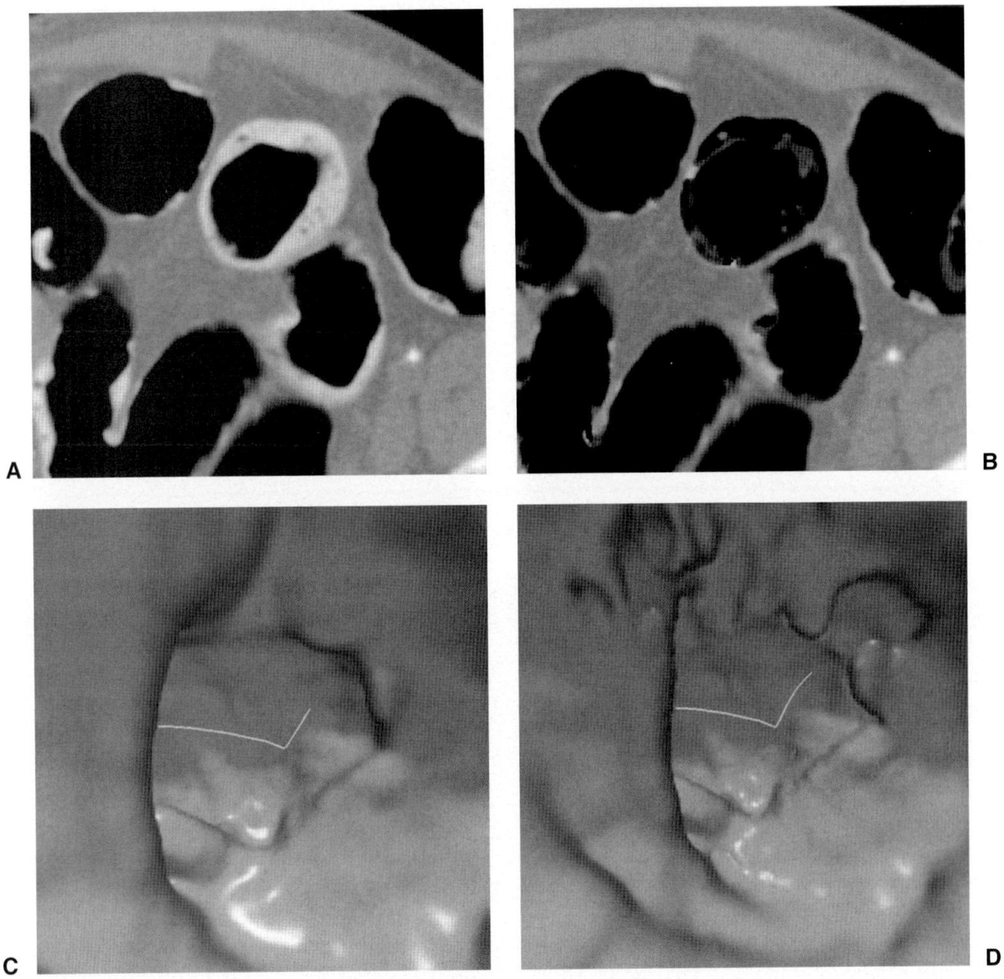

FIGURE 10.10 Heterogeneous Tagging and Electronic Subtraction. Axial images before **(A)** and after **(B)** electronic subtraction show a large amount of adherent heterogeneously tagged stool, which leaves multiple areas of artifact following removal of only the tagged material. The 3D endoluminal images before **(C)** and after **(D)** electronic subtraction show a markedly irregular wall with pseudopolypoid lesions after partial removal of tagged material.

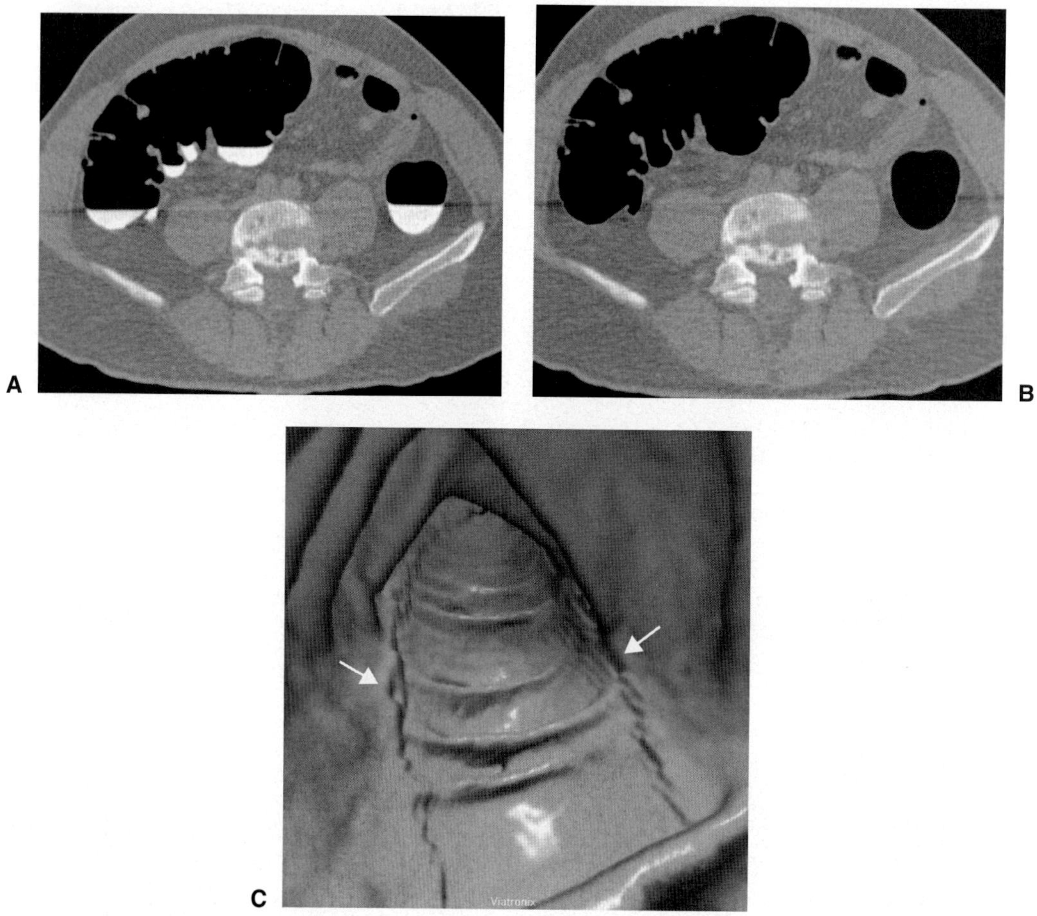

FIGURE 10.11 Rim Artifact. Axial images before **(A)** and after **(B)** electronic subtraction show adequate removal of the homogeneously tagged fluid. The most commonly encountered artifact due to electronic subtraction of fluid is a step-off around the rim of the liquid pool ("ring around the tub" appearance), which is seen on the 3D endoluminal view **(C)**.

abrupt change in pixel values.[18] These artifacts made image interpretation difficult. The authors implemented a new technique of subtraction combined with mucosal reconstruction. The subtraction algorithm modified pixels >200 HU and included the volume-averaged pixels at contrast material–air interfaces. Mucosal reconstruction was performed using special edge detection image processing techniques combined with constrained remodeling of the mucosal–air interface to reconstruct the original bowel wall. This new technique was found to produce images with reduced edge artifacts in 16 patients that allowed detection of polyps. Patients underwent a laxative-free tagging regimen consisting of 8 mL aliquots of nonionic iodinated contrast material (300 mg of iodine per milliliter) taken with meals and snacks starting 48 hours before the CT scan. Three hours before the CTC examination a final 32 mL aliquot of the contrast diluted in 700 mL of water was ingested to opacify cecal contents. Four subjects served as controls and underwent bowel cleansing with 4 L of PEG on the evening before the CTC. Low-dose CTC was performed using 3.75-mm collimation, 1.8-mm reconstruction intervals, 140 kVp, and 50 mA. Mean interpretation times for the subtracted images for two readers were 12.4 and 12.0 minutes compared with 10.4 and 10.2 minutes for the images acquired with standard cleansing. Both readers identified all five lesions measuring 10 mm and larger in this pilot study. In the study by Bielen et al. described in the previous section, electronic subtraction was applied to the image datasets using proprietary software. The authors found stair-step artifacts that occurred at curvatures. Thin haustral folds were subtracted because they were considered to be partial voxels. Image quality was suboptimal following electronic subtraction due to artifacts particularly in segments with large residual stool.

Johnson et al. evaluated three stool subtraction techniques using a phantom containing three types of simulated stool mixed with barium.[19] Results showed that a threshold of 200 HU and expansion and convolution techniques were the most effective tools for stool subtraction and minimizing artifacts. Thirty patients underwent stool tagging for CTC with evaluation of stool subtraction algorithms. CT parameters included 2.5-mm collimation, 1.25-mm reconstructions, 140 mA, and 120 kVp.

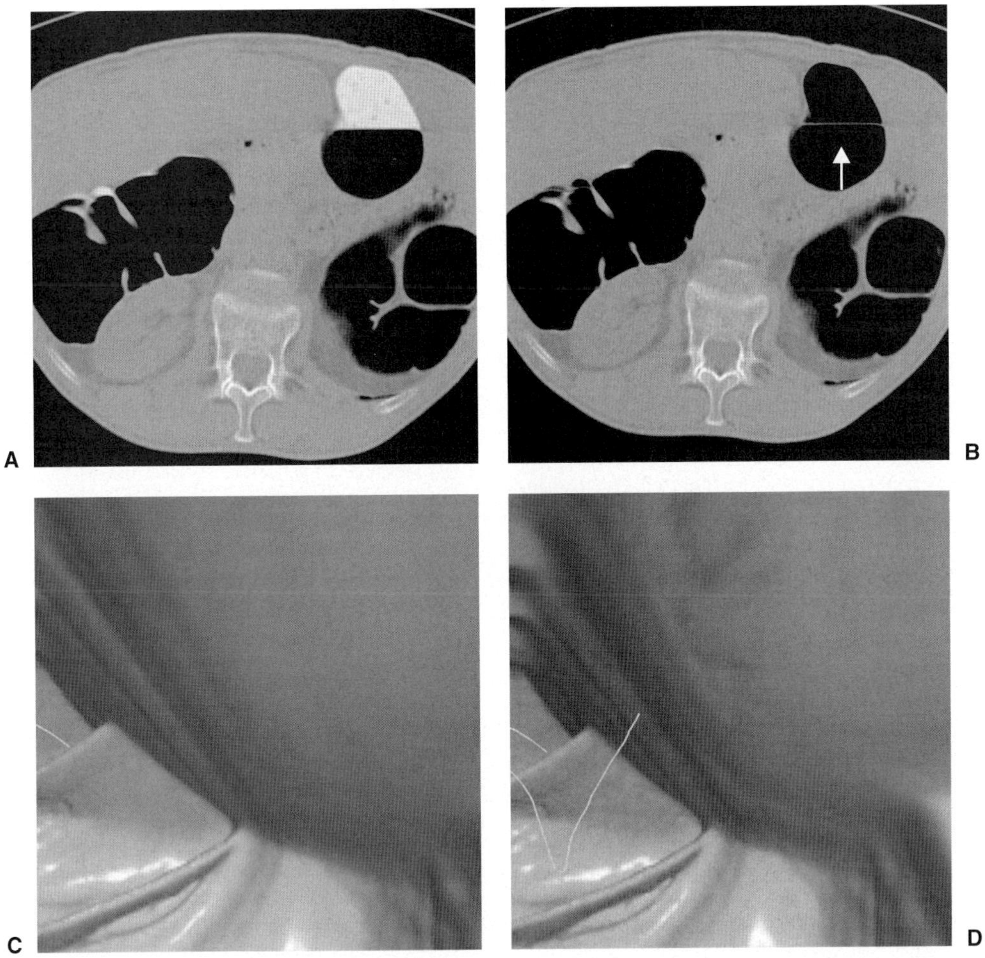

FIGURE 10.12 Incomplete Electronic Subtraction. Axial prone images before **(A)** and after **(B)** electronic subtraction show that a thin layer of untagged layering fluid remains unsubtracted. The 3D endoluminal images before **(C)** and after **(D)** electronic subtraction appear similar reflecting the ineffective removal of the thin layer of untagged layering fluid.

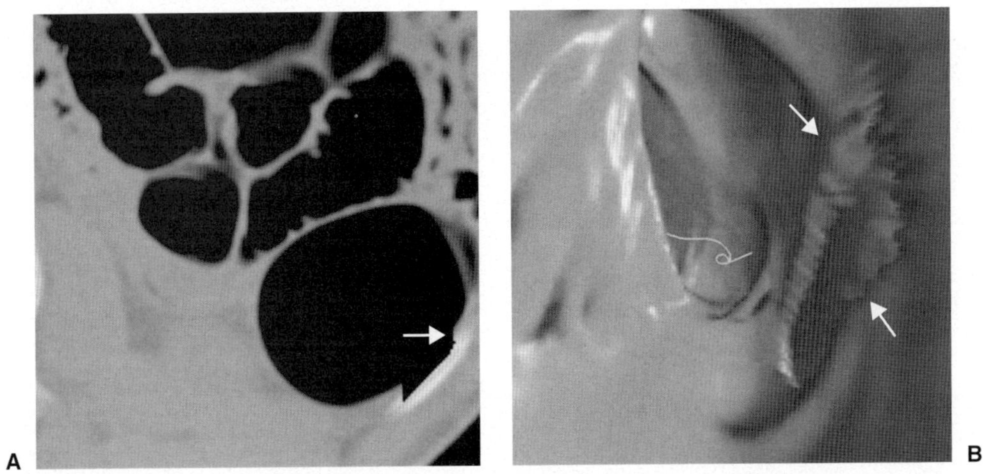

FIGURE 10.13 Electronic Subtraction of Adjacent Bone. Axial view **(A)** following electronic subtraction shows removal of tagged colonic material as well as partial removal of adjacent rib. A large irregular hole is seen in the wall on the 3D endoluminal view **(B)**, which could have caused a lesion to be missed if present along the adjacent colon wall.

The tagging regimen started 2 days before the CT scan and included ingestion of four capsules of 570 mg of barium 95% weight per volume for stool labeling. An additional 240 mL of 2.1% barium was ingested the morning of the CTC examination. Each patient ingested a total of 20.5 g of barium. Unsubtracted images were interpreted initially followed 6 weeks later by review of the unsubtracted and subtracted datasets. The sensitivity and specificity for the detection of 10 mm and larger polyps using unsubtracted images as well as for the stool-subtracted images were 90% (18/20) and 100% (4/4) respectively. It was concluded that laxative-free CTC using barium tagging has high accuracy with or without stool subtraction.

Zalis et al. compared homogeneity, adequacy, and patient acceptance of iodinated contrast versus those of barium as tagging agents for CTC combined with electronic subtraction in 68 patients.[20] Subjects were divided into three groups. Group 1 patients received seven 150 mL aliquots of 2% barium weight per volume with meals starting 2 days before the CT scan with a final 700 mL bolus 3 hours before scanning. Group 2 patients received seven 10 mL aliquots of iodinated contrast media (300 mgI/mL) with meals starting 2 days before the CT scan and a final bolus of 30 mL of contrast diluted in 700 mL of water at 3 hours before scanning. Group 3 patients ingested seven 10 mL aliquots of iodinated contrast media (300 mgI/mL) with meals starting 2 days before the CT scan, a final bolus of 30 mL of contrast diluted in 700 mL of water at 3 hours before scanning, and received 34 g of magnesium citrate the evening before the CTC. Ten control subjects received PEG solution as a laxative before CTC. CTC parameters included 3.75-mm collimation, 1.8-mm reconstruction intervals, 140 kVp, and 50 mA. Proprietary software was employed for electronic subtraction that identified and modified foci with pixel values >200 HU to render them translucent. The software contained algorithms to address volume-averaging artifacts located at the borders of opacified areas as well as to perform mucosal reconstructions after the subtraction process. Discomfort scores in Groups 1 to 3 were similar and were statistically significantly better than that of the control group who had undergone bowel cleansing with PEG. Two readers scored the readability of the subtracted images in Groups 1 and 2 to be inferior to that of Group 3 or the control group. Preparation success was also highest for Group 3. Group 1 showed a statistically significant increase in the variability of attenuation of the tagged regions. It was concluded that nonionic iodinated contrast material combined with a hyperosmotic laxative (magnesium citrate) was associated with the best qualitative and quantitative scores for readability.

REFERENCES

1. Pickhardt PJ. Translucency rendering in 3D endoluminal CT Colonography: a useful tool for increasing polyp specificity and decreasing interpretation time. *AJR Am J Roentgenol*. 2004;183:429–436.
2. O'Connor SD, Summers RM, Choi RC et al. Oral contrast adherence to polyps on CT Colonography. *J Comput Assist Tomogr*. 2006;30:51–57.
3. Fletcher JG, Johnson CD, Welch TJ, et al. Optimization of CT colonography technique: prospective trial in 180 patients. *Radiology*. 2000;216:704–711.
4. Thomeer M, Carbone I, Bosmans H, et al. Stool tagging applied in thin-slice multidetector computed tomography colonography. *J Comput Assist Tomogr*. 2003;27:132–139.
5. Lefere PA, Gryspeerdt SS, Dewyspelaere J, et al. Dietary fecal tagging as a cleansing method before CT colonography: initial results: polyp detection and patient acceptance. *Radiology*. 2002;224:393–403.
6. Gryspeerdt S, Lefere P, Dewyspelaere M, et al. Optimisation of colon cleansing prior to computed tomographic colonography. *JBR-BTR*. 2002;85:289–296.
7. Gryspeerdt S, Lefere P, Herman M, et al. CT colonography with fecal tagging after incomplete colonoscopy. *Eur J Radiol*. 2005;15:1192–1202.
8. Lefere P, Gryspeerdt S, Marrannes J, et al. CT colonography after fecal cleansing and a reduced volume of barium. *AJR Am J Roentgenol*. 2005;184:1836–1842.
9. Pickhardt PJ, Choi R, Hwang I, et al. Computed tomographic virtual colonoscopy to screen for colorectal neoplasia in asymptomatic adults. *N Engl J Med*. 2003;349:2191–2200.
10. www.acrin.org/6664_protocol.html. Accessed Jan 5, 2007.
11. Callstrom MR, Johnson CD, Fletcher JG, et al. CT colonography without cathartic preparation: feasibility study. *Radiology*. 2001;219:693–698.
12. Lefere P, Gryspeerdt S, Baekelandt M, et al. Laxative-free CT colonography. *AJR Am J Roentgenol*. 2004;183:945–948.
13. Dachman AH, Dawson DO, Lefere P, et al. Comparison of routine and unprepped CT colonography augmented by low fiber diet and stool tagging: a pilot study. *Abdom Imaging*. 2007;32:96–104.
14. Bielen D, Thomeer M, Vanbeckevoort D, et al. Dry preparation for virtual CT colonography with fecal tagging using water-soluble contrast medium: initial results. *Eur J Radiol*. 2003;13:453–458.
15. Iannaccone R, Laghi A, Catalano C, et al. Computed tomographic colonography without cathartic preparation for the detection of colorectal polyps. *Gastroenterology*. 2004; 127:1300–1311.
16. Sheppard DG, Iyer RB, Herron D, et al. Subtraction CT colonography: feasibility in an animal model. *Clin Radiol*. 1999;54:126–132.
17. Zalis ME, Hahn PF. Digital subtraction bowel cleansing in CT colonography. *AJR Am J Roentgenol*. 2001;176:646–648.
18. Zalis ME, Perumpillichira JJ, Del Frate C, et al. CT colonography: digital subtraction bowel cleansing with mucosal reconstruction- initial observations. *Radiology*. 2003; 226:911–917.
19. Johnson KT, Carston MJ, Wentz RJ, et al. Development of a cathartic-free colorectal cancer screening test using virtual colonoscopy: a feasibility study. *AJR Am J Roentgenol*. 2007;188:29–36.
20. Zalis ME, Perumpillichira JJ, Magee C, et al. Tagging-based, electronically cleansed CT colonography: evaluation of patient comfort and image readability. *Radiology*. 2006; 239:149–159.

CHAPTER 11 COMPUTER-AIDED DETECTION

Judy Yee

Computer-aided detection (CAD) has been predominantly applied to mammography for the detection of breast cancer. The first CAD products approved by the U.S. Food and Drug Administration (FDA) in the United States were for mammography.[1] Since then CAD has been applied to chest radiographs and computed tomography (CT) images for lung nodule detection. CAD of polyps and cancer on computed tomographic colonography (CTC) has also been demonstrated to be feasible and useful.

CAD for CTC has the potential to decrease interpretation time, which is important as this test is increasingly disseminated as a clinical tool and the volume of CTC studies increases. CAD also has the potential to improve both the sensitivity and specificity of CTC. Missed lesions due to human perceptual error may be detected using CAD. False positives may be excluded based on lack of detection by CAD. The variable performance of CTC in clinical trials is in part due to differences in reader experience and CAD can help to reduce inter-reader variability. The actual improvement in performance with the use of CAD likely will depend upon individual reader experience, the CT scan parameters used and the adequacy of colonic cleansing and distention.

CAD for CTC relies on three general steps: (a) segmentation of the colon from the three-dimensional (3D) data set; (b) detection of the polyp candidates; and (c) reducing false positives. CAD software typically generates a list of potential lesions with their locations that is displayed to the reader for review in order of likelihood of being a true lesion based on preset parameters. Various image displays are available that include different 2D (two dimensional) and 3D views with polyp candidates marked on them (see Figures 11.1 to 11.4). CAD interpretation schemes include its use as a primary reader and as a secondary reader. Many reviewers will interpret the entire CTC data set and then use CAD as a secondary reader to determine if there were additional lesions not detected initially. Some CAD software allow displays for concurrent interpretation of the CTC data set, which is placed adjacent to the same data set with marked potential lesions.

CAD algorithms are being evaluated using combined supine and prone image data sets to help find true polyps and to decrease the number of false positives.[2,3] Integration of CAD with tagged data sets combined with electronic cleansing is being explored as perhaps the most time-efficient and accurate method for interpretation.[4–7]

COMPUTER-AIDED DETECTION TECHNIQUES AND FEASIBILITY STUDIES

Various prototypes of CAD schemes have been developed for the detection of polyps and masses on CTC. Some algorithms extract the colonic wall surface and determine local variations in the curvature of the surface to identify polyps.[8–16] Other algorithms are based on a contour normal technique that is based on the directions of normal vectors from air to soft tissue.[17–20] These two techniques have shown high sensitivity for polyp detection but with a high false-positive rate. Still other algorithms extract a much thicker region of the colonic wall, which includes the entire polyp to decrease the number of false positives.[21–23] 3D geometric features such as volumetric shape index and curvedness may then be used to help distinguish between polyps and folds or colon wall to further improve sensitivity. Internal features of polyps may be used to help decrease the number of false positives and improve specificity.

Blake et al. evaluated the performance of a CAD algorithm for measurement of the largest linear dimension and the volume of simulated polyps in a phantom.[24] Twenty spherical and hemispherical simulated polyps within a Plexiglas phantom ranging in size between 6 mm and 25 mm were scanned using four-channel MDCT at 1.3-mm slice thickness, 0.6-mm reconstruction interval, 100 mAs (high dose), and 30 mAs (low dose). The inner surface of the phantom was derived from the CT data to calculate the maximum length and volume of each polyp. Seed filling of the lumen allowed identification of the tessellated surface between the air in the lumen and the simulated polyps. Results showed that the CAD software provided accurate measurements. Mean error for length

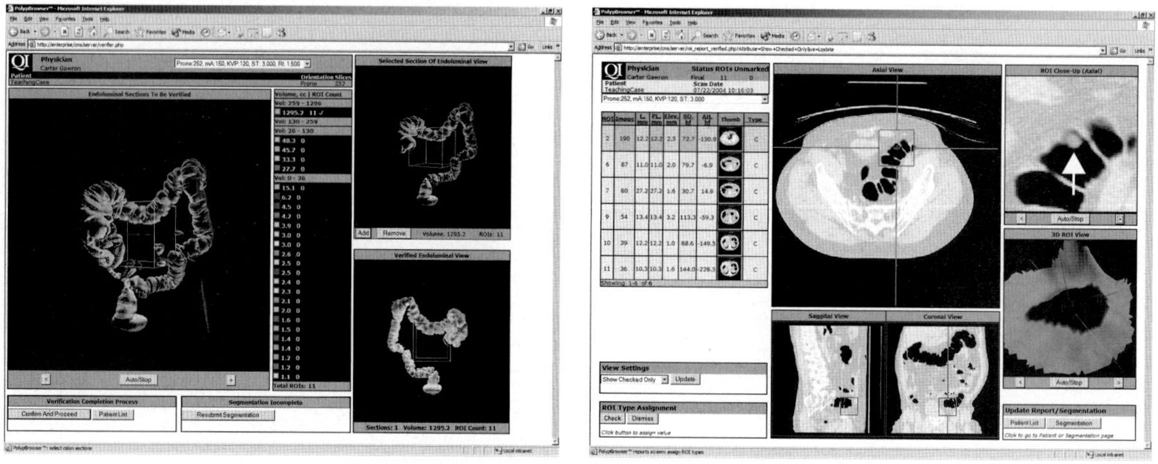

FIGURE 11.1 CAD for CTC first segments the colon from the 3D data set **(A)**. The CAD system then automatically identifies, measures, and characterizes polyp candidates and they are organized into a list of decreasing order of likelihood **(B)**. The display also includes axial, magnified axial, sagittal and coronal multiplanar images, and 3D view of the polyp candidate. (Views A and B: See also color plate.)

measurements for both spheres and hemispheres was 2%. Mean error for volume measurements was 3% for spheres and 5% for hemispheres.

Nappi et al. evaluated region-based supine-prone correspondence of CTC data sets to help reduce false positives.[2] The colon was extracted from the original CT data set by using an automated centerline-based colon segmentation method. Up to six landmarks were established for each data set and a region-growing scheme was used to divide the colon lumen into overlapping segments that matched in the supine and prone data sets. Polyp candidates detected by CAD were eliminated if contained in only one of the data sets of a patient. This method was evaluated in 121 CTC studies and results showed that there was partial or complete correspondence in 71% of cases. The sensitivity for polyp detection was 91% and there was a 19% reduction in false positives. It was concluded that supine and prone correlation of data sets can improve the specificity of CAD in CTC. Other methods for establishing supine and prone correspondence have been based on colon centerlines.[13]

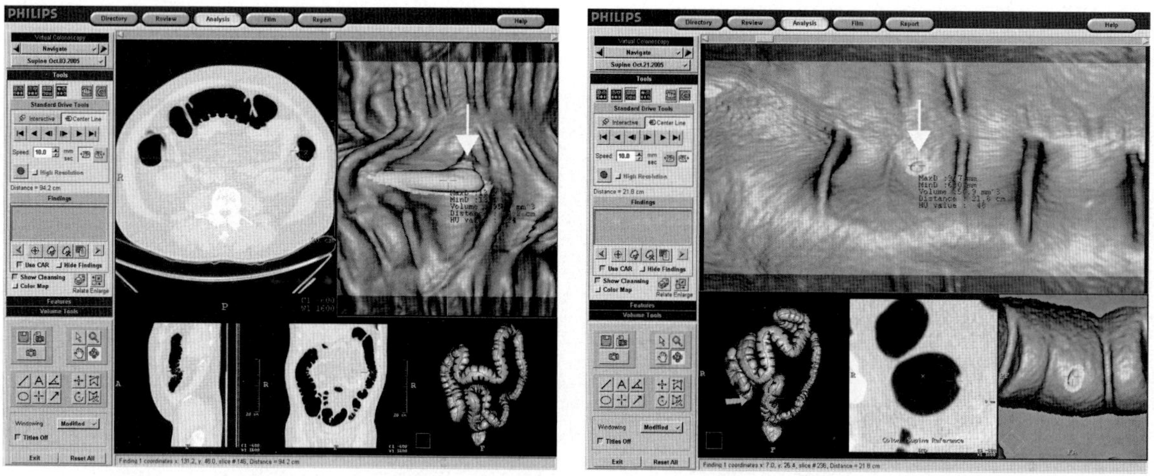

FIGURE 11.2 CAD algorithm integrated into CTC software with various image display options. A large polyp is identified in the descending colon of the first patient using a display that includes the axial image, dissection view, sagittal and coronal multiplanar reformats, and colon overview. **A:** A small polyp is detected in the sigmoid colon of the second patient using a display that includes dissection views, magnified axial view and the colon overview. **B:** Note that the CAD system provides measurements of polyp candidates automatically. (Views A and B: See also color plate.)

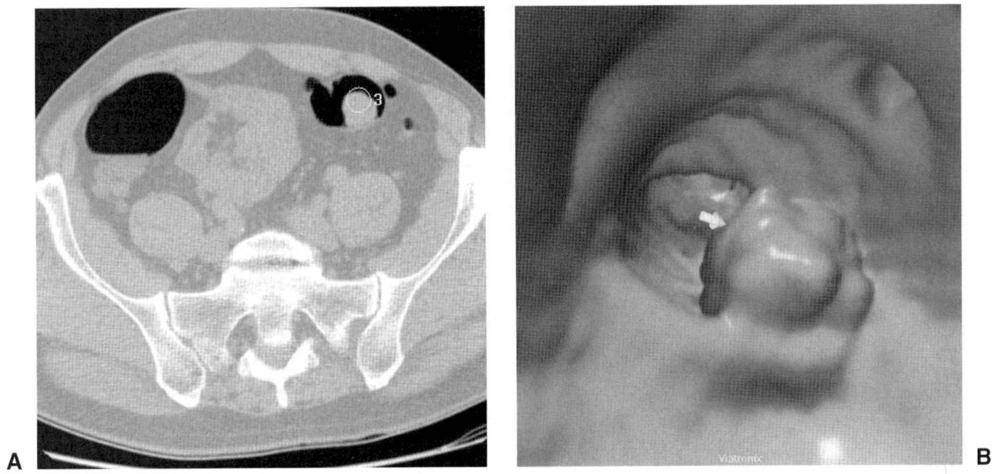

FIGURE 11.3 Large Polyp. CAD identification of a large polyp on axial **(A)** and 3D endoluminal view **(B)**.

Surface Curvature

CAD algorithms have been developed for CTC that delineate the surface of the colon wall and then polyp candidates are detected using shape criteria to determine variations in the surface curvature. The colon wall is characterized by computing its minimum, maximum, mean, and Gaussian curvatures. Additional restrictive criteria such as sphericity are then applied to exclude nonspherical shapes. The surface curvature method typically generates a small number of false positives but may have a lower sensitivity for polyp detection relative to other methods.

Summers et al. initially evaluated the surface curvature method for CTC using ten simulated colon polyps inserted into an abdominal CT scan.[8] Polyp detection was performed using a prototype detector that identified areas of the colon wall with abnormal shape. The shape-based polyp detector using a primary shape criterion of elliptic curvature of the peak subtype was able to locate six of the ten polyps. With edge profile enhancement eight of ten polyps were detected and there were no false positives. This study showed that shape analysis of colon polyps is technically feasible on CTC. A follow-up study by Summers et al. used the same shape-based algorithm measuring local variations in surface curvature but with additional filters to study 20 patients with 50 known polyps.[9] The algorithm detected lesions that protruded into the colonic lumen. The filters were additional shape criteria that included mean curvature, dimensionless ratio sphericity, and minimum polyp size. The sensitivity for detecting polyps 10 mm or larger was 64% (18/28 polyps) which increased to 71% (10/14 polyps) when considering only well-distended segments. There was a mean of six false positives per colon, which was decreased to 3.5 per

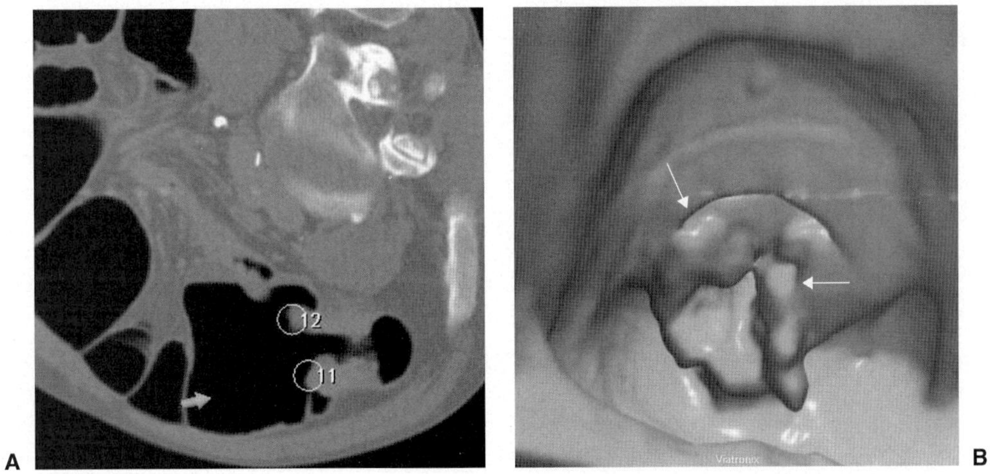

FIGURE 11.4 Carcinoma. CAD identification of a large annular carcinoma with overhanging edges on the axial image **(A)** with two separate marks. This lesion was also identified by CAD on the 3D endoluminal view with several marks **(B)**.

colon after sampling CT scan attenuation at lesion sites and discarding those lesions having an attenuation less than the threshold.

Various classifiers such as support vector machines (SVM) that use sphericity individually or with other features have been evaluated to improve sensitivity and decrease false positives generated by CAD systems.[10] Polyp segmentation based on fuzzy clustering and deformable models have also been applied to CAD to reduce false positives and to provide volumetric features for polyp classification.[11] Polyp surface shape has been evaluated by using lines of curvature to detect polyps rather than using scalar curvature of the colon wall which may cause more false positives.[12] The internal features of polyps have been used in conjunction with surface shape-based measures for colon CAD.[13] After the initial polyp candidates are identified, an ellipsoid model is placed in the lesion and the geometric and CT scan density features are extracted to help decrease false-positive detections.

Hong et al. developed a novel pipeline for CAD of colon polyps that integrates texture and shape analysis with volume rendering and conformal colon flattening.[14] After the colon surface is extracted from the CT data set, it is mapped from 3D to 2D using conformal mapping. The flattened image undergoes volume rendering and polyps are detected using a 2D clustering method. This technique is proposed to be more efficient (8 minutes to run CAD) compared to shape-based CAD methods because there is no need to compute curvature for the entire colon surface. Volumetric shape and texture features are used to reduce false positives. Using this technique 88 data sets with 123 polyps were analyzed. The sensitivity for polyp detection was 100% with approximately three false positives per data set.

Other strategies in addition to these initial shape-based algorithms have been used to reduce the number of false-positive detections such as due to the ileocecal valve and rectal catheter. Summers et al. evaluated 60 patients who underwent CTC and image analysis was performed using a CAD algorithm and an ileocecal valve recognition algorithm.[15] The thresholds used to successfully identify the ileocecal valve were a mean internal CT scan attenuation of <-124 Hounsfield Units and a volume of >1.5 cm^3. Lordanescu et al. employed a three-stage scheme to identify the rectal tube to eliminate it as a cause of false positives on CTC in 80 data sets.[16] This scheme consisted of detecting the rectal tube shaft, tracking the tube to the tip, and labeling all the voxels belonging to the rectal tube. The algorithm detected 90% of rectal tube shafts and completely tracked 72% of them. There was a 7.9% decrease in the number of false positives generated by the CAD system.

Surface Normal

A novel CAD algorithm called the *surface normal overlap method* has been applied to colon polyp detection and lung nodule detection by Paik et al.[17] The surface normal overlap method typically has a high detection rate for polyps but can generate more false positives. This method is based on the fact that normal vectors on the colon surface intersect with normals on nearby surfaces depending on the specific curvature features of the colon. Polyps have 3D shape features of a sphere and therefore have a high vector intersection concentration. Haustral folds tend to have less surface normal convergence than polyps due to their cylindrical shape. This algorithm was evaluated in eight patients who had 7 polyps 10 mm or larger and 11 polyps between 5 and 9 mm. A sensitivity of 100% was achieved for polyps 10 mm or larger, with seven false positives/colon. As the threshold was modified to decrease the number of false positives, the sensitivity for polyp detection also decreased. There was a sensitivity of 80% for large polyps with 4.6 false positives/colon. An analysis of the causes of false positives using this method revealed that 86% were due to haustral folds and 5% were due to the colon wall between adjacent loops. Less common causes of false positives were stool, rectal catheter, small bowel, and the ileocecal valve.

On the basis of the work of Paik et al., methods have been developed to help decrease false positives. Gokturk et al. applied a statistical approach using SVM for polyp identification.[18] Random orthogonal shape section was initially employed for 3D pattern processing that combined information from multiple random images to generate reliable signatures of shape and then fed these signatures to an SVM classifier for the final diagnosis. Using this approach there was a 50% increase in specificity at a constant sensitivity level. Acar et al. applied edge displacement fields to decrease false positives generated by CAD of CTC data sets and reported a 23% increase in specificity without compromising sensitivity.[19] The method simulates the way a radiologist recognizes a polyp although scrolling a cross-sectional plane through 3D CT scan data by quantifying the change in the location of edges in the 2D plane.

Sphere fitting is a method that has been employed for CTC where polyps are modeled as spherical patches. Polyp candidates are detected as sphere center clusters located in close vicinity. Folds have a cylindrical shape and their centers are spread along a line. Kiss et al. used a combination of surface normal and sphere fitting methods in a study of 18 patients with 20 polyps.[20] The sensitivity for 10 mm or larger polyps was 100% (10/10) but generated a large number of false positives (eight/case). However, if considering only the false positives for 10 mm or larger then there was a decrease to 1.9/case. The causes of false positives using this technique were colonic wall (46%), haustral folds (32%), residual stool (12%), rectal tube (7%), and the ileocecal valve (3%).

Volumetric Shape Index and Curvedness

A CAD scheme that extracts thick regions encompassing the entire colonic wall from the CT data set was developed by Yoshida et al.[21] Potential lesions are identified by using 3D geometric features called shape index and curvedness to characterize polyps, folds, and colonic wall. The volumetric shape index determines the topology of voxels and color coding is applied based on the topology. Polyps typically are bulbous and cap-like whereas folds are long and ridge-like. Volumetric curvedness represents how gently curved a structure is. Polyps have medium curvedness values whereas folds have large curvedness values. Conditional morphologic dilatation is used to extract the entire polyp. False-positive detections are decreased by analyzing the internal volumetric features of the polyp candidates.

Yoshida et al. performed a pilot study evaluating this CAD scheme on 82 data sets (41 cases) containing 18 polyps (six were 5 to 9 mm, three were 10 mm).[22] Following colon extraction as a thick contiguous layer from the volume of data, topologic shape and effective curvature were used for polyp detection. Using a per patient analysis, 89% (16/18) of polyps were detected with only two false positives/data set. Each of the two missed lesions was detected in the opposing position and therefore 100% of polyps were detected with 2.5 false positives/patient. Types of false positives by CAD were similar to those due to radiologist's perception and included prominent folds (30%), adjacent small intestine and stomach (19%), ileocecal valve (14%), residual stool (13%), rectal tube (10%), flexural pseudotumor (6%), motion artifact (3%), anorectal junction (3%), and extrinsic compression (3%).

Gradient concentration is added to decrease false positives. This technique quantifies the concentration of gradient orientations of the CT scan values within a polyp candidate and helps to differentiate polyps from folds and stool. The gradient vectors converge to a point deep in the center of a polyp whereas they converge to a line in a fold. Stool tends to be heterogeneous internally and causes gradient vectors to be directed randomly. Yoshida et al. reported performance of this CAD scheme in a study evaluating 43 patients with 12 polyps measuring 5 mm or larger.[23] Nine polyps measured between 5 and 10 mm and three polyps were >10 mm. A knowledge-guided technique was used that segments the colonic wall at a thickness of 3 to 4 mm and helps to exclude most of the extracolonic components from the segmented colon. The CAD scheme resulted in 95% sensitivity with 1.2 false positives/data set or 100% sensitivity with 2.0 false positives/data set.

COMPUTER-AIDED DETECTION PERFORMANCE

Multiple studies have been performed evaluating the sensitivity and specificity of various CAD systems for CTC. Most of the published studies have compared the performance of CAD with the performance of radiologists for colonic lesion detection. Fewer studies have evaluated the improvement in sensitivity achieved with the use of CAD as a secondary reader for CTC.

The performance of CAD using the surface curvature method has been tested in patient data sets. Summers et al. evaluated 40 patients using CTC. Twenty patients had 65 lesions with 25 polyps measuring 10 mm or larger.[25] The CTC data sets were interpreted by using a CAD algorithm based on surface curvature and by two radiologists. The sensitivity for detection of 10 mm or larger polyps was 48% (12/25) by at least one radiologist and was the same using the CAD system. However, CAD detected 4/13 large polyps that were not detected by either radiologist increasing the potential sensitivity to 64%. Sensitivity of the combination of detection with the CAD algorithm or by at least one radiologist was 89%. There was poor specificity with an average of 11 false positives/patient using CAD.

Summers et al. evaluated a similar CAD scheme in a large study of 792 patients who underwent CTC using fecal and fluid tagging with electronic subtraction of the labeled material.[26] Patients also underwent bowel cleansing with 90 mL of sodium phosphate and 10 mg of bisacodyl. The per-polyp and per-patient sensitivities for CAD based on retrospective review were both 89% (25/28) for the detection of adenomatous polyps measuring 10 mm or larger with 2.1 false positives/patient. The per-polyp sensitivity for CAD was 81% (42/52) and the per-patient sensitivity was 87% (41/47) for the detection of adenomatous polyps measuring 8 mm or larger with 6.7 false positives/patient. There were two carcinomas and both were detected by CAD with a false-positive rate of 0.7/patient. None of the five flat polyps were detected by CAD. The sensitivity of CAD in this study was not significantly different compared with that of radiologists. It was also found that for 6 mm or larger polyps, CAD sensitivity was lower for sessile polyps compared to pedunculated polyps and for polyps located on a fold versus polyps not on a fold.

CAD using the surface normal method was evaluated by Shi et al. in 36 subjects.[27] The goal of this study was to determine whether 3D viewing improves radiologists' accuracy in classifying true-positive and false-positive polyp candidates found on CAD. Forty-seven data sets were presented to four readers with 37 data sets containing at least one polyp. There were 6 polyps measuring 10 mm or larger and 23 polyps measuring 5 to 9.9 mm. Initially, only 2D images were used, but these were later supplemented with 3D views. Results showed that 3D images improved classification accuracy for three readers. Polyp size and examination quality were found to be significantly associated with accuracy. For true-positive candidates, maximum polyp width, polyp height, and preparation significantly affected accuracy. For false-positive candidates, colonic segment, attenuation, surface smoothness, distention, preparation, and true nature of candidate lesions significantly affected accuracy.

Mani et al. evaluated the feasibility of using CAD based on the surface normal method as the "first reader" in CTC.[28] In the first phase of this study, the performance of three radiologists who interpreted 41 CTC studies without CAD was recorded. In the second phase of the study, readers interpreted the same cases using a CAD list of 30 possible polyps. Results showed that the average sensitivity for the unassisted readers for the detection of polyps measuring 10 mm or larger was 63% compared to the sensitivity of 74% with the use of CAD. The per-patient analysis for the detection of large polyps showed a trend for increased sensitivity from 73% without CAD to 90% with CAD without a decrease in specificity. The average time to detection of the first polyp decreased significantly with the use of CAD whereas the total reading time was unchanged. It was concluded that CAD used as a first reader achieved similar per-polyp and per-patient sensitivities for polyp detection compared to unassisted readings. CAD was able to decrease interobserver variability.

CAD using volumetric shape index and curvedness was evaluated by Yoshida et al. who retrospectively studied 71 patients who underwent CTC and colonoscopy on the same day.[29] There were 14 patients with 15 polyps measuring 5 to 9 mm and 6 polyps measuring 10 mm or larger. CAD was applied to the data sets and resulted in 100% sensitivity with 2.0 false positives per patient using per-patient analysis and 90% sensitivity with 2.0 false positives per patient using per-polyp analysis. The authors noted that lesions that are flat or cigar shaped may not be detected or may be eliminated as a false-positive finding with the CAD scheme.

Bogoni et al. evaluated a proprietary CAD algorithm for CTC (ColonCAD; Siemens) that incorporates features based on tissue intensity, volumetric, and surface shape as well as texture characteristics.[30] Sixty-two data sets were used to test the CAD system after training the algorithm with 88 separate cases. Of the 39 polyps 18 were small, 11 were medium, and 10 were large in size. Results showed sensitivities for small, medium, and large polyp detection as 67%, 82%, and 100% respectively. The sensitivity for detecting polyps 5 mm or larger was 91%. The median false positive rate was 3 per volume.

In a study by Halligan et al., ten untrained radiologists interpreted 107 CTC cases (60 patients with 142 polyps) first without CAD and then with CAD (ColonCAR; Medicsight PLC) separated by an interval of 2 months to reduce recall bias.[31] The CAD system extracted the colon surface using a thresholding-based method and a mathematical algorithm was applied that detected protruding endoluminal objects. A sphericity filter was then used to determine polyp candidates that were presented to the reader. Following initial training of the CAD system with separate cases, a sphericity value of 0.75 was chosen for the validation phase because it identified 85% of polyps measuring 5 mm or larger with an average false positive rate of 33. With CAD 68% (41/60) of patients with polyps were identified more frequently by readers. There was no change in 18% (11/60) and 13% (8/60) were identified less frequently. There was a significant improvement in sensitivity for patients with polyps in 70% (7/10) of readers with the use of CAD. On average, 12 (9%) more polyps were detected with CAD assistance with the benefit observed due to additional medium and small polyps identified. Overall performance was suboptimal and even with CAD the average sensitivities for the detection of polyps 6 mm or larger and polyps 10 mm or larger were 38% and 51% respectively. Interpretation time decreased significantly with CAD by 1.9 minutes in patients with polyps and by 2.9 minutes for patients without polyps. It was concluded that CAD for CTC significantly increased per-patient and per-polyp detection rates and decreased interpretation times but cannot substitute for adequate reader training in CTC.

Taylor et al. performed a study comparing the sensitivity of computer-assisted reader (CAR) software with that of three expert readers using 25 cases containing 32 polyps ranging in size from 6 to 35 mm.[32] Thirteen of the cases used stool and fluid tagging. In this version of the software (ColonCAR version 1.2; Medicsight PLC) polyp candidates are highlighted for the reader at the time of primary interpretation rather than being used as a secondary reader. Polyp detection filters may also be interactively modified by the reader depending upon the case being evaluated so that there may be a trade off of decreased sensitivity for diminutive polyps in exchange for improved specificity. Therefore, the software allows filter adjustments based on various parameters that may affect performance such as CT technique, the use of tagging, and adequacy of cleansing and distention. CAR identified 81% (26/32) polyps compared with an average sensitivity of 70% for the expert readers. CAR detected 92% (11/12) polyps measuring 10 mm or larger. Almost all polyps that were missed by the three readers were detected by CAR. There was a median of 13 false positives per case, although only 9% of false positives actually required further investigation. It was also noted that significantly more false positives were generated on tagged cases compared to untagged cases (median of 16 vs. 8) and that most of the false positives were located at the fluid–air interface.

COMPUTER-AIDED DETECTION PITFALLS

Causes of false-positive detections generated by CAD systems are typically structures with a polypoid shape. The frequency with which each of these pitfalls occurs may vary depending on the specific CAD system. Common causes of false positives using CAD are various types of haustral folds (45%).[33] Specific folds that may appear polypoid are flexural pseudotumors that are sharp or bulbous folds occurring in the sigmoid or colonic flexures. Additionally converging folds or thickened folds in a poorly distended colon may be pitfalls when using CAD (see Figure 11.5). Residual stool can appear polypoid and are a common cause (20%) of false positives using

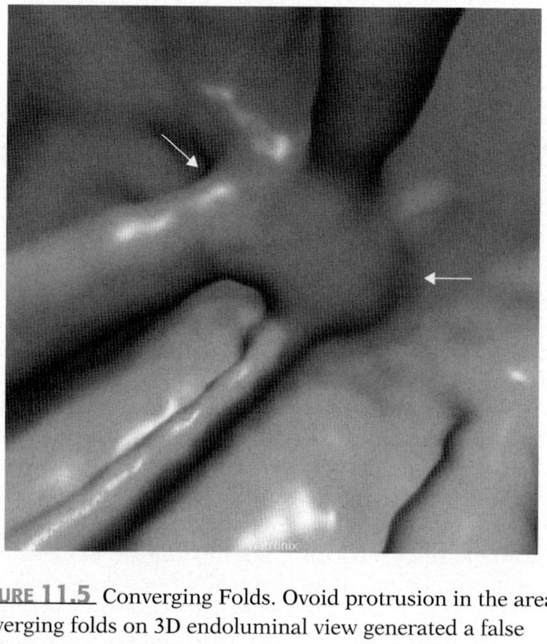

FIGURE 11.5 Converging Folds. Ovoid protrusion in the area of converging folds on 3D endoluminal view generated a false positive using a CAD system.

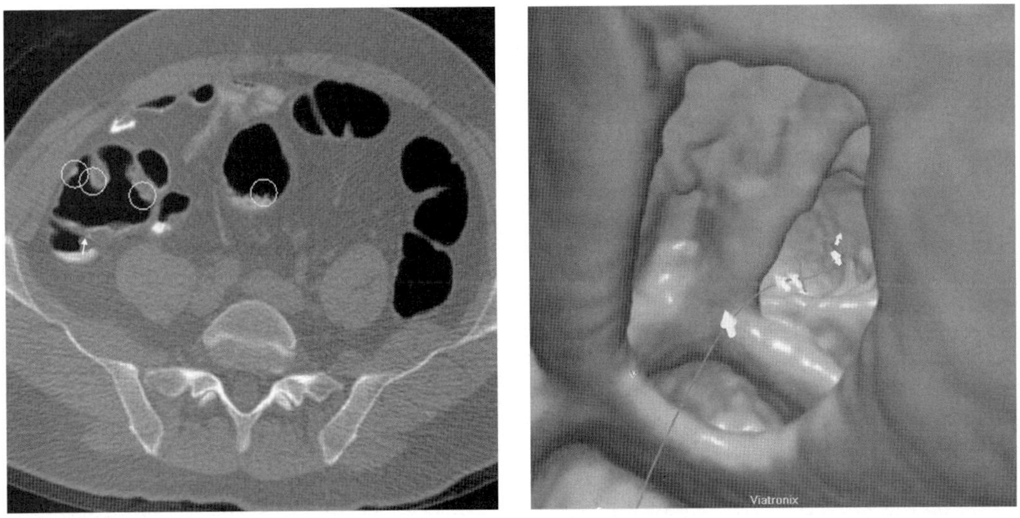

A B

FIGURE 11.6 Residual Stool. CAD identifies multiple polyp candidates with false positives due to residual stool on axial **(A)** and 3D endoluminal view **(B)**.

CAD although comparison of supine and prone views to assess mobility can help determine a true lesion (see Figure 11.6). Residual material located in the stomach and small bowel may generate false positives (15%) on CAD systems. Approximately 10% of false positives are due to the ileocecal valve, which has a polypoid appearance although the typical location and appearance can help to easily discount this as a real polyp (see Figure 11.7). Less common causes of false positives on CAD include the rectal tube, elevation of the anorectal junction by the rectal tube, and motion artifacts. Various strategies have been developed to address false-positive detections on CAD due to the ileocecal valve and the rectal tube.[15,16]

COMPUTER-AIDED DETECTION AND TAGGING

Stool and fluid tagging with oral contrast agents followed by electronic subtraction of the tagged material may help to decrease the need for purgative bowel cleansing. Reduced colonic cleansing tends to leave increased amounts of residual material that may be incompletely tagged and can be a source of false positives on CAD systems. Additionally electronic subtraction of tagged stool and fluid can leave artifacts that may also be a source of false positives. These postsubtraction artifacts tend to occur at the air–fluid interface along the colonic wall.[34]

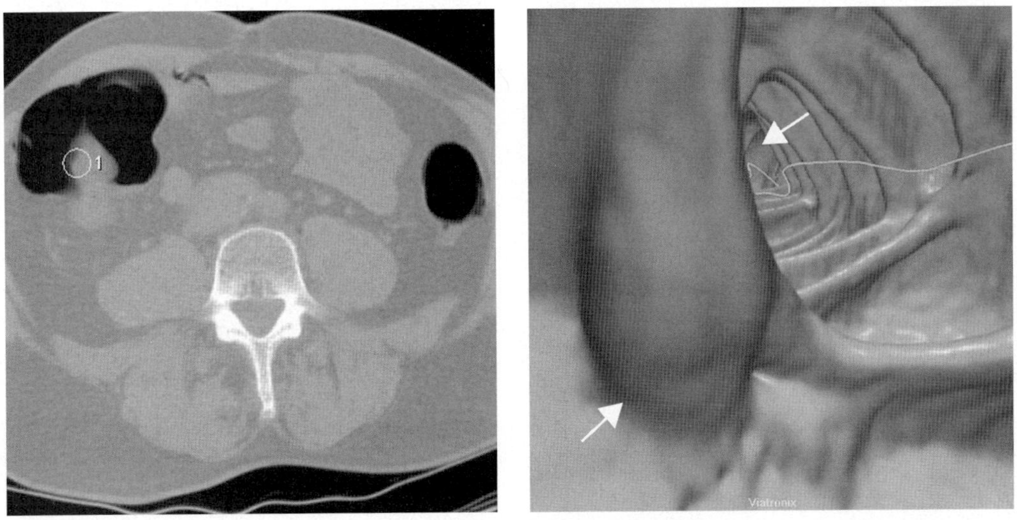

A B

FIGURE 11.7 Ileocecal Valve. CAD identifies the ileocecal valve as a polyp candidate on the axial **(A)** and 3D endoluminal view **(B)**. The reader can easily exclude this as a polyp based on the characteristic location and appearance of the ileocecal valve. The terminal ileum can be traced into the valve on the axial view.

Investigation is under way to evaluate and modify CAD systems using tagged CTC cases.

Summers et al. performed a pilot study evaluating a modified CAD system for polyp detection in 17 tagged CTC cases.[4] Patients underwent CTC following bowel cleansing with 90 mL of sodium phosphate and bisacodyl. Stool and fluid tagging were achieved by the ingestion of 500 mL of 2.1% barium and 120 mL of diatrizoate meglumine and diatrizoate sodium. Colon segmentation was performed followed by electronic subtraction of the tagged material. The CAD system was modified to detect polyps submerged in tagged fluid. Six of 22 polyps were located at the air–fluid interface and 86% (19/22) of polyps were identified by the modified CAD system. This pilot study showed that a modified CAD system can effectively detect polyps submerged in opacified fluid as well as lesions located at the air–fluid boundary.

Dehmeshki et al. modified a CAD system for CTC by changing sphericity filter values and compared tagged and untagged cases.[6] CTC was performed on 138 patients with 317 polyps who were divided into a tagged group (86) and an untagged group (52). Results showed that sensitivity was highest at low sphericity. Sensitivity for detection of polyps 6 mm or larger was 88% (144/164) and sensitivity for detection polyps 10 mm or larger was 95% (40/42) at a sphericity of 0.3. There was no difference in sensitivity for tagged and untagged cases although specificity was decreased in tagged cases at low sphericity. The number of false positives detected by the CAD system is directly impacted by the use of tagging.

Nappi et al. developed a modified CAD system using adaptive density correction (ADC) and adaptive density mapping (ADM).[2] ADC was used to minimize pseudoenhancement and ADM was used to minimize the presence of tagged material. Pseudoenhancement occurs because of the tagging agents that can artificially elevate the attenuation of polyps to >500 HU whereas polyps on untagged cases typically measure <100 HU. A new method for automated extraction of the colon wall within air-filled and tagged regions was also developed. Group 1 consisted of 32 CTC cases of patients who underwent full cathartic cleansing and Group 2 consisted of 32 CTC cases of patients who had reduced cleansing. The sensitivity of the CAD system for the detection of polyps 10 mm or larger was 94% for Group 1 with 3.6 false positives per scan and 100% for Group 2 with 4.2 false positives per scan. The modified CAD system had a 20% higher detection sensitivity compared to the conventional CAD scheme.

An alternative approach for colon CAD is the use of intravenous contrast. Luboldt et al. performed a pilot study evaluating CAD of CTC performed following the administration of 120 mL of intravenous contrast at a flow rate of 4 mL per second and a 35-second scan delay.[7] A value of 90 HU was used as the threshold for segmentation of lesions. This study showed that attenuation-based segmentation of enhancing polyps is possible although limited by insufficient enhancement of some masses.

FUTURE CHALLENGES FOR COMPUTER-AIDED DETECTION

Various CAD systems have been developed. Common challenges remain for most CAD systems that need to be addressed.[35,36] The optimal CAD system should be able to achieve high sensitivity and specificity. However, for most CAD systems there is a trade-off between sensitivity and specificity so that high sensitivity is associated with more false positives. Cancers that infiltrate the colon wall and do not protrude into the lumen may not be detected using current CAD systems. Additionally flat lesions are difficult to detect using shape-based CAD algorithms. Low-dose CT scanning techniques tend to produce noisy images and may affect the ability of CAD systems to detect lesions. The coregistration of supine and prone CT scan data sets could aid CAD systems to decrease false positives and further evaluation of this strategy is needed. Finally CAD algorithms need to be fully integrated into workstations used for CTC interpretation to facilitate efficient clinical workflow.

SUMMARY

CAD for CTC has been proved to be technically feasible and CAD systems are now available for clinical use. The role of CAD for detecting colonic lesions on CTC will likely be similar to its role in mammography where it is predominantly used as a second reader. The CAD system serves as an alert to the reader by highlighting lesion candidates that might have been overlooked during the initial read. Various CAD methods that have been used for CTC include surface curvature, surface normal, and sphere fitting methods. Geometric features such as volumetric shape index and curvedness have allowed high sensitivity and specificity for polyp detection. Existing CAD algorithms continue to be refined and large clinical trials evaluating the performance of CAD both without and with stool and fluid tagging (which may be combined with electronic subtraction) will be helpful for determining adequacy of this technique in various settings.

REFERENCES

1. Erickson BJ, Bartholmai B. Computer-aided detection and diagnosis at the start of the third millennium. *J Digit Imaging*. 2002;15:59–68.
2. Nappi J, Okamura A, Frimmel H, et al. Region-based supine-prone correspondence for the reduction of false-positive CAD polyp candidates in CT colonography. *Acad Radiol*. 2005;12:695–707.
3. Li P, Hapel S, Acar B, et al. Registration of central paths and colonic polyps between supine and prone scans in computed tomography: pilot study. *Med Phys*. 2004;31:12–23.
4. Summers RM, Franaszek M, Miller MT, et al. Computer-aided detection of polyps on oral contrast-enhanced CT colonography. *AJR Am J Roentgenol*. 2005;18:105–108.

5. Nappi J, Yoshida H. Fully automated three-dimensional detection of polyps in fecal-Tagging CT Colonography. *Acad Radiol*. 2007;14:287–300.
6. Dehmeshki J, Halligan S, Taylor SA, et al. Computer assisted detection software for CT Colonography: effect of sphericity filter on performance characteristics for patients with and without fecal tagging. *Eur Radiol*. 2007;17:662–668.
7. Luboldt W, Mann C, Tryon CL, et al. Computer-aided diagnosis in contrast-enhanced CT colonography: an approach based on contrast. *Eur J Radiol*. 2002;12(9):2236–2241.
8. Summers RM, Beaulieu CF, Pusanik LM, et al. Automated polyp detector for CT colonography: feasibility study. *Radiology*. 2000;216:284–290.
9. Summers RM, Johnson CD, Pusanik LM, et al. Automated polyp detection at CT colonography: feasibility study in a human population. *Radiology*. 2001;219:51–59.
10. Jerebko AK, Mailey JD, Franaszek M, et al. Support vector machines committee classification method for computer-aided polyp detection in CT colonography. *Acad Radiol*. 2005; 12:479–486.
11. Yao J, Miller M, Franaszek M, et al. Colonic segmentation in CT colonography-based on fuzzy clustering and deformable models. *IEE Trans Med Imaging*. 2004;23:1344–1352.
12. Zhao L, Botha CP, Bescos JO, et al. Lines of curvature for polyp detection in virtual colonoscopy. *IEEE Trans Vis Comput Graph*. 2006;12:885–892.
13. Wang Z, Liang Z, Li L, et al. Reduction of false positives by internal features for polyp detection in CT-based virtual colonoscopy. *Med Phys*. 2005;32:3602–3616.
14. Hong W, Qiu F, Kaufman A. A pipeline for computer aided polyp detection. *IEEE Trans Vis Comput Graph*. 2006;12: 861–868.
15. Summers RM, Yao J, Johnson CD. CT colonography with computer-aided detection: automated recognition of ileocecal valve to reduce number of false-positive detections. *Radiology*. 2004;233:266–272.
16. Lordanescu G, Summers RM. Reduction of false positives on the rectal tube in computer-aided detection for CT colonography. *Med Phys*. 2004;31:2855–2862.
17. Paik DS, Beaulieu CF, Rubin GD, et al. Surface normal overlap: a computer-aided detection algorithm with application to colonic polyps and lung nodules in helical CT. *IEEE Trans Med Imaging*. 2004;23:661–675.
18. Gokturk SB, Tomasi C, Acar B, et al. A statistical 3-D pattern processing method for computer-aided detection of polyps in CT colonography. *IEEE Trans Med Imaging*. 2001;20:1251–1260.
19. Acar B, Beaulieu CF, Gokturk SB, et al. Edge displacement field-based classification for improved detection of polyps in CT colonography. *IEE Trans Med Imaging*. 2002;21: 1461–1467.
20. Kiss G, Cleynenbreugel JV, Thomeer M, et al. Computer-aided diagnosis in virtual colonography via combination of surface normal and sphere fitting methods. *Eur J Radiology*. 2002;12:77–81.
21. Yoshida H, Dachman AH. Computer-aided diagnosis for CT colonography. *Semin Ultrasound CT MR*. 2004;25:419–431.
22. Yoshida H, Masutani Y, MacEneaney P, et al. Computerized detection of colonic polyps at CT colonography on the basis of volumetric features: pilot study. *Radiology*. 2002; 222:327–336.
23. Yoshida H, Nappi J. Related three-dimensional computer-aided diagnosis scheme for detection of colonic polyps. *IEEE Trans Med Imaging*. 2001;20:1261–1274.
24. Blake ME, Soto JA, Hayes RA, et al. Automated volumetry at CT colonography: a phantom study. *Acad Radiol*. 2005; 12:608–613.
25. Summers RM, Jerebko AK, Franaszek M, et al. Colonic polyps: complementary role of computer-aided detection in CT colonography. *Radiology*. 2002;225:391–399.
26. Summers RM, Yao J, Pickhardt PJ, et al. Computed tomographic virtual colonoscopy computer-aided polyp detection in a screening population. *Gastroenterology*. 2005; 129:1832–1844.
27. Shi R, Schraedley-Desmond P, Napel S, et al. CT colonography: influence of 3D viewing and features of polyp candidate on interpretation using computer aided detection. *Radiology*. 2006;239:768–776.
28. Mani A, Napel S, Paik D, et al. CT colongraphy: feasibility of computer-aided polyp detection in a "First Reader" paradigm. *J Comput Assist Tomogr*. 2004;28:318–326.
29. Yoshida H, Nappi J, MacEneaney P, et al. Computer-aided diagnosis scheme for detection of polyps at CT colonography. *Radiographics*. 2002;22:963–979.
30. Bogoni L, Cathier P, Dundar M, et al. Computer-aided detection (CAD) for CT colonography: a tool to address a growing need. *Br J Radiol*. 2005;78:S57–S62, Spec No. 1.
31. Halligan S, Altman DG, Mallett S, et al. Computed tomographic colonography: assessment of radiologist performance with and without computer-aided detection. *Gastroenterology*. 2006;131:1690–1699.
32. Taylor SA, Halligan S, Burling D, et al. Computer-assisted reader software versus expert reviewers for polyp detection on CT colonography. *AJR Am J Roentgenol*. 2006;186: 696–702.
33. Yoshida H, Dachman AH. CAD techniques, challenges, and controversies in computed tomographic colonography. *Abdom Imaging*. 2005;30:26–41.
34. Zalis ME, Perumpillichira JJ, Del Frate C, et al. CT colonography: digital subtraction bowel cleansing with mucosal reconstruction- initial observations. *Radiology*. 2003;226: 911–917.
35. Perumpillichira JJ, Yoshida H, Sahani DV. Computer-aided detection for virtual colonoscopy. *Cancer Imaging*. 2005;5:11–16.
36. Summers RM. Challenges for computer-aided diagnosis for CT colonography. *Abdom Imaging*. 2002;27:268–274.

APPENDIX A: SAMPLE VIRTUAL COLONOSCOPY PREPARATION INSTRUCTIONS

VIRTUAL COLONOSCOPY PREPARATION INSTRUCTIONS (PLEASE READ ALL OF THE INSTRUCTIONS)

Supplies:

Make sure you have ALL of the following laxatives before starting the preparation.

1. One 10 oz bottle of magnesium citrate
2. *Four* 5 mg bisacodyl oral tablets
3. One 10 mg bisacodyl suppository (DO NOT keep this in your pocket or anywhere warm—it will melt and become unusable.)

The day before the test: (specify day and date)

Do not eat *any* solid food all day. You can *only* have clear liquids such as water, tea, coffee, juice, soda, broth, and jello.

Drink 1 glass of clear liquid each hour until bedtime. Over the course of the day, drink at least 2 quarts of liquids.

At 5:00 PM, drink 10 oz of magnesium citrate. The laxative may begin working within 30 minutes or it may take up to 3 hours.

At 7:30 PM, take *all four* 5 mg oral bisacodyl tablets with one large (8 oz) glass of water. Do not chew the tablets. Bisacodyl tablets generally produce bowel movements in 6 to 12 hours.

After midnight, do not eat or drink *anything*.

The day of the exam: (specify day and date)

Do not eat or drink *anything*.

In the morning, at least 2 hours before the time of your examination, unwrap the 10 mg bisacodyl suppository and discard the foil or wrapper. While lying on your side with your leg raised, insert the suppository into the rectum and gently push in as far as possible.

Report to the Radiology Front Desk.

Just before CT scan, check that your rectum is empty by attempting one more evacuation.

Special precautions:

In general, you should continue to take any routine prescribed medications during the preparation.

If you take blood pressure or heart medication, prednisone or other steroids, take them before 7 AM with a sip of water on the day of the test.

If you are taking INSULIN, the dosage many need to be adjusted the day prior and the morning of the test. Contact your physician for instructions regarding dosage.

Call your doctor if you have kidney disease.

INDEX

Note: Page numbers in italics indicate figures; those followed by *t* indicate tables.

D

E